WORD BOOKS FROM SAUNDERS

Sloane: *The Medical Word Book*, 2nd edition

Sloane: *Medical Abbreviations and Eponyms*

DeLorenzo: *Pharmaceutical Word Book*

Tessier: *The Surgical Word Book*

Sloane and Dusseau: *A Word Book in Pathology and Laboratory Medicine*

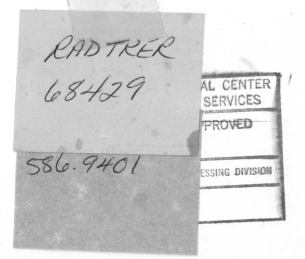

A WORD BOOK IN RADIOLOGY

with anatomic plates and tables

SHEILA B. SLOANE

Formerly President, Medi-Phone, Inc.
Author, The Medical Word Book;
A Word Book in Pathology and Laboratory Medicine;
and Medical Abbreviations and Eponyms

1988

W. B. SAUNDERS COMPANY
Harcourt Brace Jovanovich, Inc.

Philadelphia   London   Toronto   Montreal   Sydney   Tokyo

W. B. SAUNDERS COMPANY

Harcourt Brace Jovanovich, Inc.

West Washington Square
Philadelphia, PA 19105

Library of Congress Cataloging-in-Publication Data
Sloane, Sheila B.
    A word book in radiology.

    1. Radiology, Medical—Dictionaries. I. Title. [DNLM:
    1. Radiology—terminology. WN 15 S634w]

RC78.S58   1988   616.07′57′0321   87-23335

ISBN 0-7216-2100-7

Editor: Dudley Kay
Developmental Editor: Frances T. Mues
Designer: Patti Maddaloni
Production Manager: Bill Preston
Manuscript Editor: Terry Russell
Illustration Coordinator: Lisa Lambert

A Word Book in Radiology
With Anatomic Plates and Tables   ISBN   0-7216-2100-7

Last digit is the print number: 9   8   7   6   5   4   3   2   1

To John
With Love and Appreciation

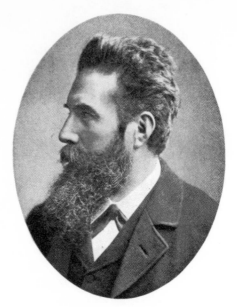

Wilhelm Conrad Roentgen
1845–1923

PREFACE

In 1895, Wilhelm Conrad Roentgen, a distinguished physicist with no pretensions to medical knowledge, discovered a new ray that was to become the most valuable diagnostic tool ever devised by man. In a paper entitled "On a New Kind of Rays," Roentgen said, "The justification for calling by the name rays the agent which proceeds from the wall of the discharging apparatus, I derive in part from the entirely regular formation of shadows, which are seen when more or less transparent bodies are brought between the apparatus and the fluorescent screen or the photographic plate. I have observed, and in part photographed, many shadow pictures of this kind, the production of which has a particular charm. I possess, for instance, photographs . . . of the shadows of the bones of the hand; the shadow of a covered wire wrapped on a wooden spool; of a set of weights enclosed in a box; of a compass in which the magnetic needle is entirely enclosed by metal; of a piece of metal whose lack of homogeneity becomes noticeable by means of the x-ray." Modestly, Professor Roentgen called these x-rays but, upon the insistence of several friends who immediately saw their usefulness, they were renamed Roentgen rays. Despite his award of the Nobel Prize in 1901 and his worldwide fame, Roentgen remained a simple and retiring person who began to dislike all publicity, especially when in his later years his discovery was falsely imputed to an assistant. He died in 1923, a lonely and embittered man neglected by a younger generation of physicists indifferent to his nobility of character and the greatness of his achievement. Imagine Roentgen's amazement if he were alive today. The advances made in the field of radiology since his early discovery are phenomenal. Ultrasound, diagnostic imaging, ionizing radiation, nuclear medicine, diagnostic interventional radiology, nuclear magnetic resonance, all would be beyond his wildest imagining.

Radiology presents unique problems to the transcriptionist, the medical records librarian, and the medical secretary because of its individual and immense vocabulary. Its individuality springs from a scientific underpinning in anatomy, physiology, optics, and physics, and its immensity from the circumstance that almost all diseases and disorders of man have been studied roentgenologically. Hence, it is the purpose of this book to provide for those who deal with radiologic terminology a simple means for quickly finding and correctly spelling the elusive term. The vocabulary does not attempt to be complete, but rather includes words and phrases most frequently used in the practice of radiology. Words in quotation marks are terms used exclusively in radiology and are, therefore, included in this text. Some examples are "pencil-like" deformity, "popcorn" calcification, and "Mercedes-Benz" sign.

The book is divided into three major parts. The first is an alphabetically arranged Vocabulary that includes radiation, roentgenology and resonance imaging. New syndromes have been included, particularly those relating to radiology of the hand. Terms pertaining to interventional radiology as well as conventional radiology are included. Both simple and difficult words are listed within the vocabulary. Simple words that are meaningful in combination with other words are given. For example, donor, cassette, and element are listed with the appropriate subentries peculiar to the terminology of radiology. Most, but not all, subentries are entered as separate terms to further expedite the search for a given word. The second part comprises Anatomy with 48 plates of human structure and detailed tables of arteries, bones, ligaments, muscles, nerves, and veins. The third and concluding part of the book includes six Appendices giving data of especial use to the medical transcriptionist, secretary, nurse, technician, or student.

Many references have been used in the compilation of this book, all of which have helped to make this listing current and accurate. Of these sources several stand out for their authority and comprehensiveness. They are

Meschan: Roentgen Signs in Diagnostic Imaging, Volumes I, II, and III, 2nd Edition, W. B. Saunders, 1985

Dorland's Illustrated Medical Dictionary, 26th Edition, W. B. Saunders, 1981

Poznanski: The Hand in Radiologic Diagnosis, Volumes I and II, 2nd Edition, W. B. Saunders, 1984

Moss, Gamsu, and Genant: Computed Tomography of the Body, W. B. Saunders, 1983

Hilton, Edwards, and Hilton: Practical Pediatric Radiology, W. B. Saunders, 1984

Ballinger: Merrill's Atlas of Radiographic Positioning and Radiologic Procedures, Volumes I, II, and III, 5th Edition, C. V. Mosby, 1982

Felson: Chest Roentgenology, W. B. Saunders, 1973

People as well as reference sources have been of help to me in the long course of bringing the book to completion. I should like to express my sincere appreciation to Dr. David Shaw of Winthrop Breon Laboratories for his expert guidance in the listing of the numerous contrast media used in various radiological studies. I offer my deepest gratitude to my husband, John Dusseau, for the organization and compilation of the Tables that appear in the Anatomy section, and to Hazel Hacker for her expertise in their final preparation. As with my other books, the editorial and production staffs of the W. B. Saunders Company have been of unstinting assistance, and I thank my copy editor, Terry Russell, and Wynette Kommer.

The intent of this book is to provide in one volume the basic vocabulary of the practice of radiology. It is hoped that this effort will, in some measure, give the reader easier access to the sought-after word.

SHEILA B. SLOANE

CONTENTS

PART I

VOCABULARY

Radiation, Roentgenology and Resonance Imaging

A – anterior
Å – angström
AAPM – American Association of Physicists in Medicine
Ab – antibody
abdomen
abdominal
abdominoaortic
abdominopelvic
abducens
abducent
abduction
aberrant
aberration
    chromatic a.
    chromatid-type a.
    chromosome a.
    commatic a.
abetalipoproteinemia
ABL –
    anthropologic base line
    anthropomorphic base line
abnormality
    chromosome 18 a.
    sex chromosome a.
abortion
above a selected threshold
ABPA – allergic bronchopulmonary aspergillosis
ABR – American Board of Radiology

abrasion
Abrodil
abruptio placentae
abscess
    abdominal a.
    amebic a.
    appendiceal a.
    Brodie's a.
    cerebral a.
    cortical a.
    epidural a.
    epiploic a.
    fungal a.
    gangrenous a.
    gas-forming a.
    hepatic a.
    iliopsoas a.
    intra-abdominal a.
    intrahepatic a.
    intramammary a.
    intraperitoneal a.
    intrarenal a.
    manubriosternoclavicular a.
    mesenteric a.
    multiloculated a.
    pararenal a.
    pelvic a.
    periapical a.
    periappendiceal a.
    pericholecystic a.
    pericolonic a.

abscess *(continued)*
    perigraft a.
    perihepatic a.
    perinephric a.
    perirenal a.
    perisigmoidal a.
    psoas a.
    pulmonary a.
    pyogenic a.
    renal a.
    retromammary a.
    retroperitoneal a.
    retropharyngeal a.
    sacrococcygeal a.
    splenic a.
    streptococcal a.
    subcutaneous a.
    subdiaphragmatic a.
    subdural a.
    subhepatic a.
    subphrenic a.
abscessogram
abscopal
absorbance
absorbed
    a. dose
    a. dose rate
    a. fraction
absorbent
absorber
absorptiometer
absorptiometry
absorption
    bone radiation a.
    a. coefficient
    a. line
    photoelectric a.
    a. unsharpness

absorption *(continued)*
    a. x-ray spectrum
a.c. – alternating current
Acacia
acalculous
acanthiomeatal line
acanthion
acanthioparietal
acanthus
ACAT – automated computer-
    ized axial tomography
accelerating potential
acceleration
accelerator
    atomic a.
    electronic linear a.
    linear a.
acceptor
accessory
accommodation
ACD – annihilation coinci-
    dence detection
acetabular
acetabulum (acetabula)
acetanilidoiminodiacetic acid
acetic
    a. acid
    a. anhydride
acetrizoate
acetrizoic acid
acetylated
acetylation
acetylcholine
acetylcysteine
a.c. generator
achalasia
acheiria
Achilles' tendon

achondrogenesis
achondroplasia
acidophilic
acidosis
     renal tubular a.
acinar-like
acinus (acini)
aclasis
     diaphyseal a.
     tarsoepiphyseal a.
aconitine tincture
acoustic
     a. enhancement
     a. impedance
     a. interface
     a. labyrinth
     a. meatus
     a. mismatch
     a. nerve
     a. neuroma
     a. shadow
a.c. power supply
acquired immune deficiency
     syndrome
ACR – American College of
     Radiology
acral-renal association
acrobrachycephaly
acrocallosal syndrome
acrocephalopolysyndactyly
acrocephalo-synankie
acrocephalosyndactyly
     Pfeiffer's a.
     Saethre-Chotzen a.
acrodysostosis
acrodysplasia
acroedema
acrofacial

acromegaly
acromelia
acromelic
acromesomelic
acrometagenesis
acromial
acromioclavicular
acromiocoracoid
acromiohumeral
acromion process
acromioscapular
acromiothoracic
acromutilation
acro-osteolysis
acropachy
acro-pectoro-vertebral dysplasia
ACTH – adrenocorticotropic
     hormone
actinic radiation
actinium
actinogen
actinogenesis
actinogram
actinograph
actinography
actinokymography
actinomycosis
actinon
actinopraxis
actinoscopy
activated
     a. atom
     a. water
activity (curie)
ACTR – American Club of
     Therapeutic Radiologists
acuity
"acute abdomen"

acute renal failure
acute tubular necrosis
a.c. voltage
acyanotic
AD –
> above diaphragm
> absorbed dose

adactyly
adamantinoma
adaptation
adapters
ADC – analog-to-digital con-
> verter

A/D converter
Addison's plane
adduction
adductor
adenitis
adenoacanthoma
adenoameloblastoma
adenocarcinoma
adenochondroma
adenofibroma
adenohypophyseal
adenohypophysis
adenohypophysitis
adenoid
> a. cystic carcinoma

adenoleiomyofibroma
adenolipoma
adenolymphoma
adenoma
> acidophilic a.
> basophilic a.
> benign a.
> bronchial a.
> chromophobic a.
> cortical a.

adenoma *(continued)*
> oxyphil a.
> pituitary a.
> pleomorphic a.
> a. sebaceum
> thyroid a.
> villous a.

adenomatoid
adenomatosis
adenomatous
> a. coli

adenomyofibroma
adenomyoma
adenomyomatosis
adenomyosarcoma
adenomyosis
adenomyxoma
adenomyxosarcoma
adenopathy
> hilar a.
> mediastinal a.

adenosarcoma
adenosine
> a. deaminase deficiency
> a. diphosphate
> a. triphosphate

adenosquamous
adenovirus
ADH – antidiuretic hormone
adherent
adhesion
> interthalamic a.

adhesive
ADI – atlanto-dens interval
adiabatic fast passage
adipose
aditus
> a. ad antrum

aditus *(continued)*
    a. ad pelvis
    a. laryngis
    a. orbitae
    a. vaginae
adjuvant
    Freund's a.
Administration of Radioactive
    Substances Advisory
    Committee
adnexa
ADP – adenosine diphosphate
adrenal
    a. arteriography
    a. cortex
    a. gland
    a. hyperplasia
    a. hypertension
    a. hypofunction
    a. imaging
    Marchand's a.'s
Adrenalin
adrenaline
adrenocortical
adrenocorticotropic hormone
adrenogenital
adrenogram
Adrian-Crooks type cassette
adult respiratory distress syndrome
advanced life support
adynamic
AEC –
    Atomic Energy Commission
    automatic exposure control
aeration

Aerobacter
aeroesophagography
aerophagia
aerosol inhalation studies
afferent
    a. loop syndrome
AFP – adiabatic fast passage
afterglow
Ag – silver
agammaglobulinemia
aganglionosis
agar
AgBr – silver bromide
AGC – automatic gain control
agenesis
aggregated
aglossia-adactyly syndrome
agnogenic myeloid metaplasia
AHRA – American Hospital
    Radiology Administrators
AIDS – acquired immune deficiency syndrome
ainhum
AIP – American Institute of
    Physics
air
    a. alveologram
    a. arthrography
    a. bronchogram sign
    a. cap sign
    a. contrast radiography
    a. core transformer
    a. crescent sign
    "a. dome" sign
    a. dose
    a. drift
    a. embolism
    extraperitoneal a.

air *(continued)*
    extrapleural a.
    a. fog
    free a.
    a. gap technique
    a. insufflation
    intraperitoneal a.
    intrapleural a.
    a.-space disease
    a.-wall ionization chamber
airflow obstruction diseases
airway
    a. obstruction
    patent a.
    pulmonary a.
AIUM – American Institute of Ultrasound in Medicine
AIVV – anterior internal vertebral veins
akinesis
Al – aluminum
ala (alae)
alactasia
alar scapula
Albers-Schönberg
    method
    position
Albert's position
Albright's osteodystrophy
albumin
    iodinated I 125
    serum a.
    iodinated I 131 aggregated a.
    iodinated I 131
    serum a.
    macroaggregated a.

albumin *(continued)*
    a. microsphere
alcoholism
aldosterone
aldosteronism
aldosteronoma
Alexander's method
algebraic reconstruction technique
algorithm
    Cooley-Tukey a.
aliasing
alignment
alimentary
alkaline
    a. phosphatase
alkalosis
alkaptonuria
allergic
    a. bronchopulmonary aspergillosis
allergy
allowed beta transition
alloxan
alloy
allylamine
alnico
alpha
    a.-1-antitrypsin deficiency
    a. chamber
    a. decay
    a. particle
    a. radiation
    a. ray
    a. threshold
ALS – advanced life support
alternation

alternator
alumina
aluminum
alveobronchiolitis
alveolar
    a. canals
    a. cell carcinoma
    a. duct
    a. emphysema
    a. infiltrate
    a. microlithiasis
    a. nodule
    a. pattern
    a. process
    a. proteinosis
    a. ridge
    a. sac
alveolitis
"alveolization"
alveolocapillary
alveologram
alveololabial
alveololingual
alveolonasal
alveolopalatal
alveoloplasty
alveolus (alveoli)
alymphoplasia
    thymic a.
AMA – American Medical Association
ambient
amebiasis
amebic
amelia
ameloblastic
    a. fibroma
    a. sarcoma

ameloblastoma
    melanotic a.
    pituitary a.
amenorrhea
American Association of Physicists in Medicine
American Board of Radiology
American Club of Therapeutic Radiologists
American College of Radiology
American Hospital Radiology Administrators
American Institute of Physics
American Institute of Ultrasound in Medicine
American Medical Association
American Registry of Diagnostic Medical Sonographers
American Registry of Radiologic Technologists
American Rheumatism Association
American Roentgen Ray Society
American Society of Radiologic Technologists
American Society of Registered Technologists
American Standards Association
americium
amidotrizoic acid
amine precursor uptake and decarboxylation cell tumor
amino acids
γ – aminobutyrate
aminophylline

aminopterin
Amipaque
ammeter
    filament a.
ammonium thiosulfate
amniography
amnion
amniotic sac
A-mode – amplitude modulation
amorphous
amp – ampere
amperage
amphiarthrodial
amphiarthrosis
amphoric
amphoteric
amplification
amplifier
    buffer a.
    gradient power a.
    image a.
    linear a.
    nuclear pulse a.
    pulse a.
    voltage a.
amplifying systems
amplitude modulation
ampulla (ampullae)
    a. of Vater
amputation
a.m.u. – atomic mass unit
amygdala
amygdaloid
amyloid
amyloidoma
amyloidosis
    interstitial a.

amyloidosis *(continued)*
    pulmonary a.
    tracheal a.
amyoplasia
    a. congenita
amyotrophic lateral sclerosis
anaerobe
anaerobic
anal
    a. atresia
    a. canal
    a. fissure
analgesia
analgia
analog
    a. computations
    a. photo
    a. rate meter
    a.-to-digital converter
analogous
analysis
    activation a.
    basic volume image a.
    chemical a.
    correlation a.
    least-squares a.
    neutron activation a.
    quantitative a.
    quantitative bone mineral a.
    regression a.
    saturation a.
analyzer
anaphylactoid
anaphylaxis
anaplasia
anaplastic
anastomosis (anastomoses)

anatomic
anatomy
ancillary
Anderson's method
Andrén's method
anechoic
anemia
    aplastic a.
    Blackfan-Diamond a.
    Cooley's a.
    erythroblastic a.
    Fanconi's a.
    hemolytic a.
    hypochromic-
      microcytic a.
    hypoplastic a.
    iron deficiency a.
    Mediterranean a.
    megaloblastic a.
    myelophthisic a.
    myelosclerotic a.
    osteosclerotic a.
    pernicious a.
    pyruvate kinase defi-
      ciency a.
    sickle cell a.
anencephalic
anencephaly
anesthesia
anesthetic
aneurysm
    abdominal aortic a.
    aortic a.
    arteriovenous a.
    cirsoid a.
    fusiform a.
    Galen's vein "a."
    innominate a.

aneurysm *(continued)*
    Pott's a.
    racemose a.
    Rasmussen's a.
    syphilitic a.
    thoracic a.
    varicose a.
    ventricular a.
aneurysmal
Anger camera
angina
    exudative a.
    Ludwig's a.
    a. pectoris
    Prinzmetal's a.
angioblastic
angioblastoma
angiocardiogram *(see* angiocar-
    diography)
angiocardiography
    first-pass radionuclide a.
    intravenous a.
    radionuclide a.
    selective a.
    venous a.
angiocardiokinetic
Angioconray
angiodysplasia
angioendothelioma
angiofibroma
Angiografin
angiogram *(see* angiography)
angiography
    abdominal a.
    biliary a.
    cardiac a.
    carotid a.
    cerebral a.

angiography *(continued)*
    digital subtraction a.
    first-pass isotope a.
    four-vessel a.
    hepatic a.
    magnification a.
    multigated a.
    nuclear a.
    peripheral a.
    pulmonary a.
    radionuclide a.
    renal a.
    subtraction a.
    three-vessel a.
    vertebral a.
    vertebrobasilar a.
    visceral a.
angiolipoma
angiology
angiolymphangioma
angioma
angiomatosis
    encephalotrigeminal a.
angiomyolipoma
angiomyoma
angioneurotic
angio-osteohypertrophic syn-
    drome
angioplasty
    percutaneous translu-
      minal a.
angiosarcoma
angioscintigraphy
angiotensin
Angiovist
angle
    basal a.
    a. board

angle *(continued)*
    Boogaard's a.
    branching a.
    cardiophrenic a.
    cerebellopontine a.
    costophrenic a.
    facial a.
    hepatic a.
    iliac a.
    lumbosacral a.
    naso-pineal a.
    phrenicoverte-
      bral a.
    scapho-lunate a.
    sphenoid a.
    splenic a.
    sternal a.
    subcarinal a.
    talocalcaneal a.
    tuber a.
Angström unit
angular
angulation
    caudad a.
    cephalic a.
    lumbosacral a.
    volar a.
angulator
anhydrase
    carbonic a.
anhydride
anion
aniridia
anisura
ankylodactyly
ankyloglossia superior
ankylosing
    a. spondylitis

ankylosis
    glossopalatine a.
annihilation coincidence detec-
    tion
annular
    a. lesion
    a. phased arrays
    a. sclerosis
annulus
    a. fibrosus
anode
    a. cooling curve chart
    rotating a.
    stationary a.
    a. thermal capacity
anomalad
    Robin's a.
anomalous
anomaly
anonychia
anorchidism
anosteogenesis
anoxia
antagonist
antalgic
anteflexion
antegrade
    a. perfusion pressure
      measurement
    a. pyelography
anterior
    a. arch
    a. junction line
    a. pararenal space
anteroposterior
anteroseptal
anteversion
anthrax

anthropologic base line
anthropometry
anthropomorphic base line
antibiotic
antibody
    antinuclear a.
anticoagulant
anticoagulation
anticoincidence circuit
anticonvulsant
antidiuretic hormone
antigenic
antihypertensives
anti-inflammatory
antimony trisulfide
antineoplastic
antineutrino
antinuclear
antiparticle
antiproton
antiseptic
antisera
antitrypsin
antral
    a. remnant syndrome
    a. web
antrum (antra)
    cardiac a.
    ethmoid a.
    frontal a.
    gastric a.
    Highmore's a.
    mastoid a.
    maxillary a.
    pyloric a.
    tympanic a.
    a. of Willis
anuria

anus (anus)
>   imperforate a.
>   preternatural a.
>   a. vestibularis
>   vulvovaginal a.

aorta (aortas, aortae)
>   abdominal a.
>   ascending a.
>   descending a.
>   dextropositioned a.
>   overriding a.
>   thoracic a.
>   ventral a.

aortic
>   a. aneurysm
>   a. arch
>   a. atresia
>   a. dissection
>   a. knob
>   a. laceration
>   a. leaflet
>   a. lumen
>   a. murmur
>   a. node
>   a. pulmonic lymph node
>   a.-pulmonic window
>   a. regurgitation
>   a. root
>   a. rupture
>   a. sac
>   a. stenosis
>   a. triangle
>   a. valve

aorticopulmonary
aorticorenal
aortitis
aortocaval
aortocoronary

aortoduodenal
aortofemoral
aortogram (*see* aortography)
aortography
>   abdominal a.
>   arch a.
>   catheter a.
>   lumbar a.
>   renal a.
>   retrograde a.
>   selective visceral a.
>   thoracic a.
>   translumbar a.
>   venous a.
>   visceral a.

aortoiliac
AP – anteroposterior
aperture
apex (apices)
aphthous
apical
>   a. cap
>   a. dystrophy
>   a. murmur
>   a. pleura

apices
aplasia
>   pectoral a.

aplastic
apnea
aponeurosis
>   abdominal a.
>   bicipital a.
>   crural a.
>   epicranial a.
>   falciform a.
>   lingual a.
>   palmar a.

aponeurosis *(continued)*
- perineal a.
- pharyngeal a.
- plantar a.
- subscapular a.
- supraspinous a.
- temporal a.
- vertebral a.

apophyseal

apophysis (apophyses)
- basilar a.
- cerebral a.
- genial a.
- iliac crest a.
- odontoid a.
- pterygoid a.
- ring a.

apoplexy
- pituitary a.

appearance
- "applecore-like" a.
- "ball-in-hand" a.
- "beaded" a.
- "beaked" a.
- "beaten brass" a.
- "bone within bone" a.
- "bubble-like" a.
- "candle dripping" a.
- "cobblestone" a.
- "coiled-spring" a.
- "cotton ball" a.
- "cotton-wool" a.
- double-bubble a.
- drumstick a.
- "frayed string" a.
- "ground glass" a.
- "hair-standing-on-end" a.

appearance *(continued)*
- "hammered brass" a.
- "hot-cross-bun" a.
- "inverse comma" a.
- "jail bars" a.
- "kernal of pop-corn" a.
- "lacelike" a.
- "leafless tree" a.
- "light bulb" a.
- "moth-eaten" a.
- "onion skin" a.
- "pancake" a.
- "panda" a.
- "picture frame" a.
- "popcorn-like" a.
- "pruned-tree" a.
- "punched out" a.
- "railroad track" a.
- "rugger jersey" a.
- "saber shin" a.
- "sandwich" a.
- "scottie dog" a.
- "shell of bone" a.
- "soap bubble" a.
- "spadelike" a.
- "sunburst" a.
- "sun-ray" a.
- "Swiss Alps" a.
- "trefoil" a.
- "weblike" a.
- "wineglass" a.
- "wormy" a.

appendiceal

appendicitis

appendicolith

appendicolithiasis

appendicular

appendix (appendices)
    retrocecal a.
"apple core" lesion
"applecore-like" appearance
APPM – antegrade perfusion
    pressure measurement
apposition
Apresoline
APS – anterior pararenal space
APT – automatic peak tracking
APUDoma – *a*mine *p*recursor
    *u*ptake and *d*ecarboxyla-
    tion cell tumor
apyrogenicity
aqua
aqueduct
    cerebral a.
    fallopian a.
    a. of Sylvius
aqueous
AR – aortic regurgitation
ARA – American Rheumatism
    Association
arachnodactyly
arachnoid
    a. canal
    a. cyst
    a. villi
arachnoiditis
arborization
Arcelin's method
arch
    anterior a.
    aortic a.
    a. aortography
    fallopian a.
    longitudinal a.
    lumbar a.

arch *(continued)*
    lumbocostal a.
    posterior a.
    pubic a.
    subpubic a.
    superciliary a.
    transverse a.
    vertebral a.
    zygomatic a.
architecture
archival storage
arcing
arcuate
ARDMS – American Registry
    of Diagnostic Medical
    Sonographers
ARDS – adult respiratory dis-
    tress syndrome
area
    Broca's a.
areae gastricae
areola
areolar
ARF – acute renal failure
argentaffinoma
argon
armadillo
armature
Armillifer
    A. armillatus
Arnold-Chiari malforma-
    tion
Arnold's canal
array processor
arrays
    annular phased a.
    linear phased a.
    linear sequenced a.

arrested hydrocephalus occlusus
arrhythmia
        atrial a.
        ventricular a.
ARRS – American Roentgen
        Ray Society
ARRT – American Registry of
        Radiologic Technolo-
        gists
ARSAC – Administration of
        Radioactive Substances
        Advisory Committee
arsenic
ART – algebraic reconstruction
        technique
arterial
        a. embolization
        a. murmur
        a. occlusion
        a. occlusive disease
        a. phase
        a. puncture
arteriogram (*see* arterio-
        graphy)
arteriography
        adrenal a.
        aortofemoral a.
        brachial a.
        brachiocephalic a.
        carotid a.
        catheter a.
        celiac a.
        cerebral a.
        coronary a.
        digital a.
        femoral a.
        hepatic a.

arteriography *(continued)*
        magnified carotid a.
        magnified vertebrobasi-
            lar a.
        mesenteric a.
        percutaneous carotid a.
        peripheral a.
        "pruned-tree" a.
        pulmonary a.
        renal a.
        selective a.
        splenic a.
        superior mesenteric a.
        vertebral a.
        vertebrobasilar a.
        visceral a.
        wedge a.
arteriole
arteriosclerosis
        cerebral a.
        coronary a.
        hyaline a.
        hypertensive a.
        nodular a.
        a. obliterans
        peripheral a.
        presenile a.
        senile a.
arteriosclerotic
arteriosus
        patent ductus a.
arteriovenous
        a. shunt
arteritis (arterides)
        giant cell a.
        granulomatous a.
        pulmonary a.
        Takayasu's a.

artery (*see* Part II, Table of
    Arteries)
arthritis
        cricoarytenoid a.
        degenerative a.
        enteropathic a.
        erosive a.
        exudative a.
        gonococcal a.
        hypertrophic a.
        Jaccoud's a.
        juvenile rheumatoid a.
        psoriatic a.
        pyogenic a.
        radiocarpal a.
        Reiter's a.
        rheumatoid a.
        septic a.
        subtalar a.
        syphilitic a.
        tuberculous a.
        venereal a.
        vertebral a.
"arthritis mutilans"
arthrodesis
arthrodial
arthrodynia
arthrodysplasia
arthroempyesis
arthroereisis
arthrogenous
arthrogram (*see* arthrography)
arthrography
        air a.
        double-contrast a.
        opaque a.
        "vacuum" a.

arthrogryposis
        a. multiplex congenita
arthrokatadysis
arthrokleisis
arthrolith
arthrolithiasis
arthrology
arthromeningitis
arthroncus
arthronosos
        a. deformans
arthro-onychodysplasia
arthro-ophthalmopathy
arthropathy
        Jaccoud's a.
        neurogenic a.
        neuropathic a.
arthrophyte
arthroplasty
arthropneumography
arthropneumoroentgenography
arthroscintigram
arthroscintigraphy
arthrosclerosis
arthrosis
articular
        a. cartilage
        a. facet
        a. fracture
        a. pillar
        a. process
        a. surface
        a. tubercle
articulate
articulated process
articulation
        apophyseal a.

articulation *(continued)*
    atlanto-occipital a.
    cervicothoracic a.
    costomanubrial a.
    incudostapedial a.
    lumbosacral a.
    sternoclavicular a.
    temporomandibular a.
    tibiofibular a.
artifact
    geometric a.
    nonlinear a.
artifactual
artificial
    a. permanent magnet
    a. radioactive isotope
aryepiglottic
arytenoid
ASA – American Standards
    Association
asbestos
asbestosis
ascariasis
ascending
ascites
    exudative a.
    loculated a.
ascitic
ASD – atrial septal defect
asepsis
aseptic
ASIS – anterior superior iliac
    spine
aspergillosis
    allergic bronchopulmon-
      ary a.
    bronchopneumonic a.

aspergillosis *(continued)*
    pulmonary a.
Aspergillus
    A. fumigatus
asphyxia
asphyxiating
    a. thoracic dysplasia
aspirate
aspiration
    a. biopsy
    CT guided a.
    cytologic a.
    meconium a.
    mineral oil a.
    a. pneumonia
    a. pneumonitis
    pulmonary a.
    a. syndromes
    a. transducer
asplenia
ASRT –
    American Society of
      Radiologic Technolo-
      gists
    American Society of Reg-
      istered Technologists
assay
    erythropoietin a.
assimilation
Association of University
    Radiologic Technologists
Association of University Ra-
    diologists
AST – above a selected thresh-
    old
astatine
asterion

asthenia
asthma
asthmatic
astragalocalcanean
astragaloscaphoid
astragalotibial
astragalus
astroblastoma
astrocyte
     fibrous a's
     plasmatofibrous a's
     protoplasmic a's
astrocytoma
     juvenile pilocytic a.
asymmetric
asymmetry
asymptomatic
asynchronous
asystole
ataxia
atelectasis
atelosteogenesis
atherogenesis
atheromatous
atherosclerosis
atherosclerotic
atlantoaxial
atlanto-dens interval
atlantoepistrophic
atlantomastoid
atlanto-occipital
atlanto-odontoid
atlas
     Greulich-Pyle a.
atlas (C-1 vertebra)
atloido-occipital
ATN – acute tubular necro-
     sis

atom
     activated a.
     excited a.
     helium a.
     hydrogen a.
     inert a's
     ionized a's
     Na a's
     potassium a.
     a. smasher
     stripped a.
     tagged a.
atomic
     a. accelerator
     a. energy
     a. mass
     a. mass unit(s)
     a. nucleus
     a. number
     a. orbit
     a. shell
     a. spectrum
     a. theory
     a. volume
     a. weight
Atomic Energy Commission
atomization
atomizer
     jet–high pressure a.
     spinning disk a.
     two-stream impact jet a.
     ultrasonic a.
atony
ATP – adenosine triphosphate
atresia
     anal a.
     aortic a.
     biliary a.

atresia *(continued)*
>bronchial a.
>choanal a.
>duodenal a.
>esophageal a.
>follicular a.
>glottic a.
>intestinal a.
>mitral a.
>pulmonary a.
>pyloric a.
>tricuspid a.

atretic
atrial
>a. arrhythmia
>a. fibrillation
>a. flutter
>a. infarction
>a. myxoma
>a. obstruction
>a. septal defect
>a. tachycardia

atrioventricular
atrioventricularis communis
atrium (atria)
atrophic
atrophy
>mucosal a.
>Sudeck's a.

atropine
attenuation
>a. coefficient
>a. value

attenuator
attic
atypical
auditory
>a. canal

auditory *(continued)*
>a. meatus
>a. nerve
>a. ossicle
>a. tube
>a. vesicle

Auger's
>effect
>electron

AUR – Association of University Radiologists
auricle
auricula (auriculae)
>a. atrii
>a. cordis
>a. dextra cordis
>a. sinistra cordis

auricular
auriculoinfraorbital
AURT – Association of University Radiologic Technologists
auscultation
auscultatory
autofluoroscope
autogenous
autologous
>a. labelled leukocytes

automatic
>a. collimation
>a. exposure control
>a. gain control
>a. line voltage compensator
>a. peak tracking
>a. pressure injector
>a. processing system
>a. serial changer

autonomic nervous system
autonomous
autoradiograph
autoradiographic
autoradiography
      contact a.
      dip-coating a.
      film-stripping a.
      thick-layer a.
      two-emulsion a.
autoregulation
autoregulatory
autosomal
autotomogram
autotomography
autotransformer
autotrepanation
auxiliary
AV –
    arteriovenous
    atrioventricular
avalanche
      Townsend's a.
avascular
average
      a. deviation
      a. gradient
      a. life
      a. power

Avogadro's number
avulsion
axial
      a. plane
      a. resolution
      a. skeleton
      a. transverse tomogra-
        phy
axilla (axillae)
axillary
      a. node
      a. prolongation
      a. space
axiolateral
axiopetrosal
axis
      celiac a.
      longitudinal a.
      vertical a.
      X a.
      Y a.
axis (C-2 vertebra)
axon
Azetylpromazine
azotemia
azygoesophageal
      a. recess
azygography
azygos

B
b

B – Bucky (film in cassette in Potter-Bucky diaphragm)
tomogram with oscillating Bucky

β – beta particle

Ba – barium

bacillus
Friedländer's b.

background
b. activity
b. count
b. density
b. erase
b. radiation

backscatter

"backwash ileitis"

bacteremia

bacteria

bacterial

bacteriologic

bacterium

bacteriuria

bagassosis

Baker's cyst

ball-and-socket joint

"ball catcher's" view

"ball-in-hand" appearance

ballistic milliampere

balloon
b. catheterization
b. dilatation

balloon (continued)
b. image data
intra-aortic counterpulsation b.
b. tamponade

ballooning

Ball's method

balsa wood block

"bamboo" spine

band
Ladd's b's

bandwidth

bank resistors

BAP – brightness area product

barbiturate

baritosis

barium
b. enema
b. fluorochloride
hydrophilic nonflocculating b.
b. lead sulfate
b. meal study
b. platinocyanide
b. strontium sulfate
b. sulfate
b. swallow
b. vaginography

barium ($^{137}_{56}$Ba, atomic number 56)

barn

barotrauma

"barrel chest"
barreling distortion
Barrett's
    epithelium
    esophagus
Bartholin's duct
Barton's fracture
Bart's abdomino-peripheral an-
    giography unit
basal
    b. angle
    b. cell carcinoma
    b. cistern
    b. foramina
    b. ganglia
    b. kyphosis
    b. neck fracture
base
    b. density
    b. fog
    orbital b.
baseball
    "b. bat" shape
    b. finger
basic volume image analysis
basilar
    b. impression
    b. processes
    b. vein
basiocciput
basion
basket cells
"basket guidewire"
$BaSO_4$ – barium sulfate
basophilic
basoverticle
bathrocephaly
Batson's plexus

"bat's wing" shadow
battery
Bayes' theorem
Bayler-Pinneau method
"bayonet" deformity
BBB – blood-brain barrier
BCD – binary coded decimal
BD – below diaphragm
BDM – border detection
    method
BE – barium enema
bead chain cystography
"beaded" appearance
beak sign
"beaked" appearance
"beaking" of brainstem
beam
    b. barrier
    central b.
    b. CT scanner
    electron b.
    b. flattening filter
    b. monitor
    primary b.
    b. quality comparison
    b. restrictor
    b. therapy
    useful b.
    x-ray b.
beamsplitter
"beaten brass" appearance
Béclère's
    method
    position
BEI – butanol-extractable io-
    dine
bellomedullary
Bell's brachydactyly

Benadryl
Benassi's
        method
        position
benign
Bennett's fracture
Benoist's penetrometer
benzoate
benzoic acid
berkelium
Berteil's projection
Bertel's method
Bertin's column
berylliosis
beryllium
BES – British engineering system
        tem
beta
        b. decay
        b. detection
        b. emission
        b. emitter
        b.-oxybutyric acids
        b. particle
        b. radiation
        b.-ray spectrometer
        b. transition
Betadine
betatron
BEV – billion electron volts
bevatron
bezoar
biarticular
biaxial
bicarbonate
Bichat's canal
bicipital
biconcave

bicondylar
bicornuate
bicuspid
bicycle ergometer
bifid
bifurcate
bifurcation
bilateral
Bilbao-Dotter tube
bile
        b. duct
        b. leakage
        b. salt breath test
        b. salts
biliary
        b. atresia
        b. calculi
        b. canal(s)
        b. canaliculi
        b. cirrhosis
        b. decompression
        b. duct
        b. enteric fistula
        b. obstruction
        b. stenosis
        b. system
        b. tract
Biligrafin
Biligram
Biliodyl
bilirubin
Bilivistan
bilocular
biloma
Bilopaque
Biloptin
bimalleolar
bimastoid

bimolecular
binary coded decimal
binding
 b. energy
 ionic b.
 protein b.
binocular stereoscope
bioassay
 erythropoietin b.
biochemical
bioenergetics
biologic
biological half-life
biomedical
biomolecular
biophysics
biopsy
 aspiration b.
 bronchial brush b.
 CT directed b.
 CT guided b.
 cytologic b.
 endoscopic duodenal b.
 large-bore b.
 percutaneous liver b.
biosynthesis
biparietal
bipartite
bipedal
biphasic
biplane
 b. film changer
 b. screening
bird-headed dwarfism
bisacodyl tannex
bismuth
bit CT

"bite sign"
bite-wing
biventer
biventricular
 b. dilatation
 b. enlargement
 b. failure
Blackett-Healy
 method
 position
Blackfan-Diamond anemia
black pleura sign
bladder
 b. calculi
 b. diverticulum
 neurogenic b.
 b. sphincter dyssynergia
 urinary b.
blanking
blastoderm
Blastomyces
 B. dermatitidis
blastomycosis
bleb
blind loop syndrome
Blineau's projection
blink mode
Bloch's equations
block
 alveolar-capillary b.
 balsa wood b.
 b. vertebra
blood
 b. -brain barrier
 b. count
 b. flow study
 b. pool imaging

blood *(continued)*
    b. pool scan
    b. volume measurements
blooming focal spot
"blow-out"
    b.-o. fracture
    b.-o. view projection
BLS – basic life support
"blue bloater"
Blumensaat's line
blurring
B-mode – brightness modulation
BNA – Basle Nomina Anatomica
BOBA – beta-oxybutyric acids
Bochdalek's
    hernia
    valve
body
    b. atomic number (human)
    carotid b.
    ciliary b.
    b. composition
    Howell-Jolly b's
    pineal b.
    b. section radiography
    b. tonicity disturbance
    vitreous b.
    b. wasting
    b. water
Bohr's
    equation
    radius
    theory

Boltzmann's distribution factor
bolus
bombardment
bond
    chemical b.
    covalent b.
    valence b.
bonding
bone (*see* Part II, Table of Bones)
    b. age radiograph
    b. marrow scanning
    b. radiation absorption
    b. scan
    b. seeker
"bone within bone" appearance
Boogaard's angle
"book cassette"
booster circuit
border
    b. detection method
    b. sign
Bordetella
    B. pertussis
boron
bossa
    parietal b.
bosselated
bosselation
botryoid
botryoides
Bouchard's node
bound
    b. electron
    b. tissue water
bougie

boutonnière deformity
bovine serum albumin
bowel
"bowing" sign
Bowman's capsule
"bowtie filter"
"boxer's" fracture
BPD – bronchopulmonary dys-
    plasia
Bracco
brachial
        b. plexus
brachiocephalic
brachiocephaly
brachiocubital
brachycephalic
brachycephaly
brachydactyly
        Bell's b.
        Christian's b. syndrome
        Mohr-Wriedt's b.
brachyesophagus
brachymelia
brachymesophalangism
brachymesophalangy
brachymetacarpalia
        cryptodontic b.
brachymetacarpalis
brachymorphic
brachytelephalangy
brachytherapy
bradycardia
bradykinin
Bragg's
        curve
        equation
        peak
        spectrometer

brain
        blood-b. barrier
        b. death
        b. scan
brainstem
"braking" radiation
branch
branchial
        b. arch syndrome
branching
        b. angle
        b. decay
        b. fraction
        b. point
        b. ratio
branchiogenic
breast
        fatty b.
        fibrofatty b.
        fibroglandular b.
        funnel b.
        pigeon b.
breeder reactor
bregma
bregmatomastoid
bremsstrahlung [Ger] –
        breaking or stopping ra-
        diation
        b. process
        b. radiation
brevicollis
BRH – Bureau of Radiological
        Health
bridge circuit
brightness area product
brightness modulation
brimstone liver
British engineering system

British thermal unit
broad-beam scattering
Broca's area
Broden's
      method
      position
Brodie's
      abscess
      joint
Brodney's clamp
"broken bough" pattern
bromide
bromine
brominized oil
Bromsulphalein
bronchi (*see* bronchus)
bronchial
      b. adenoma
      b. asthma
      b. atresia
      b. brush biopsy
      b. brushing
      b. hyperreactivity
      b. obstruction
      b. pneumonia
      b. rupture
      b. tree
bronchiectasis
      bronchiolar b.
      cylindrical b.
      cystic b.
      reversible b.
      saccular b.
      varicose b.
bronchiectatic
bronchiogenic
bronchiolar
bronchiole

bronchiolectasis
bronchiolitis
      b. obliterans
bronchioloalveolar
bronchitis
bronchogenic
bronchogram (*see* bronchography)
bronchography
      Cope-method b.
      inhalation b.
      percutaneous transtracheal b.
broncholith
broncholithiasis
bronchomalacia
bronchopleural
bronchopneumonia
bronchopneumonic
bronchopulmonary
      b. dysplasia
bronchoradiography
bronchoscopy
      fiberoptic b.
      nonfiberoptic b.
bronchospasm
bronchostenosis
bronchus (bronchi)
      anomalous b.
      basal segmental b.
      fractured b.
      lobar b.
      lower lobe b.
      main stem b.
      middle lobe b.
      patent b.
      segmental b.
      subsegmental b.

bronchus *(continued)*
    upper lobe b.
bronze liver
"brown" tumor
Brucella
Brunner's gland
BSA – bovine serum albumin
B-scan
BSP – Bromsulphalein
BTR – Biomation transient recorder
BTU – British thermal unit
"bubble-like" appearance
buccal
bucket handle fracture
buckling
bucks
Bucky's
    diaphragm
    grid
    table
    tray
    wallstand
Budd-Chiari syndrome
Budin's joint
bulbar
bulbomedullary
bulbospinal
bulbospiral
bulbourethral
bulbous
bulboventricular
bulla (bullae)
    emphysematous b.
    ethmoid b.
    b. mastoidea
    b. ossea

bullous
bumper fracture
bunamiodyl
bunion
Bureau of Radiological Health
Burkitt's lymphoma
burrowing
bursa
    ischial b.
    omental b.
    subacromial-subdeltoid b.
    suprapatellar b.
    trochanteric b.
bursitis
    iliopsoas b.
    trochanteric b.
"burst" fracture
busulfan
butanol-extractable iodine
"butterfly"
    b. distribution
    b. lesion
    b. pattern
    b. shadow
    b. vertebrae
buttock
"button"
    Kistner tracheal b.
    b. sequestrum
    tracheal "B"
buttressing
butyl-iminodiacetic acid
bypass
    cardiac b.
    jejunoileal b.

Cc

C. –
    capacitance
    cathode
    Celsius
    centigrade
    clonus
    coulomb
c. –
    capacitor
    curie
CABBS – computer assisted blood background subtraction
CABG – coronary artery by-pass graft
cable
    cathode c.
CAD – coronary artery disease
cadmium
    c. zinc sulfide
café au lait spots
cage
    Faraday's c.
CAHEA – Committee on Allied Health, Education and Accreditation
Cahoon's method
caisson disease
cal – calorie
calcaneal
calcaneoapophysitis
calcaneoastragaloid
calcaneocavus
calcaneocuboid

calcaneofibular
calcaneonavicular
calcaneoplantar
calcaneoscaphoid
calcaneotibial
calcaneovalgocavus
calcaneus
calcar
calcareous
calcarine
calcific
    c. density
    c. shadows
    c. tendonitis
calcification
    abdominal c.
    annular c.
    cartilage c.
    conglomerate c.
    costochondral c.
    ectopic c.
    "eggshell" c.
    heterotopic c.
    intracranial c.
    joint c.
    "mulberry-type" c.
    non-neoplastic c.
    pancreatic c.
    "parentheses-like" c.
    pericardial c.
    "popcorn" c.
    prostatic c.
    punctate c.
    stippled c.

31

calcification *(continued)*
>   thoracic c.
>   thrombus c.
>   valvular c.
>   vascular c.

calcified

calcimine

calcinosis
>   interstitial c.
>   tumoral c.
>   c. universalis

calcitonin

calcium
>   c. chloride
>   c. endocrine regulation
>   c. gluconate
>   c. ioglycamate
>   ipodate c.
>   milk-of-c.
>   oragrafin c.
>   c. phosphate
>   c. pyrophosphate dihy-
>   drate

calcium
>   c. tungstate

calcium $^{40}_{20}$Ca, atomic
>   number 20

calculi *(see calculus)*

calculogram

calculography

calculus (calculi)
>   biliary c.
>   renal c.
>   "staghorn calculi"
>   ureteral c.

Caldwell-Moloy method

Caldwell's
>   method

Caldwell's *(continued)*
>   position
>   projection

calibrate

calibration
>   E-dial c.

calibrator
>   digital isotope c.
>   radioisotope c.

calices

caliculus

caliectasis

californium

caliper
>   direct reading c.
>   pelvimetry c.

calix (calices)

callosal

callous

callus
>   buttressing c.
>   exuberant c.
>   c. formation

calor

calorie

calvaria

calvarial

calvarium

Calvé's vertebra plana

calyceal

calyces

calyx (calyces)

camera
>   Anger c.
>   cine c.
>   gamma c.
>   Isocon c.
>   Medx c.

camera *(continued)*
    multicrystal c.
    multiformat c.
    Orthicon television c.
    pinhole c.
    positron scintillation c.
    radioisotope c.
    scintillation c.
    television c.
    c. tube
    video display c.
Cameron's method
Camp-Coventry position
Camper's line
Camp-Gianturco method
campomelic
Camp's grid cassette
camptobrachydactyly
camptodactyly
camptomicromelic
Campylobacter
    C. jejuni
canal
    abdominal c.
    accessory palatine c's
    adductor c.
    alimentary c.
    alveolar c's
    anal c.
    arachnoid c.
    archinephric c.
    Arnold's c.
    atrioventricular c.
    auditory c.
    Bichat's c.
    biliary c's
    carotid c.
    carpal c.

canal *(continued)*
    cerebrospinal c.
    cervical c.
    cochlear c.
    condylar c.
    craniopharyngeal c.
    crural c.
    entodermal c.
    ethmoid c.
    eustachian c.
    femoral c.
    haversian c.
    hypoglossal c.
    infraorbital c.
    inguinal c.
    lacrimal c.
    mandibular c.
    medullary c.
    nasolacrimal c.
    nasopalatine c.
    neural c.
    optic c.
    petromastoid c.
    portal c.
    pterygoid c.
    pterygopalatine c.
    pudendal c.
    pyloric c.
    sacral c.
    semicircular c's
    sphenopalatine c.
    sphenopharyngeal c.
    spinal c.
    supraciliary c.
    supraoptic c.
    tubal c.
    umbilical c.
    urogenital c's

canal *(continued)*
    uterine c.
    uterocervical c.
    ventricular c.
    Volkmann's c.
    vomerobasilar c.
    vomerovaginal c.
    vulvar c.
    vulvouterine c.
    zygomaticotemporal c.
canalicular
canaliculus (canaliculi)
cancellous
cancer
Candida albicans
candidiasis
"candle dripping" appearance
Cannon's ring
cannula
cannulate
cannulation
canthomeatal
canthus (canthi)
Cantor's tube
capacitance
capacitive reactance
capacitor
    c. discharge system
    electrical c.
capacity
capillary
    c. blockade perfusion
      scan
    c. phase
    renal c.
    c. telangiectasia
    c. wedge pressure
capital

capitate
capitatum
capitellum
capitopedal
capitular
capitulum (capitula)
    c. costae
    c. fibulae
    c. humeri
    c. mallei
    c. mandibulae
    c. ossis metacarpalis
    c. ossis metatarsalis
    c. radii
    c. stapedis
    c. ulnae
capsula (capsulae)
capsular
capsule
    adipose c.
    fibrous c.
    Bowman's c.
    Gerota's c.
    Tenon's c.
capsulitis
    adhesive c.
    idiopathic c.
capture
    cross section c.
    electron c.
    gamma-ray c.
    resonance c.
caput (capita)
    c. medusae
carbon
    c. dioxide
    c. monoxide
    c. tetrachloride

carbon $_6^{12}$C, atomic number 6
carbonate
carbonic
    c. anhydrase
carboxyl carbons
carbuncle
carcinogen
carcinogenesis
carcinoid
carcinoma
    adenoid cystic c.
    adenosquamous c.
    alveolar cell c.
    anaplastic c.
    basal cell c.
    bile duct c.
    bronchogenic c.
    cavitary c.
    cervical c.
    embryonal cell c.
    endometrial c.
    esophageal c.
    gastric c.
    hepatocellular c.
    islet cell c.
    jejunal c.
    laryngeal c.
    linitis plastica c.
    medullary c.
    metastatic c.
    mucinous c.
    mucoepidermoid c.
    nevoid basal cell c.
    oat cell c.
    obstructive c.
    pancreatic c.
    polypoid c.
    renal cell c.

carcinoma *(continued)*
    "spindle cell" c.
    squamous c.
    squamous cell c.
    subglottic c.
    subungual
      epidermoid c.
    supraglottic c.
    thyroid c.
    transglottic c.
    transitional cell c.
      stage A
      stage B1
      stage B2
      stage C
      stage D1
      stage D2
    uterine c.
    vaginal c.
    verrucous c.
carcinomatosis
carcinomatous
cardboard film holder
cardia
cardiac
    c. antrum
    "c. asthma"
    c. asystole
    c. blood pool imaging
    c. catheterization
    c. cycle
    c. herniation
    c. imaging
    c. incisura
    c. murmur
    c. notch
    c. orifice
    c. output

cardiac *(continued)*
    c. shunt detection
    c. silhouette
    c. sphincter
    c. tamponade
    c. thrombus
    c. ventricle
cardioangiography
cardioaortic
cardiocele
cardiochalasia
cardiocirculatory
cardiocirrhosis
Cardio-Conray
cardiodiaphragmatic
cardiodiosis
cardioesophageal
cardiogenesis
cardiogenic shock
Cardiografin
cardiohepatic
cardiohepatomegaly
cardiolith
cardiology
    nuclear c.
    quantitative c.
cardiomalacia
cardiomegaly
cardiomelic syndrome
cardiomyopathy
    atrophic c.
    congestive c.
    hypertrophic c.
    obstructive c.
    restrictive c.
cardionecrosis
cardionephric
cardioneural

cardiopathy
cardiopericarditis
cardiophrenic
cardiopulmonary
    c. arrest
    c. resuscitation
cardiopyloric
cardiorenal
cardioscan
cardiospasm
cardiothoracic
cardiotoxicity
cardiovalvular
cardiovascular
    c. monitoring
    c. nuclear medicine
    c. support
    c. system
    c. ultrasonography
carditis
    rheumatic c.
    streptococcal c.
    verrucous c.
caries
carina (carinae)
carinal
C-arm
"Carman-Kirklin meniscus"
    sign
Carnoy's solution
caroticocavernous
carotid
    c. arteriography
    c. artery
    c. body
    c. canal
    c. occlusion
    c. siphon

carpal
>   c. age
>   c. angle
>   c. canal
>   c. center
>   c. collapse
>   c. dislocation
>   c. fracture
>   c. fusion
>   c. joint
>   c. necrosis
>   c. ossification
>   c. subluxation
>   c. synostosis
>   c. tunnel syndrome
>   c. width

carpe bossu
carpocarpal
carpometacarpal
carpopedal
carpophalangeal
carpoptosis
carpotarsal
carpus
carrier
>   c.-free radioisotope

Carr-Purcell sequence
cartilage
>   accessory c.
>   alar c.
>   articular c.
>   arytenoid c.
>   conchal c.
>   corniculate c.
>   costal c.
>   cricoid c.
>   cuneiform c.
>   diarthrodial c.

cartilage *(continued)*
>   hyaline c.
>   c. inhibitor
>   innominate c.
>   interosseous c.
>   intervertebral c.
>   laryngeal c.
>   semilunar c.
>   septal c.
>   thyroid c.
>   triangular c.
>   vomeronasal c.
>   xiphoid c.

cartilaginous
>   c. annulus fibrosis
>   c. exostosis
>   c. joint
>   c. labrum
>   c. ossification

caruncle
caruncula (carunculae)
cascade
>   c. stomach

caseous
cassette
>   Adrian-Crooks type c.
>   Camp's grid c.
>   c. changer
>   grid c.
>   multisection c.
>   c. tunnel
>   c. unloader
>   Wisconsin kV.p test c.

cast
>   "egg" c's
>   ellipsoidal c.
>   spheroidal c.
>   "c. syndrome"

CAT –
   chlormerodrin accumula-
      tion test
   computerized axial tomog-
      raphy
   computer assisted tomog-
      raphy
catabolism
catalyst
cataphoresis
cataract
"catarrhal mastoiditis"
catecholamine
catenary system
cathartic
catheter
   aortic flush pigtail c.
   c. aortography
   c. arteriography
   central venous
      pressure c.
   French polyethylene c.
   Grollman pigtail c.
   Grüntzig balloon-tip c.
   headhunter c.
   c. induced thrombosis
   Ingram's trocar c.
   intraluminal c.
   intraperitoneal c.
   nasogastric c.
   pigtail angiographic c.
   radiopaque c.
   retrograde c.
   Ring-McLean c.
   sheathed c.
   sidewinder c.
   Simmons c.
   subclavian c.

catheter *(continued)*
   Swan-Ganz c.
   trocar c.
   umbilical c.
   Von Sonnenberg's c.
catheterization
   balloon c.
   cardiac c.
   Seldinger's c.
cathode
   c. cable
   hot c.
   c. ray
   c. ray tube
cation
catphantom
cauda (caudae)
   c. cerebelli
   c. epididymidis
   c. equina
   c. helicis
   c. nuclei caudati
   c. pancreatis
caudad
caudocranial
Causton's method
cavernolith
cavernous
cavitary
cavitation
cavity
   abdominal c.
   abdominopelvic
   buccal c.
   dorsal c.
   glenoid c.
   Meckel's c.
   medullary c.

cavity *(continued)*
>   orbital c.
>   pelvic c.
>   pericardial c.
>   peritoneal c.
>   pleural c.
>   tympanic c.
>   ventral c.

cavogram
cavography
cavovalgus
cavum (cava)
>   c. septum pellucidum
>   c. vergae

cavus foot
cb – cardboard or plastic film holder without intensifying screens
CBF – cerebral blood flow
CBG – corticosteroid-binding globulin
c.c. – cubic centimeter
CCI – Cronqvist cranial index
CCK-PZ – cholecystokinin-pancreozymin
CCT – cranial computed tomography
CCU – coronary care unit
Cd – cadmium
CDC – chenodeoxycholic acid
CDH – congenital dislocation of hip
cecal
cecum
celiac
celiocentesis
cell
>   ethmoidal air c's

cell *(continued)*
>   Kupffer's c.
>   osteoprogenitor c.
>   polygonal c.
>   reticuloendothelial c.
>   spindle c.

cellulitis
>   submandibular c.

Celsius
cementifying
cementoma
centesis
centigrade
centigray
centimeter
centimeter-gram-second system
central
>   c. beam
>   c. lobe
>   c. nervous system
>   c. ray
>   c. sulcus
>   c. venous pressure catheter

centrencephalic
centrifugal force
centrifuge
centrilobular
centripetal force
centrum
>   c. semiovale

cephalad
cephalic
cephalocaudad
>   c. instability

cephalocaudal
cephalohematoma

cephalometry
   fetal c.
   ultrasonic c.
cephalopelvic
   c. disproportion
cephalopelvimetry
cephalopolydactyly
   Greig's c.
cephalopolysyndactyly
ceramidase
cerebellar
   c. hemisphere
   c. hemorrhage
   c. notch
   c. tonsil
   c. vermis
cerebellomedullary
cerebellopontine
cerebellorubrospinal
cerebellospinal
cerebellotegmental
cerebellothalamic
cerebellum
cerebral
   c. abscess
   c. angiography
   c. apophysis
   c. aqueduct
   c. arteriography
   c. arteriosclerosis
   c. blood flow
   convexities
   c. cortex
   c. fossa
   c. gigantism
   c. gyri
   hemisphere

cerebral *(continued)*
   c. infarction
   c. nuclei
   c. palsy
   c. peduncle
   c. pneumography
   c. radionuclide angiog-
      raphy
   c. sulci
   c. ventricle
cerebritis
cerebro-hepato-renal syndrome
cerebrospinal fluid
cerebrovascular
cerebrum
Cerenkov's radiation production
cerium
ceruloplasmin
cervical
   c. canal
   c. carcinoma
   c. curve
   c. hydrocele
   c. lymph node
   c. myelogram
   c. puncture
   c. rib
   c. spine
   c. trachea
   c. tunnel
   c. vertebra
   c. vesicle
cervico-occipital
   c.-o. junction
cervicothoracic
   c. sign

cervix
          c. uteri
cesium (with barium 137m)
^{14}C-glycine-labelled bile salt
          breath test
^{14}C-glycocholic acid tests
CGS – centimeter-gram-second
CGy – centigray
"chain" cystourethrography
chalasia
"chalky" radiography
chamber
          alpha c.
          ion c.
          ionization c.
          multiwire propor-
            tional c.
          pocket c.
          spark c.
          Wilson's c.
Chamberlain's
          line
          method
Chance's fracture
changeover switch
changer
          Puck cutfilm c.
channel
          collateral c's
          c. of Lambert
characteristic
          c. curve
          c. peak
          c. radiation
          c. spectrum
          c. x-ray
characterization

charcoal
Charcot's
          joint
          spine
charger
          Sanchez-Perez
            cassette c.
Chassard-Lapiné
          method
          position
          projection
Chauffeur's fracture
Chaussé's
          method
          projection
          view
cheirolumbar
cheiromegaly
cheirospasm
chemical
          c. analysis
          c. behavior
          c. bond
          c. dosimeter
          c. element
          c. energy
          c. fog
          c. pneumonitis
          c. potential energy
          c. shift
chemodectoma
chemoreceptor
chemotherapeutic
chemotherapy
chemotoxic
chenodeoxycholic acid
Cherenkov's counter

"cherubism"
chest-abdomen sign
CHF – congestive heart
    ailure
Chiari's malformation
chiasma
        optic c.
chiasmatic
Chiba needle
chickenpox
chisel fracture
^{14}C-lactose breath test
Chlamydia
chlorambucil
chloride
chlorine
chlormerodrin
        c. accumulation test
        c.-cysteine complex
        c. Hg 197
        c. Hg 203
chloromycetin
chlorpromazine
choana (choanae)
choanal
choanoid
choke coil
cholangiocarcinoma
cholangiogram (*see* cholan-
    giography)
cholangiographic
cholangiography
        delayed operative c.
        endoscopic retrograde c.
        intraoperative c.
        intravenous c.
        operative c.
        oral c.

cholangiography *(continued)*
        percutaneous hepatobili-
            ary c.
        percutaneous transhe-
            patic c.
        postoperative c.
        retrograde c.
        transabdominal c.
        transhepatic c.
        T-tube c.
cholangiopancreatography
        endoscopic retrograde c.
cholangiotomogram
cholangitis
        c. lenta
        sclerosing c.
Cholebrine
cholecalciferol
cholecystangiography
cholecystectomy
cholecystitis
        acalculous c.
        emphysematous c.
cholecystocholangiography
cholecystocolic
cholecystoenteric
cholecystogogue
cholecystogram
cholecystographic
cholecystography
        intravenous c.
        oral c.
cholecystokinin-pancreozymin
cholecystopaques
cholecystosis
cholecystosonography
choledochal
choledochogram

choledochograph
choledochography
choledocholithiasis
choledochus
cholegraphy
choleliths
cholelithiasis
cholescintigram
cholescintigraphy
 radionuclide c.
cholestasis
cholesteatoma
 renal c.
 suprasellar c.
cholesterol
cholesterolosis
choline
Cholografin
 C. meglumine
 C. methylglucamine
Cholovue
chondral
chondrification
chondritis
chondroangiopathia calcificans
 congenita
chondroblastoma
chondrocalcinosis
chondrodysplasia
 Conradi-Hünermann c.
  punctata
 giant cell c.
 Grebe's c.
 metaphyseal c.
 myotonic c.
 c. punctata
chondrodystrophia
 c. calcificans congenita

chondrodystrophia *(continued)*
 c. fetalis
chondroectodermal
 c. dysplasia
chondrolysis
chondroma
 periosteal c.
 juxtacortical c.
chondromalacia
chondromatosis
 synovial c.
chondromatous
chondrometaplasia
chondromyoma
chondromyxoid
chondromyxoma
chondromyxosarcoma
chondronecrosis
chondro-osseous
chondro-osteodystrophy
chondroplasia
 metaphyseal c.
chondrosarcoma
Chopart's
 fracture-dislocation
 joint
chordae tendineae
chordoma
chorea
choriocarcinoma
chorion
choroid
 c. plexus
Christian's brachydactyly syndrome
chromaffin
chromaffinomatosis
chromate

chromatic
chromatid-type aberration
chromatoelectrophoretic
chromatogram
chromatographic
chromatography
chromic phosphate P 32
chromium
      c. Cr 51 serum albumin
chromophobe
chromosomal
      18p c. abnormality
chromosome
      ring B c.
      c. 18 abnormality
chronic obstructive pulmonary
    disease
CHRS - cerebro-hepato-renal
    syndrome
churning
chyle
chylocyst
chylopericarditis
chylopericardium
chyloperitoneum
chylopneumothorax
chylothorax
chylous
chyluria
chylus
chyme
Ci - curie
cicatricial
cicatrix (cicatrices)
CID - cytomegalic inclusion
    disease
cilia
ciliary

cine
    c. camera
    c. CT scan
    c. study
cineangiocardiography
cineangiograph
cineangiography
cinebronchography
cinedensigraphy
cinefluorography
cinefluoroscopy
cinematography
cinematoradiography
cinemicrography
cinephlebography
cineradiography
cineroentgenofluorography
cineroentgenography
cineurography
cingulate
cingulum (cingula)
circadian
    c. rhythm
circle
    c. of confusion
    c. of Willis
circuit
    anticoincidence c.
    booster c.
    c. breaker
    closed c.
    coincidence c.
    constant potential c.
    c. diagram
    direct current c.
    external c.
    filament c.
    magnetic c.

circuit *(continued)*
    parallel c.
    photoelectric c.
    phototube output c.
    primary x-ray c.
    rectifying c.
    self-rectified c.
    series c.
    three-phase c.
    c. x-ray
circuitry
circular
    c. striation
    c. tomography
circulation
circulatory
circumcardiac
circumcaval
circumduction
circumferential
circumflex
circumlinear
circumscribed
cirrhosis
    biliary c.
    Laennec's c.
    macronodular c.
    muscular c.
    xanthomatous biliary c.
cirsoid
cistern
    basal c.
    cerebellomedullary c.
    chiasmatic c.
    interpeduncular c.
    subarachnoidal c.
    c. of Sylvius
    terminal c's

cisterna (cisternae)
    c. ambiens
    c. cerebellomedullaris
    c. chiasmatis
    c. chyli
    c. fossae lateralis cerebri
    c. interpeduncularis
    c. magna
    perinuclear c.
    s. pontis
    c. venae magnae cerebri
cisternal
    c. injection
    c. puncture
cisternogram
cisternography
    radionuclide c.
cisternomyelography
citrate
CK – creatine kinase
clamp
    Brodney's c.
clasmocytic
clasmocytoma
classification
    Salter-Harris c.
clastogenic
claudication
claustrum (claustra)
clavicle
clavicular fracture
claw
    c. hand
    c.-like finger
    c. toe
"clay shoveler's" fracture

clearing time
Cleaves'
    method
    position
cleft
    c. hand
    laryngotracheoeso-
      phageal c.
    c. lip
    c. palate
    c. vertebra
cleidocranial
    c. dysostosis
    c. dysplasia
Clements-Nakayama position
"Cleopatra" projection
click-murmur syndrome
clinodactyly
    factitious c.
    traumatic c.
clinoid
clivus
cloaking
Cloquet's node
closed core transformer
Clostridium
    C. perfringens
clostridium (clostridia)
cloud
    c. chamber
    electron c.
cloverleaf
    c. deformity
    c. skull
clubbing
clubfoot
Clutton's joints
clysis

Clysodrast
cm – centimeter
CML – chronic myelocytic leu-
    kemia
$CMRO_2$ – cerebral metabolic
    oxygen consumption
CMV – cytomegalovirus
CNS – central nervous system
Co – cobalt
coagulation
coalescence
coalition
    tarsal c.
coarctation
coarsening
coaxial cable
cobalt
    c. 60
"cobblestone" appearance
Cobb's
    measurement
    method
$^{14}CO_2$ breath tests
Coccidioides
    C. immitis
coccidioidomycosis
    subglottic c.
coccydynia
coccygeal
coccyx
cochlea
cochlear
^{58}Co-cyanocobalamin
coded-aperture imaging
"codfish" vertebra
Codman's triangle
coefficient
    absorption c.

coefficient *(continued)*
- attenuation c.
- conversion c.
- effective mass attenuation c.
- linear absorption c.
- linear attenuation c.
- mass absorption c.
- partition c.

coeur en sabot
coffin
coherence
coherent scattering
cohesion
''coiled-spring'' appearance
coil
- Gianturco c's
- Golay c's
- quadruple c.

coincidence
- c. circuit
- c. counting
- c. loss
- positron c.
- c. sum peak

coinlike
Colbert's method
Colcher-Sussman method
colchicine
cold
- c. area
- c. lesion
- c. spot

colic
- c. flexure
- c. valve

colitis
- amebic c.

colitis *(continued)*
- bacterial c.
- cathartic c.
- c. cystica profunda
- granulomatous c.
- infectious c.
- ischemic c.
- milk-induced c.
- mucous c.
- pseudomembranous c.
- radiation c.
- ulcerative c.
- whipworm c.

collagen
collagenase
collagenation
collagenitis
collagenoblast
collagenous
collapse
- bronchiectatic c.
- compression c.
- contraction c.
- inspiratory c.
- lobar c.
- obstructive c.
- pulmonary c.
- vascular c.

''collar button'' ulceration
collateral
- c. air drift
- c. channels
- c. flow
- c. ligament
- c. ventilation

collecting
- c. system
- c. tubule

Colles' fracture
colliculus (colliculi)
collimate
collimation
collimator
    automatic c.
    converging c.
    detector c.
    diverging c.
    focusing c.
    high energy c.
    high resolution c.
    high sensitivity c.
    multihole c.
    parallel-hole c.
    pin-hole c.
    single-hole c.
    slant hole c.
    source c.
    thick septa c.
    thin septa c.
colliquation
colliquative
collision
colloid
colloidal gold
colon
    ascending c.
    descending c.
    iliac c.
    "lead pipe" c.
    pelvic c.
    sigmoid c.
    transverse c.
colonic
    c. angiodysplasia
    c. distention
    c. ileus

colonic *(continued)*
    c. lymphangioma
    c. perforation
    c. polyp
colonoscopy
colorectal
colorimetric
colorimetrically
colostomy
colovesical
colpocephaly
columella
column
    Bertin's c.
    ilioischial c.
    iliopubic c.
    vertebral c.
columnar
comatose
combined transmission-
    emission scintiphoto
commatic aberration
comminuted fracture
comminution
commissure
    habenular c.
Committee on Allied Health,
    Education and Accredita-
    tion
Committee of Radiation from
    Radioactive Medicinal
    Products
common
    c. bile duct
    c. hepatic duct
communicating
    c. hydrocele
    c. hydrocephalus

commutator
    c. ring
compact bone
comparison view
compartment
    pararenal c.
    perirenal c.
    vascular c.
compartmental analysis
compensating filter
compensator
    line voltage c.
    space-charge c.
complement
    c. deficiency
complemental
complex
    chlormerodrin-
      cysteine c.
    Eisenmenger's c.
composite
compound
    c. fracture
    Hurler-Scheie c.
    c. molecule
    c. scanning
    unsaturated c's
compression
    abdominal c.
    c. collapse
    c. cone
    c. device
    digital c.
    c. fracture
    "pancake" c.
    c. technique
    ureteric c.
    vascular c.

Compton's
    edge
    effect
    electron
    scattering photon
    scatter radiation
    wavelength
computed
    c. myelogram
    c. myelography
    c. tomography
computer
    c. assisted tomography
computerized
    c. axial tomography
    c. radiotherapy
    c. tomography
CON – Certificate of Need
concave
concavity
concavoconcave
concavoconvex
concentric
concept
    "ring of bone" c.
concha (conchae)
    ethmoidal c.
    nasal c.
    sphenoidal c.
concretion
condenser
conductance
conductivity
    electrical c.
    thermal c.
conductor
condylar fracture
condylarthrosis

condyle
condyloid
condyloma (condylomata)
condylomatoid
condylomatous
condylus (condyli)
cone
     c. epiphysis
     medullary c.
     c.-shaped configuration
coned-down view
configuration
     closed fist c.
     cone-shaped c.
     cylindrical c.
     donut c.
     horseshoe c.
     ''sawtooth'' c.
     sigmoid-shaped c.
     ''wooden shoe'' c.
confluence
confluent
congenital
     c. adrenal hyperplasia
     c. analgia
     c. constricting bands
     c. contractural arachno-
       dactyly
     c. contracture
     c. curve
     c. hepatic fibrosis
     c. hyperuricosuria
     c. hypoplastic anemia
     c. malformation
     c. metacarpotalar syn-
       drome
     c. nystagmus
     c. osteoporosis

congenital *(continued)*
     c. pulmonary venolobar
       syndrome
     c. renal dysplasia
     c. scoliosis
congestion
congestive
     c. cardiomyopathy
     c. heart failure
conglomerate
conical
coniosis
conjoined
conjugata
     c. vera obstetrica
conjugate
     c. diameter
     glucuronide c.
conjugated
     c. hyperbilirubinemia
conjunctiva
conjunctival
connective tissue disease
connector
conoid
Conradi-Hünermann chondro-
     dysplasia punctata
Conray
console
     direct-display c.
     operator c.
consolidation
constant
     decay c.
     dipolar coupling c.
     longitudinal time c.
     permeability c.
     Planck's c.

constant *(continued)*
    c. potential circuit
    c. potential system
    spin-lattice relaxation
      time c.
    spin-spin relaxation
      time c.
constipation
    psychogenic c.
constriction
constrictor
    c. pharyngis
contagion
contagious
contamination
    renal medullary c.
contiguous
continuous wave
    c. w. resonance
continuum
contour
    ''cupid's bow'' c.
contracted
contractility
contracting
    c. skull
contraction
contractural
contracture
    congenital c.
    distal c.
    Dupuytren's c.
    extension c.
    flexion c.
    joint c.
    c. postischemia
    Volkmann's c.
contralateral

contrast
    c. enhancement
    c. resolution
    short scale c.
    subject c.
contrast media
    Abrodil
    acetrizoate
    acetrizoic acid
    amidotrizoic acid
    Amipaque
    Angioconray
    Angiografin
    Angiovist
    barium sulfate
    benzoic acid
    Biligrafin
    Biligram
    Biliodyl
    Bilivistan
    Bilopaque
    Biloptin
    bismuth
    Bracco
    brominized oil
    bunamiodyl
    calcium
    Cardio-Conray
    Cardiografin
    cerium
    Cholebrine
    Cholografin
    Cholovue
    Clysodrast
    Conray
    Cystografin
    Cystokon
    diaginol

contrast media *(continued)*
  diatrizoate
  diatrizoic acid
  diodine
  diodone
  Diodrast
  Dionosil
  diprotrizoate
  Duografin
  Duroliopaque
  dysprosium
  Endobile
  Endografin
  Ethiodane
  ethiodized oil
  Ethiodol
  ethyliodophenylundecyl
  gadolinium
  Gastrografin
  glucagon
  Hexabrix
  Hippuran
  Hypaque
  Hytrast
  Intropaque
  iobenzamic acid
  iobutoic acid
  iocarmate meglumine
  iocarmic acid
  iocetamate
  iocetamic acid
  iodamic acid
  iodamide
  iodatol
  iodecol
  iodide
  iodipamide
  iodized oil

contrast media *(continued)*
  iodoalphionic acid
  iodohippurate
  iodomethamate
  iodophendylate
  iodophthalein
  iodopyracet
  iodoxamate
  iodoxamic acid
  iodoxyl
  ioglicate
  ioglicic acid
  ioglucol
  ioglucomide
  ioglunide
  ioglycamic acid
  ioglycamide
  iogulamide
  iohexol
  iomide
  Iopamidol
  iopanoate
  iopanoic acid
  iophendylate
  iophenoxic acid
  ioprocemic acid
  iopromide
  iopronic acid
  iopydol
  iopydone
  iosefamate
  iosefamic acid
  ioseric acid
  iosulamide
  iosumetic acid
  iotasul
  ioteric acid
  iothalamate

contrast media *(continued)*
- iothalamic acid
- iotrol
- iotroxamide
- iotroxic acid
- ioxaglate
- ioxaglic acid
- ioxithalamate
- ioxithalamic acid
- iozomic acid
- ipodate
- ipodic acid
- Isopaque
- Isovue
- Kinevac
- Lipiodol
- Liquipake
- magnesium
- manganese chloride
- meglumine
- methiodal
- methylglucamine
- metrizamide
- metrizoate
- metrizoic acid
- Micropaque
- Microtrast
- Monophen
- Myodil
- Neo-Iopax
- Niopam
- Novopaque
- Nyegaard
- Omnipaque
- Orabilex
- Oragrafin
- Oravue
- Osbil

contrast media *(continued)*
- Pantopaque
- phenobutiodyl
- phentetiothalein
- potassium bromide
- Praestholm
- Priodax
- propyliodone
- Raybar 75
- Rayvist
- Renografin
- Reno-M-30
- Reno-M-60
- Reno-M-Dip
- Renovist
- Renovue
- Retro-Conray
- Salpix
- sincalide
- Sinografin
- Skiodan
- Skiodan Acacia
- sodium
- Solu-Biloptin
- Solutrast
- Steripaque-BR
- Steripaque-V
- Telebrix
- Telepaque
- Teridax
- tetrabromophenol-phthalein
- tetraiodophenolphthalein
- Thixokon
- thorium dioxide
- thorium tartrate
- Thorotrast
- triiodobenzoic acid

contrast media *(continued)*
  Triosil
  tyropanoate
  tyropanoic acid
  Umbradil
  Urografin
  Uromiro
  Uropac
  Urovision
  Vasiodone
"contrecoup" fracture
contusion
  myocardial c.
  pulmonary c.
conus
  c. medullaris
conventional
  c. single-phase system
  c. theory of current
convergence lines
conversion
  c. coefficient
  c. factor
  internal c.
converter
  analog-to-digital c.
  digital-to-analog c.
  image c.
  rotary c.
convex
convexity
convexobasia
convexoconcave
convexoconvex
convoluted
convolutional
convolution/deconvolution

convulsions
convulsive fracture
coolant
Cooley's anemia
Cooley-Tukey algorithm
Coolidge's
  transformer
  tube
cooling system
"Cooper's droop"
COPD – chronic obstructive pulmonary disease
Cope-method bronchography
copper
copper-7 intrauterine device
copper-T intrauterine device
coprecipitation
coprolith
cor
  c. adiposum
  c. dextrum
  c. pendulum
  c. pulmonale
  c. sinistrum
  c. triatriatum
  c. triloculare
  c. venosum
  c. villosum
coracobrachialis
coracoclavicular
coracoid
Corbin's technique
cord
  genital c.
  hepatic c.
  lumbosacral c.
  medullary c.
  nephrogenic c.

cord *(continued)*
    spermatic c.
    spinal c.
    umbilical c.
    vocal c.
cordiform
core iron
corkscrew
    c. esophagus
    c. pattern
cornea
corniculate
cornu (cornua)
cornucommissural
coronal
coronary
    c. arteriography
    c. arteriosclerosis
    c. artery disease
    c. spasm
coronoid
cor pulmonale
corpus (corpora)
    c. callosum
    c. luteum
    c. uteri
corpuscular
    c. radiation
correlation time
corresponding ray
cortex (cortices)
    adrenal c.
    cerebral c.
    homotypical c.
    piriform c.
    renal c.
    subchondral c.
    visual c.

cortical
    c. bone loss
    c. destruction
    c. hyperostosis
    c. lucency
    c. mineralization
    c. sclerosis
    c. striation
    c. thickness
corticobulbar
corticocerebellar
corticomedullary
corticoperiosteal
corticopontine
corticorubral
corticospinal
corticosteroid
    c.-binding globulin
corticosteroidism
corticothalamic
cortisol
cortisone
cosmic
    c. radiation
    c. ray
cosmotron
costal
    c. cartilage
    c. groove
    c. margin
    c. process
costicartilage
costicervical
costispinal
costocartilage
costocervical
costochondral
costochondritis

costoclavicular
costocoracoid
costomanubrial
costophrenic
costopleural
costoscapular
costosternal
costotransverse
costovertebral
costoxiphoid
"cotton ball" appearance
Cotton's fracture
"cotton-wool" appearance
cotyloid
cotylopubic
cotylosacral
cough fracture
coulomb
Coulomb's
    force
    law
Coumadin
count density
counter
    boron c.
    Cherenkov's c.
    c. electromotive force
    gamma well c.
    Geiger c.
    Geiger-Müller c.
    ionization c.
    proportional c.
    radiation c.
    scintillation c.
    whole-body c.
counterbalance
counterpulsation balloon
    intra-aortic c. b.

countershock
counting rate meter
coupling
    c. agent
    c. constants
covalent bond
Cowper's duct
coxa
    c. magna
    c. valga
    c. vara
coxsackievirus
Coyle's trauma position
^{11}C-palmitate
CPAP – continuous positive
    airway pressure
CPB – competitive protein
    binding
cpm – cycles per minute
CPPD – calcium pyrophos-
    phate dihydrate
CPR – cardiopulmonary resus-
    citation
cps – cycles per second
CR – central ray
Craig needle
craniad
cranial
    c. computed tomogra-
        phy
cranioaural
craniobuccal
cranio-carpo-tarsal dyspla-
    sia
craniocaudad
craniocaudal
craniocele
craniocerebral

craniodiaphyseal
    c. dysplasia
cranioectodermal
    c. dysplasia
craniofacial
    c. dysplasia
craniograph
craniography
craniolacunia
craniomalacia
craniomeningocele
craniometaphyseal
    c. dysplasia
craniopathy
craniopharyngeal
craniopharyngioma
craniosacral
craniospinal
craniostat
craniostenosis
craniostosis
craniosynostosis
craniotelencephalic
    c. dysplasia
craniotelencephaly
craniotrypesis
craniovertebral
cranium
^{51}Cr-chloride
^{51}Cr-chromate-labelled red cell
    technique
crease
    inframammary c.
    simian c.
creative kinase
crepitation
crepitus
crescendo

crescentic
crest
    iliac c.
    intertrochanteric c.
    c. voltmeter
cretinism
^{51}Cr-heated RBC's
cribriform
"cricket bat" shape
cricoarytenoid
cricoesophageal
cricoid
    c. ring
cricopharyngeal
cricopharyngeus
cricothyroid
cri du chat syndrome
crinkle mark
crista (cristae)
    c. falciformis
    c. galli
    c. lacrimalis
    c. transversa
critical mass
^{51}Cr-labelled red cells
Crohn's
    duodenitis
    granulomatous enteritis
    ileitis
    jejunitis
Cronqvist's cranial index
Crookes' tube
crossed coil designs
cross-fire treatment
crosshatch grid
cross-sectional plane
croup
Crouzon's dysostosis

"crowfoot" sign
CRRMP – Committee of Radiation from Radioactive Medicinal Products
CRT – cathode ray tube
cruciform
crura (*see* crus)
crural
crus (crura)
    c. commune
    diaphragmatic c.
Cruveilhier's joint
cryoglobulinemia
cryostable
    c. magnet
cryostat
cryothermometer
crypt
    c's of Lieberkühn
cryptococcosis
Cryptococcus
cryptodontic
cryptophthalmos
cryptopodia
cryptorchidism
cryptoscope
    Satvioni's c.
cryptoscopy
crystal
    piezoelectric c's
    sodium chloride c.
crystalline
CSF – cerebrospinal fluid
C syndrome
CT –
    computerized tomography
    computed tomography

CT
    body scanner
    disc
    guided biopsy
    scan
    slice thickness
CTMM – metrizamide-assisted computed tomography
^{14}C triolein breath test
Cu – copper
cubic
    c. centimeter
    c. image matrix
cubitocarpal
cubitoradial
cubitus
    c. valgus
    c. varus
cuboid
cuboidal
cuboideonavicular
cuff
    musculotendinous c.
    rotator c.
cul-de-sac
Culiner's theory
culture
cumulative
cuneate
cuneiform
cuneocuboid
cuneometatarsal
cuneonavicular
cuneoscaphoid
cuneus (cunei)
"cupid's bow" contour
cupping
cupula

curie
Curie's law
curium
current
    alternating c.
    c. density
    direct c.
    eddy c.
    electric c.
    filament c.
    generated c.
    induced c.
    ionization c.
    c. meter
    pulsating c.
    rectified c.
    saturation c.
    single-phase c.
    c. stabilizer
    three-phase c.
    undirectional c.
curvature
curve
    Bragg's c.
    cervical c.
    characteristic c.
    compensatory c.
    concave forward c.
    congenital c.
    convex forward c.
    extravertebral c.
    Hurter and Driffield
      photographic c.
    idiopathic c.
    isodose c.
    kyphotic c.
    lordotic c.
    lumbar c.

curve *(continued)*
    neuromuscular c.
    sacral c.
    secondary c.
    thoracic c.
    thoracolumbar c.
    time density c.
curvilinear
cut
    tomographic c.
cutaneous
Cutie Pie
cutis
cut-off sign
c.v. – coefficient of variation
CVCT – cardiovascular com-
    puted tomography scanner
CVP – central venous pressure
CW – continuous wave
CXR – chest x-ray
cyanocobalamin
    c. Co 57
    c. Co 58
    c. Co 60
cyanosis
cyanotic
CYBER 170/720
Cybex ergometer
cycle
    cardiac c.
    Krebs c.
    pentose c.
    c's per second
    QRS c.
cyclic
cyclophosphamide
cyclotron radiation
cycon

cylinder
cylindrical
cylindroma
cyst

    alveolar c.
    arachnoid c.
    aryepiglottic c.
    Baker's c.
    branchial cleft c.
    branchiogenic c.
    bronchogenic c.
    calcified renal c.
    choledochal c.
    colloid c.
    dentigerous c.
    dermoid c.
    diaphragmatic c.
    duplication c.
    echinococcal c.
    echinococcus c.
    enterogenous c.
    ependymal c.
    epidermoid c.
    epidural c.
    epithelial c.
    gastrogenic c.
    hemorrhagic c.
    hepatic c.
    hydatid c.
    intestinal duplication c.
    intracranial c.
    intramedullary c.
    intrapericardial c.
    leptomeningeal c.
    lymphangiectatic c.
    mediastinal c.
    multilocular renal c.
    neurenteric c.

cyst *(continued)*

    pancreatic c.
    parenchymal c.
    pericardial c.
    perinephric c.
    peripelvic c.
    porencephalic c.
    primordial c.
    pulmonary c.
    radicular c.
    renal c.
    retention c.
    serous c.
    splenic c.
    subchondral c.
    subglottic c.
    synovial c.
    theca lutein c.
    thymic c.
    thyroglossal duct c.
    thyroid c.
    unifocal c.
    urachal c.
    vitelline c.
cystadenocarcinoma
cystadenoma
cystectomy
cysteine
cystic

    adenoid c. carcinoma
    c. angiomatosis
    c. bronchiectasis
    c. differentiated ne-
      phroblastoma
    c. duct
    c. fibrosis
    c. gastritis
    c. kidney

cystic *(continued)*
    c. lymphangioma
    c. pattern
cysticercosis
cysticsolid
cystinosis
cystitis
    bacterial c.
    catarrhal c.
    c. emphysematosa
    c. follicularis
    c. glandularis
    c. papillomatosa
Cystografin
cystogram *(see* cystography)
cystography
    bead chain c.
    radionuclide c.
    retrograde c.
    triple-voiding c.
Cystokon
cystoperitoneal
    c. shunt

cystoscopic
cystoscopy
cystourethrogram *(see* cysto-
    urethrography)
cystourethrography
    "chain" c.
    expression c.
    isotope voiding c.
    micturition c.
    radionuclide voiding c.
    retrograde c.
    voiding c.
cystoureterogram
cystoureterography
cytologic
cytologist
cytology
cytomegalic
    c. inclusion disease
cytomegalovirus
cytopathologist
cytopathology
cytotoxic

$\overline{D}$ – mean dose
D or ^2_1H – deuterium
DAC – digital-to-analog con-
    verter
dacryocystography
dactyledema
dactylion

dactylitis
    tuberculous d.
"dagger" sign
Dalkon shield intrauterine de-
    vice
dartos
DAS – data acquisition system

dashboard fracture
data
      d. acquisition system
      ferrokinetic d.
datacamera
datum (data) (*see* data)
daughter
      d. element
      d. nucleus
      d. nuclide
Davis' method
daylight system
db – decibel
d.c. – direct current
DDC – direct display console
DE – dose equivalent
dead man switch
debility
de Broglie's wavelength
decade scaler
decalcification
decay
      alpha d.
      beta d.
      branching d.
      d. constant
      exponential d.
      isomeric d.
      d. mode
      nuclear d.
      positron d.
      d. product
      radioactive d.
      d. scheme
deceleration
decibel
decidua
deciduous

decision matrix
decompression
decontamination
deconvolution analysis
decubitus
decussation
deep therapy
de-excitation
defecation
defecography
defect
      atrial septal d.
      fibrous cortical d.
      filling d.
      "napkin-ring" d.
      septum primum d.
defibrillation
defibrillator
defibrination
deficiency
      acid ceramidase d.
      adenosine deaminase d.
      alpha-1-antitrypsin d.
      complement d.
      copper d.
      disaccharidase d.
      enterokinase d.
      galactosidase d.
      glucocerebrosidase d.
      glucose-6-phosphate de-
         hydrogenase d.
      β-glucuronidase d.
      growth hormone d.
      homogentisic acid oxi-
         dase d.
      hypoxanthine-guanine
         phosphoribosyltrans-
         ferase d.

deficiency *(continued)*
    IgA d.
    myeloperoxidase d.
    purine nucleoside phos-
       phorylase d.
    pyruvate kinase d.
    radial ray d.
    terminal d.
    transverse d.
deflation
deflection
deformity
    "bayonet" d.
    boutonnière d.
    cloverleaf d.
    clubfoot d.
    coxa valga d.
    coxa vara d.
    "Erlenmeyer flask" d.
    Hill-Sachs d.
    Kirner's d.
    Klippel-Feil d.
    kyphotic d.
    lobster claw d.
    Madelung's d.
    "pencil-in-cup" d.
    "penciling" d.
    "pencil-like" d.
    pes cavus d.
    "rat tail" d.
    recurvatum d.
    "shepherd's crook" d.
    Sprengel's d.
    swan-neck d.
    trigger finger d.
    ulnar drift d.
    valgus d.
    varus d.

degassing
degeneration
degenerative
deglutition
dehiscence
dehydration
delay circuit
delimitation
delineated
delineation
delta
    d. mesoscapulae
    d. phalanx anomaly
    d. ray
    d. winding
demagnetization
    adiabatic d.
demarcated
demarcation
    no line of d.
    "shell-like" d.
dementia
demifacet
demilune
demineralization
demyelinating
demyelinization
denatured
dendrite
dendritic
denervation
dens (dentes)
densitometer
densitometry
    quantitative CT d.
density
    background d.
    base d.

density *(continued)*
    calcific d.
    d. equalization
      filter
    hydrogen d.
    inherent d.
    ionization d.
    d. latitude
    pulmonary d.
    radiographic d.
    d. resolution
    spin d.
densography
dentate
dentigerous
dentition
dentoalveolar
dentoalveolitis
dentofacial
denture
6-deoxy-1-galactose
deoxygenated
deoxyribonucleic acid
Department of Health, Education and Welfare
Department of Health and Social Security (UK)
depression
depth
    d. dose
    d. of focus
    d. perception
de Quervain's thyroiditis
dermal
dermatan sulfate
dermatitis
    caterpillar d.
    radiation d.

dermatoarthritis
    lipoid d.
dermatofibroma
dermatofibrosarcoma
dermatofibrosis
dermatoglyphic
dermatomyositis
dermis
dermoid
desferrioxamine
desmoid
desmoplastic
desquamative
destructive
detection
    gastropulmonary aspiration d.
detector
    collimated scintillation d.
    crystalline phosphor d.
    dielectric track d.
    radiation d.
    semiconductor d.
    tissue-equivalent d.
    x-ray d.
detergent
dethyroidism
detrusor
    d. sphincter dyssynergia
Deuel's halo sign
deuterium
deuteron
deuteropathy
deviation
    left axis d.
    mean d.
    radial d.

deviation *(continued)*
    tracheal d.
    ulnar d.
device
    compression d.
    Pigg-O-Stat immobiliza-
        tion d.
dexamethasone
dextral
dextran
dextroangiocardiogram
dextrocardia
dextrocardiogram
dextrocerebral
dextrogastria
dextrogram
dextromanual
dextropedal
dextropositioned
dextrorotatory
dextrosinistral
dextroversion
dextroverted
DHSS – Department of Health
    and Social Security (UK)
DI – diagnostic imaging
diabetes
    lipotrophic d.
    d. mellitus
diabetic
diabrosis
diacondylar
diaginol
diagnosis
Diagnost 120 (Philips)
diagnostic imaging
diagonal
diagrammatic radiography

dialysis
diamagnetic shift
diamagnetism
diaphoresis
diaphragm
    Bucky's d.
    Potter-Bucky d.
diaphragma
    d. sellae
diaphragmatic
diaphyseal
    d. aclasis
    d. dysplasia
    d. sclerosis
    d. tuberculosis
diaphysis (diaphyses)
diapositive
diarrhea
diarthric
diarthrodial
diarthrosis (diarthroses)
diastasis
diastematomyelia
diastematopyelia
diastereomerism
diastereomers
diastole
diastolic
diastrophic
    d. dwarfism
    d. dysplasia
diatomite
diatrizoate
    d. meglumine
    d. sodium
diatrizoic acid
DIC – disseminated intravascu-
    lar coagulation

dicheiria
dichotomous
dicondylar
Dicopac test
dielectric
    d. hysteresis
    d. loss
    d. track detector
diencephalon
diethylenetriamine pentaacetic
    acid
diethyl-iminodiacetic acid
diethyltriamine pentaacetic acid
differential diagnosis
differentiated
differentiation
diffraction
    d. grating
    d. waves
diffuse
    d. fibrosing alveolitis
    d. goiter
    d. idiopathic skeletal
        hyperostosis
    d. interstitial pulmonary
        fibrosis
diffusion
digastric
digestive system
digital
    d. fluoroscopy
    d. subtraction angiogra-
        phy
    d. vascular imaging
digitate
digitization
digitotalar
Digitron computer

diglucuronide
dihydroxycholecalciferol
    1,25-d.
    24,25-d.
diisofluorophosphate
diisopropyl-iminodiacetic
    acid
Dilantin
dilatation
dimelia
dimer
        ionic d's
        nonionic d's
2,3-dimercaptosuccinic acid
dimerization
Dimer-X
dimethylacetanilide iminodi-
        acetic acid
dimethylnitrosamine
dimethylsuccinic acid
dimethylterephalate
diminution
dimming circuit
diode
diodine
diodone
Diodrast
Dionosil
DIP –
        desquamative interstitial
            pneumonitis
        distal interphalangeal
            (joint)
diphenhydramine
2, 5-diphenyloxazole
diphosphonate
diphtheria
diplococci

diploë
venous d.
diplogram
diploic
d. lake
d. vein
dipolar interaction
dipole
diprotrizoate
dipyramidole
direct
d. current
d. Fourier transforma-
tion imaging
d. mapping sequence
d. radiation
disaccharidase
disarticulation
disc, disk
CT d.
floppy d.
herniated d.
intervertebral d.
intra-articular d.
lumbar d.
lumbosacral d.
magnetic d.
Molnar d.
d. space
video d.
Winchester's d.
discitis, diskitis
discogram, diskogram
discography, diskography
discoid
d. lupus erythemato-
sus
discovertebral

discrete
d. Fourier transformation
d. x-ray
discriminator
disease (*see* Part III, Eponymic
Diseases and Syndromes)
DISH – diffuse idiopathic skeletal hyperostosis
disharmonic
DISI – dorsiflexion intercalated
segment instability
DISIDA – diisopropyl-iminodiacetic acid
disinfectant
disintegration
nuclear d.
radioactive d.
spontaneous d.
disk (*see* disc)
dislocation
carpal d.
carpometacarpal d.
congenital hip d.
d.-dissociation
d. fracture
lunate d.
Monteggia's d.
perilunate d.
scaphoid-capitate frac-
ture-d.
scaphoid-lunate d.
slice fracture d.
subglenoid d.
transscaphoid peri-
lunate d.
vertebral d.
disodium etidronate
dispersion

displacement
display
    A-mode d.
    B-mode d.
    d. matrix
    M-mode d.
    d. monitor
    static image d.
    d. system
disproportion
    cephalopelvic d.
dissection
disseminated
    d. intravascular coagu-
      lation
    d. lipogranulomatosis
dissemination
dissociation
    scapho-lunate d.
distance
    "teardrop" d.
distention
    colonic d.
    gaseous d.
distortion
    geometric d.
    pin-cushion d.
    radiographic d.
distraction
distribution
    Boltzmann's d.
    "butterfly" d.
    depth dose d.
    gaussian d.
    maxwellian d.
    Poisson's d.
    spatial dose d.
    d. transformer

diuresis
diuretic
divergence
diverticula (*see* diver-
    ticulum)
diverticulitis
diverticulosis
diverticulum (diverticula)
    acquired d.
    bladder d.
    bronchogenic d.
    calyceal d.
    esophageal d.
    "Hutch" d.
    jejunal d.
    laryngeal d.
    Meckel's d.
    pharyngeal d.
    pharyngoesophageal d.
    pituitary d.
    Rokitansky's d.
    supradiaphragmatic d.
    tracheal d.
    Zenker's d.
D-max – maximum density
DMNA – dimethylnitrosamine
DMSA – dimethylsuccinic acid
DMT – dimethylterephalate
DNA – deoxyribonucleic acid
Dodge's principle
Doerner-Hoskins distribution
    law
doigt en lorgnette
dolichocephalic
dolichocephaly
dolichoectasia
dolor
dominance

dominant
donor
Dooley, Caldwell and Glass
    method
DOOR syndrome – deafness-
    onychodystrophy-osteo-
    dystrophy-retardation
    syndrome
dopamine
Doppler
    effect
    ultrasonography
    ultrasound
dorsal
    d. root ganglia
dorsalis
    d. pedis
dorsiflexion
dorsispinal
dorsoanterior
dorsocephalad
dorsointercostal
dorsolateral
dorsolumbar
dorsomedian
dorsomesial
dorsonasal
dorsonuchal
dorsoplantar
dorsoposterior
dorsoradial
dorsosacral
dorsoscapular
dorsoventrad
dorsoventral
dorsum
    d. pedis
    d. sellae

dosage rate
dose
    air d.
    absorbed d.
    cumulative d.
    depth d.
    doubling d.
    d. equivalent radiation
    erythema d.
    d. estimate
    exit d.
    genetically significant d.
    integral d.
    lethal d.
    maximum permis-
       sible d.
    mean d.
    nominal single d.
    organ tolerance d.
    permissible d.
    radiation absorbed d.
    d. rate
    d. reciprocity theorem
    skin d.
    threshold d.
    tissue tolerance d.
    tumor lethal d.
dosimeter
    chemical d.
    pencil d.
    pocket d.
    thermoluminescent d.
    ultraviolet fluorescent d.
    Victoreen d.
dosimetric
dosimetrist
dosimetry
    pion d.

"dots and dashes"
dot scan
Dotter tube
double
> d.-bonded carbon
> d.-bubble appearance
> d.-bubble shadow
> "d.-bubble" sign
> d.-contrast arthrogram
> d.-contrast arthrography
> d.-contrast barium enema
> d.-contrast study
> d. exposure
> d. focus tube
> d. lesion sign
> d.-pole single throw
> d. track sign
> "d. wall" sign

doubling
> d. dose
> d. time

douche
"doughnut"
> d. kidney
> d. lesion
> d. sign
> d. transformer

Douglas' pouch
DPR – dynamic planar reconstructor
d.p.s.t. – double-pole single throw
Dracunculus
> *D. medinensis*

drainage
DRG – dorsal root ganglia

drip-infusion
> d-i. pyelography
> d-i. urography

"dromedary hump"
droop
> "Cooper's d."

dropsy
"drowned lung"
"drowned newborn syndrome"
drum crest
drumhead
drumstick appearance
drusen
dryer system
DSA – digital subtraction angiography
DSR – dynamic spatial reconstructor
DSV – diameter of the spherical volume
DTPA – diethylenetriamine pentaacetic acid
dual-contrast study
Duchenne's dystrophy
duct
> alveolar d.
> Bartholin's d.
> bile d.
> common bile d.
> common hepatic d.
> Cowper's d.
> cystic d.
> ejaculatory d.
> endolymphatic d.
> excretory d.
> extrahepatic biliary d.
> hepatic d.
> intrahepatic bile d.

duct *(continued)*
    nasofrontal d.
    nasolacrimal d.
    omphalomesenteric d.
    pancreatic d.
    parotid d.
    Rivinus' d.
    seminal d.
    Stensen's d.
    sublingual d.
    submandibular d.
    submaxillary d.
    thoracic d.
    thyroglossal d.
    Wharton's d.
    Wirsung's d.
ductography
    peroral retrograde pan-
      creaticobiliary d.
ductule
ductulus (ductuli)
ductus
    d. choledochus
    d. deferens
    d. parotideus
    patent d. arteriosus
"dumbbell"
    d. lesion
    d. shape
dumping syndrome
Duncan-Hoen method
Dunlap, Swanson and Penner
    method
duodenal
    d. bulb
    d. ulcer
duodenitis
    Crohn's d.

duodenocholangeitis
duodenogastric
duodenogram
duodenography
    hypotonic d.
duodenojejunal
duodenum
Duografin
duplication
    d. cyst
    esophageal d.
    gastric d.
    intestinal d.
    renal d.
    tracheal d.
Dupuytren's
    contracture
    fracture
dural
dura mater
Duroliopaque
DUST – disproportionate upper
    septal thickening
Duverney's fracture
DVI – digital vascular imaging
DVT – deep vein thrombosis
dwarfism
    bird-headed d.
    campomelic d.
    camptomicromelic d.
    diastrophic d.
    dyssegmental d.
    Laron's d.
    megepiphyseal d.
    mesomelic d.
    metatropic d.
    microcephalic d.
    osteoglophonic d.

dwarfism *(continued)*
    polydystrophic d.
    psychosocial d.
    short-limbed d.
    thanatophoric d.
dye
    d.-dilution method
    halogenated phenol-
      phthalein d.
    rose bengal d.
dymelia
dynamic
    d. ileus
    d. magnetic field
    molecular d's
    d. planar reconstructor
    d. spatial reconstructor
    d. volume imaging
Dynapix
dyne
dynode
dysarthria
dysarthrosis
dysautonomia
dyscephaly
dyschondroplasia
dyschondrosteosis
dyscrasia
    lipoid d.
dysdactyly syndrome
dysencephalia splanchnocystica
dyserythropoiesis
dysfunction
dysgammaglobulinemia
dysgenesis
dysgerminoma
dysharmonic
dyshormonogenesis

dyskinesis
dysmaturity
dysmelia
dysmorphism
    digitotalar d.
dysmotility
dysosteosclerosis
dysostosis
    acrofacial d.
    cheirolumbar d.
    cleidocranial d.
    craniofacial d.
    Crouzon's d.
    mandibulofacial d.
    metaphyseal d.
    d. multiplex
    oro-digito-facial d.
    osteo-onycho-d.
dyspepsia
dysphagia
dysplasia
    acromesomelic d.
    acro-pectoro-
      vertebral d.
    asphyxiating thoracic d.
    bronchopulmonary d.
    campomelic d.
    chondroectodermal d.
    cleidocranial d.
    congenital renal d.
    cranio-carpo-tarsal d.
    craniodiaphyseal d.
    cranioectodermal d.
    craniofacial d.
    craniometaphyseal d.
    craniotelencephalic d.
    diaphyseal d.
    diastrophic d.

dysplasia *(continued)*
- ectodermal d.
- epiphyseal d.
- d. epiphysialis hemimelica
- faciocardiomelic d.
- fibrous d.
- focal dermal d.
- frontometaphyseal d.
- frontonasal d.
- hip d.
- Kniest's d.
- mammary d.
- mandibuloacral d.
- metaphyseal d.
- metatropic d.
- monostotic fibrous d.
- oculo-auriculo-vertebral d.
- oculo-dento-osseous d.
- onycho-osteo-arthro d.
- oto-spondylo-megaepiphyseal d.
- parastremmatic d.
- polyostotic fibrous d.

dysplasia *(continued)*
- pseudoachondroplastic d.
- renal d.
- spondyloepiphyseal d.
- spondylometaphyseal d.
- ventriculoradial d.

dysplastic
dyspnea
dysprosium
dysproteinemia
dysraphia
dysraphism
dyssegmental
dyssynergia
dystelephalangy
dystopic
dystrophy
- apical d.
- reflex sympathetic d.
- thoracic-pelvic-phalangeal d.

dysuria
dystrophy
- Duchenne's d.
- muscular d.
- reflex sympathetic d.

E – kidney extraction efficiency
EAA – extra-alveolar air collections
EAM – external auditory meatus

earth screens
Ebstein's malformation
eburnation
ECAT – emission computer-assisted tomography

eccentric
eccentricity
ECG – electrocardiogram
ECG-gating – electrocardi-
    ographic-gating
echinococcal
echinococcosis
Echinococcus
        E. alveolaris
        E. granulosus
echinococcus
echo
echocardiogram
echocardiography
        two-dimensional e.
echoencephalography
echogenicity
echogram
        renal e.
        retroperitoneal e.
echolaminography
echo-planar imaging
echovirus
ECT – emission computed
    tomography
ectasia
        communicating cavern-
            ous e.
        vascular e.
ectatic
ectodermal
        e. dysplasia
ectopia
ectopic
        e. ACTH production
        e. calcification
        e. infusion
        e. kidney

ectopic *(continued)*
        e. ossification
        ''e. pinealomas''
        e. pregnancy
        e. thyroid
        e. ureter
ectrodactyly
ectromelia-ichthyosis syndrome
ECW – extracellular
    water
eddy current
edema
        angioneurotic e.
        gastrointestinal e.
        interstitial e.
        laryngeal e.
        nephrotic e.
        pulmonary e.
edematous
edentulous
edge
        Compton's e.
        e. enhancement
        e. gradient
        e. packing
        e. response function
E-dial calibration
Edison's
        effect
        flouroscope
EDR –
        effective direct radiation
        electrodermal response
EDTA – ethylenediamine te-
    traacetic acid
EDTMP – ethylenediamine tet-
    ramethylene phosphoric
    acid

EEC syndrome – ectrodactyly-
    ectodermal dysplasia–
    clefting syndrome
EEG – electroencephalogram
effacement
effect
    Auger's e.
    biological e.
    Compton's e.
    Doppler e.
    Edison's e.
    heel e.
    isotope e.
    Mach e.
    Overhauser's e.
    photoelectric e.
    photographic e.
    piezoelectric e.
    radiographic e.
    Volta's e.
    Warburg's e.
    "washboard" e.
effective
    e. atomic number
    e. area
    e. current
    e. focal spot
    e. half-life
    e. mass attenuation coef-
        ficient
    e. renal plasma flow
    e. voltage
efferent
effluents
    radioactive e.
effusion
    extraperitoneal e.
    hemorrhagic e.

effusion (continued)
    interlobar e.
    intraperitoneal e.
    pericardial e.
    pleural e.
egesta
"egg" casts
"eggshell" calcification
EHDP – ethylene hydroxydi-
    phosphonate
Eindhoven's magnet
einsteinium
Eisenmenger's complex
ejaculatory
ejection
    e. fraction
    e. murmur
elastic collision
electric
    e. current
    e. field
    e. field strength
    e. flux
    e. generator
    e. lines of force
electrical
    e. alternans
    e. capacitor
    e. charge
    e. condenser
    e. conductivity
    e. conductor
    e. contact
    e. countershock
    e. energy
    e. field
    e. force
    e. hazard

electrical *(continued)*
- e. impulse
- e. intensity
- e. phase
- e. potential
- e. power
- e. resistance

electrocardiogram
electrocardiographic-gating
electrocardiography
electrocoagulation
electroconvulsive
electrode
- focusing e.

electrodermal
electrodynamics
electrodynamometer
electroencephalogram
electrokymogram
electrokymograph
electroluminescent
electrolyte
electromagnet
- iron-core e.
- e. video tape

electromagnetic
- e. energy
- e. field
- e. induction
- e. radiation
- e. spectrum
- e. unit
- e. wave

electromagnetism
electrometer
- dynamic-condenser e.
- vibrating-reed e.

electromotive force
electron
- Auger's e.
- e. beam
- e. beam tube
- bound e.
- e. capture
- e. cloud
- Compton's e.
- excited e.
- free e.
- e. flow
- e. gun
- e. linear accelerator
- e. multiplier tube
- negative e.
- e. orbit
- orbital e.
- oscillating e.
- e. paramagnetic resonance
- e. -positron pair
- e. radiography
- recoil e.
- secondary e.
- e. spin resonance
- e. theory
- e. transition
- e. tube
- e. valence
- e. -volt

electronic
- e. circuit
- e. device
- e. grid
- e. subtraction
- e. timer

electronneutrino
electrophoresis
electrophoretically
electroscope
electrostatic
    e. force
    e. imaging
    e. induction
    e. law
    e. method
    e. repulsion
    e. unit
element
    chemical e.
    daughter e.
    parent e.
    radioactive e.
elephantiasis
ELF – extremely low frequency
elfin facies syndrome
ellipse sign
ellipsoid
ellipsoidal
elliptical
Elon
elongation
Elscint Excel 905 scanner
elutriation
emaciation
Embden-Meyerhof glycolytic pathway
emboli (*see* embolus)
embolic
embolism
    air e.

embolism *(continued)*
    coronary e.
    fat e.
    pulmonary e.
embolization
    arterial e.
    arteriographic e.
    therapeutic e.
    transhepatic e.
embolus (emboli)
    neoplastic e.
    pulmonary e.
    thrombotic e.
    tumor e.
embryology
embryonal
embryonic
embryopathy
    fetal anticoagulant e.
    fetal warfarin e.
emesis
emetic
emf – electromotive force
EMI – Electric and Musical Industries (scanner)
EMI CT 500 scanner
eminence
    arcuate e.
    frontal e.
    iliopubic e.
    intercondylar e.
    parietal e.
    thenar e.
eminentia
    e. arcuata
EMI 7070 scanner
emissary

emission
- beta e.
- e. computed tomography
- filament e.
- negatron e.
- photoelectric e.
- secondary e.
- thermionic e.
- e. tomography

emitter

emphysema
- alveolar e.
- atrophic e.
- bullous e.
- centrilobular e.
- compensatory e.
- gangrenous e.
- glass blower's e.
- hypoplastic e.
- idiopathic unilobar e.
- interlobular e.
- interstitial e.
- lobar e.
- lobular e.
- panacinar e.
- panlobular e.
- paracicatricial e.
- paraseptal e.
- pulmonary interstitial e.
- senile e.

emphysematous
- e. bulla
- e. cholecystitis
- e. cystitis
- e. gastritides
- e. gastritis
- e. vaginitis

"empty" sella

empyema
- pneumococcal e.
- postpneumonectomy tuberculous e.
- streptococcal e.
- subdural e.
- "technical" e.

emu – electromagnetic unit

emulsification

emulsion
- nuclear e.

enantiomeric

enantiomerism

enantiomers

enarthritis

enarthrodial

enarthrosis

en bloc

encapsulated

encapsulation

encephalitis

encephalo-arteriography

encephalocele

encephalocystocele

encephalogram

encephalography

encephalolith

encephaloma

encephalomeningitis

encephalomeningocele

encephalometry

encephalomyelitis
- e. disseminata

encephalomyelopathy

encephalon

encephalopathy

encephalotrige-
    minal
enchondroma
enchondromatosis
enchondromatous
enchondrosarcoma
enchondrosis
encoding
encroachment
encrustation
encysted
endarteritis
    e. calcificans cerebri
    e. obliterans
    e. proliferans
endaural
endemic
Endobile
endobronchial
endocardial
endocarditis
    bacterial e.
    infective e.
    Löffler's e.
    subacute bacterial e.
endocardium
endochondral
endocrine
endocrinopathy
endoergic
Endografin
endolarynx
endolymphatic
endometrial
endometriosis
endometrium
endomyocardial
endoprosthesis

endoscopic
    e. duodenal biopsy
    e. retrograde cholan-
      giography
    e. retrograde cholangio-
      pancreatography
endoscopy
endosteal
    e. sclerosis
endosternum
endosteum
endothelial
endothelioma
endothoracic
endotoxin
endotracheal
endouterine
enema
    barium e.
    cleansing e.
    double-contrast
      barium e.
    opaque e.
    single-contrast
      barium e.
energy
    atomic e.
    binding e.
    chemical potential e.
    e. dependence
    electrical potential e.
    electromagnetic e.
    e. frequency
    gravitational potential e.
    kinetic e.
    mechanical potential e.
    nuclear e.
    photon e.

energy *(continued)*
    potential e.
    quantum e.
    radiant e.
    radiation e.
    e. resolution
    e. spectrum
    thermal e.
    e. wavelength
    x-ray e.
enhancement
    acoustic e.
    contrast e.
enophthalmos
enostosis
en plaque
ensiform process
Entamoeba
    E. histolytica
enteral
enteric
enteritis
    bacterial e.
    Crohn's granuloma-
      tous e.
    eosinophilic e.
    infectious e.
    regional e.
enterobiliary
enterocele
enterochromaffin
enteroclysis
enterococcus (enterococci)
enterocolic
enterocolitis
    bacterial e.
    infectious e.
    necrotizing e.

enterocolitis *(continued)*
    pseudomembranous e.
enterocutaneous
enterocyst
enterocystocele
enterocystoma
enteroepiplocele
enterogastritis
enterogenous
enterohepatitis
enterohydrocele
enteroinvasive
enterokinase
enterolith
enterolithiasis
enteropathic
enteropathogenic
enteropathy
enteropeptidase
enteroptosis
enterospasm
enterostenosis
enterotoxigenic
enterotoxin
enterovenous
enterovesical
enterovirus
enthesis
enthesitis
entodermal
entrapment
    peripheral e.
enucleation
enuresis
envelope
    e. feedback
    glass e.
enzyme

eosinophilia
    Löffler's e.
eosinophilic
eparterial
epaxial
EPEC – enteropatho-
    genic *Escherichia coli*
ependyma
ependymal
ependymitis
ependymoblast
ependymoblastoma
ependymoma
epibronchial right
    pulmonary artery
    syndrome
epicardial
epicardium
epicerebral
epicondylar
epicondyle
epicondylic
    e. ridge
epicondylitis
epicranial
epidemiology
epidermal
epidermoid
epidermoidoma
epidermolysis
    e. bullosa
epididymis
epididymitis
epididymography
epididymo-orchitis
epididymovesiculography
epidural
    e. abscess

epidural *(continued)*
    e. cyst
    e. fat
    e. hematoma
    e. space
epidurography
epigastric
epigastrium
epiglottic
epiglottiditis
epiglottis
epiglottitis
epilepsy
epileptiform
    e. seizure
epiloia
epinephrine
epiphora
epiphyseal
    e. acrodysplasia
    e. dysgenesis
    e. dysplasia
    e. growth plate
    e. necrosis
    e. plate line
    e. vessel
epiphysiolysis
epiphysis (epiphyses)
    capital e.
    cone e.
    distal humeral e.
    femoral e.
    ivory e.
    slipped capital femoral e.
    stippled e.
epiphysitis
    vertebral e.
epiplocele

epiploenterocele
epiploic
epipyramis
epispadias
epistaxis
epithelioglandular
epithelioma
epithelium
    Barrett's e.
    columnar e.
epithermal
epitransverse
epitympanic
    e. recess
    e. space
EPR –
    electron paramagnetic res-
        onance
    epitympanic recess
equation
    Bloch's e's
    Bohr's e.
    Bragg's e.
    Fick's e.
    Hamiltonian e.
    Larmor's e.
    Schroedinger's e.
    Stewart-Hamilton e.
    transformer e.
equilibrium
    e. gated format
    radioactive e.
    secular e.
    e. study
    thermal e.
· equinus
equivalent
    e. capacitance

equivalent *(continued)*
    e. resistance
    e. roentgen
equivocal
eraserophagia
Erasmo's method
erbium
ERCP – endoscopic retrograde
    cholangiopancreatography
ERF – edge response function
erg – a centimeter-gram-
    second (CGS) unit of
    work or energy
ergocalciferol
ergometer
    cybex e.
ergonovine maleate
"Erlenmeyer flask" deformity
ERPF – effective renal plasma
    flow
eructation
eruption
    Kaposi's varicelliform e.
erythema
    e. doubling
    e. fugax
    e. multiforme
    e. nodosum
    toxic e.
erythroblastic
erythroblastosis fetalis
erythrocyte
erythrogenesis
    e. imperfecta
erythrokinetic study
erythroleukemia
    Friend's e.
erythromelalgia

erythropoietin
Escherichia coli
esophageal
    e. atresia
    e. carcinoma
    e. diverticulum
    e. duplication
    e. dysmotility
    e. hiatus
    e. lung
    e. obstruction
    e. reflux
    e. rupture
    e. spasm
    e. ulcer
    e. varices
    e. web
esophagectasia
esophagitis
esophagobronchial
esophagocele
esophagogastric
esophagography
esophagomalacia
esophagopleural
esophagoscopy
esophagospasm
esophagraphy
esophagus
    Barrett's e.
    corkscrew e.
ESR –
    electron spin resonance
    erythrocyte sedimentation
      rate
Essex-Lopresti's fracture
esthesioneuroblastoma
estrogen

esu – electrostatic unit
Ethiodane
ethiodized oil
Ethiodol
ethmoid
ethmoidal
    e. air cells
    e. concha
    e. labyrinth
    e. notch
    e. sinuses
ethmoidomaxillary
ethyl alcohol
ethylenediamine tetraacetic
    acid
ethylenediamine tetramethylene
    phosphoric acid
ethylene glycol
ethylene hydroxydiphosphonate
ethyliodophenylundecyl
etiology
E trisomy
EU – excretory urography
Euler's number
eunuchoidism
europium
eustachian
euthyroid
eutonic
eutopic
eV – electron volt
evagination
Evan's method
eventration
eversion
Ewing's
    sarcoma
    tumor

exanthema
exanthematous
excitation
excited
      e. atom
      e. electron
      e. state
excreta
excretion
excretory
excursion
      respiratory e.
exfoliative
exit dose
exoccipital
exocrine
exophthalmos
exophytic
exostosis (exostoses)
      cartilaginous e.
      subungual e.
      "turret" e.
expansile process
expectoration
expiration
expiratory
exponent
exponential
exposure
      e. angle
      e. dose
      e. dose rate
      double e.
      e. meter
      overcouch e.
      radiation e.
      e. rate
      e. time

exposure *(continued)*
      e. timer
exstrophy
extension
extensor
external
exteroceptive
extra-alveolar air collections
extra-articular
extracapsular
extracardiac
extracellular
extracerebral
extracorticospinal
extraduodenal
extradural
extraesophageal
extragastric
extrahepatic
extralobar
extraluminal
extramedullary
extramural
extraocular
extraoral
extraosseous
extraperitoneal
extrapleural
      e. sign
extrapolate
extraprostatic
extrapyramidal
extrarenal
extrathoracic
extrauterine
extravasation

extravascular
extravertebral
extremity
extrinsic

extrusion
exudate
exudative
E-zero offset

f

F –Fahrenheit
filament
fuse
f –
    farad
    frequency
fabella (fabellae)
facet
      articular f.
      clavicular f.
      malleolar f.
faceted
faceting
facial
facies
faciocardiomelic
      f. dysplasia
facio-digito-genital syndrome
factitious
factor
      Boltzmann's f.
      conversion f.
      geometric f.
      geometry f.
      intensification f.
      intrinsic f.

factor *(continued)*
      magnification f.
      power f.
      quality f.
      rheumatoid f.
Fahrenheit
falciform
falcine
fallopian
      f. aqueduct
      f. arch
      f. artery
      f. ligament
      f. tube
Fallot's tetralogy
fallout
      radioactive f.
falx
      f. cerebri
familial
      f. acrocephalosyndac-
        tyly
      f. adenomatosis coli
      f. carpal necrosis
      f. chromaffinomatosis
      f. dysautonomia

86   FAMILIAL – FEMORAL

familial *(continued)*
  f. idiopathic osteoar-
    thropathy
  f. multiple exostosis
  f. osteoectasia
Fanconi's
  anemia
  pancytopenia
farad
Faraday's
  cage
  law
farmer's lung
fascia (fasciae)
  bulbar f.
  diaphragmatic f.
  endothoracic f.
  Gerota's f.
  iliac f.
  lateroconal f.
  perirenal f.
  psoas f.
  quadratus lumborum f.
  renal f.
  Tenon's f.
  transversalis f.
  Zuckerkandl's f.
fasciagram
fasciagraphy
fascial
fascicle
fascicular
fasciculation
fasciitis
fast Fourier transformation
fast single slice method
fat
  f. absorption breath test

fat *(continued)*
  f. embolism
  epidural f.
  extraperitoneal f.
  extrarenal f.
  orbital f.
  f. pad sign
  pararenal f.
  peribiliary f.
  perirenal f.
  properitoneal f. stripe
fatigue fracture
fatty
  f. acid resonance
  f. infiltration
  f. meal
faucial
faux (fauces)
FDA – Food and Drug Administration
feather analysis
feathery
febrile
fecal
fecalith
feces
^{59}Fe citrate
feet per second
Feist-Mankin position
Feist's method
femora
femoral
  f. arteriography
  f. canal
  f. condyle
  f. epiphysis
  f. head
  f. neck

femoral *(continued)*
>   f. shaft
>   f. torsion
>   f. triangle

femorocele
femoroiliac
femoropatellar
femorotibial
femur (femora)
femur-fibula-ulna syndrome
fenestra (fenestrae)
>   f. choledocha
>   f. cochleae
>   f. rotunda
>   f. vestibuli

fenestral
fenestrated
fenestration
Ferguson's
>   measurement
>   method

fermium
ferric
>   f. chloride
>   f. hydroxide

ferritin
ferrokinetic
ferromagnetic relaxation
ferrous citrate Fe 59
fetal
>   f. alcohol syndrome
>   f. aminopterin
>   f. anticoagulant embryopathy
>   f. Dilantin syndrome
>   f. folic acid antagonist syndrome
>   f. hydantoin syndrome

fetal *(continued)*
>   f. methotrexate
>   f. thalidomide
>   f. warfarin embryopathy

fetid
fetogram
fetography
fetus
FEV_1 – forced expiratory volume (in one second)
fever
>   Mediterranean f.

FF – filtration fraction
FFD – focal film distance
FFT – fast Fourier transformation
FFU syndrome – femur-fibula-ulna syndrome
fiber
>   Sharpey's f's

fibercolonoscope
fibergastroscope
fiber-illuminated
fiberoptic
fiberoptics
fiberscope
fiberscopic
"fibrillar"
fibrillation
>   atrial f.
>   ventricular f.

fibrin ball
fibrinogen
fibroadenoma
fibroadenosis
fibroangioma
fibroangiomatous
fibroareolar

fibroatrophy
fibroblastic
fibroblastoma
fibrocalcific
fibrocarcinoma
fibrocartilage
fibrocartilaginous
fibrocaseous
fibrocavitary
fibrocellular
fibrochondroma
fibrocollagenous
fibrocyst
fibrocystic
fibrocystoma
fibrodysplasia
    f. ossificans
    f. ossificans progressiva
fibroelastic
fibroelastosis
    endocardial f.
fibroepithelioma
fibrofatty
fibrogenesis
    f. imperfecta ossium
fibrogenic
fibroglandular
fibroglia
fibroglioma
fibroid
fibrolipoma
fibrolipomatosis
fibroma
    ameloblastic f.
    cementifying f.
    chondromyxoid f.
    desmoplastic f.
    nonossifying f.

fibroma *(continued)*
    nonosteogenic f.
    ossifying f.
fibromatoid
fibromatosis
    juvenile hyaline f.
    Stout's f.
fibromatous
fibromembranous
fibromuscular
fibromyalgia
fibromyitis
fibromyoma
    f. uteri
fibromyositis
fibromyxoma
    odontogenic f.
fibromyxosarcoma
fibronuclear
fibro-osseous
fibro-osteoma
fibropapilloma
fibroplasia
    retrolental f.
fibropurulent
fibrosarcoma
fibrosclerosis
fibrosing
fibrosis
    cartilaginous annulus f.
    congenital hepatic f.
    cystic f.
    diatomite f.
    endomyocardial f.
    graphite f.
    idiopathic pulmonary f.
    idiopathic retroperito-
      neal f.

fibrosis *(continued)*
    interstitial f.
    mediastinal f.
    neoplastic f.
    nodular subepidermal f.
    panmural f.
    perianeurysmal f.
    periureteric f.
    postfibrinous f.
    progressive portal f.
    proliferative f.
    pulmonary f.
    replacement f.
    retroperitoneal f.
    root sleeve f.
    submucosal f.
    f. uteri
fibrositis
    capsular f.
fibrothorax
fibrotic
fibrous
    f. cortical defect
    f. dysplasia
    f. histiocytoma
    f. xanthoma
fibrovascular
fibroxanthoma
fibula
fibular
fibularis
fibulocalcaneal
Fick's
    equation
    law
    position
    principle
FID – free induction decay

field
    absolute f.
    alternating f.
    f. coil
    dynamic magnetic f.
    electrical f.
    f. emission x-ray system
    f. focusing nuclear magnetic resonance
    f. of force
    f. gradient
    f. intensity
    f. line
    magnetic f.
    pulsed radiofrequency f.
    f. size
    static magnetic f.
    f. strength
    f. of view
filament
    ammeter f.
    f. circuit
    f. current
    f. emission
    f. saturation
    f. stabilizer
    thorinated tungsten f.
    f. transformer
    f. voltage
filariasis
filling defect
film
    acetate f.
    f. badge
    f. base
    f. bin
    comparison f.

film *(continued)*
- f. contrast
- f. corner cutter
- f. defects
- f. density calibration
- f. dispenser
- f. emulsion
- expiratory f.
- gamma f.
- f. graininess
- grid f.
- f. hangers
- lateral decubitus f.
- overpenetrated f.
- plain f.
- f. processing
- prone f.
- rapid processing f.
- f. ring
- f. screen contact test tool
- screen type f.
- f. sensitivity
- sequential f.
- serial f.
- single emulsion f.
- f. speed
- stress f.
- f. subtraction
- f. tube distance
- x-ray f.

film changer
- Schonander f. c.

filter
- compensating f.
- density equalization f.
- inherent f.
- radiography f.

filter *(continued)*
- spatial f.
- Thoraeus' f.
- Wedge's f.
- Wratten's 6B f.

filtered back projection

filtration
- f. fraction
- glomerular f.
- inherent f.

filum (fila)
- f. terminale

fimbria (fimbriae)

fimbriated

finger
- baseball f.
- claw-like f.
- drop f.
- fifth f.
- mallet f.
- f. pads
- trigger f.
- webbed f's

"fingerprint" pattern

Finnish type nephrosis

first-pass isotope angiography

first-pass radionuclide angio-cardiography

Fischgold's
- bimastoid line
- biventer line

"fish" vertebra

Fisk's method

fission

fissure
- anal f.
- azygos lobe f.
- calcarine f.

fissure *(continued)*
>interhemispheric f.
>interlobar hepatic f.
>intersegmental he-
>>patic f.
>intrapulmonary f.
>longitudinal f.
>orbital f.
>parieto-occipital f.
>petrosquamous f.
>petrotympanic f.
>pulmonary f.
>sylvian f.
>f. of Sylvius
>transverse f.

fistula (fistulas or fistulae)
>aortoduodenal f.
>arteriovenous f.
>biliary-enteric f.
>bronchopleural f.
>cholecystocolic f.
>cholecystoen-
>>teric f.
>colovesical f.
>esophagopleural f.
>gastrocolic f.
>sigmoid-vesicle f.
>thyroglossal f.
>tracheoesophageal f.
>tracheoinnominate f.

fistulogram
fistulography
fistulous
fixation
fixer solution
fixing time
flaccid
flaccidity

flail
>f. chest
>f. joint
>f. valve

"flank stripe"
flatulence
flatus
Fleischner's
>line
>method
>position

flexion
flexor
flexure
>colic f.
>duodenojejunal f.
>hepatic f.
>splenic f.

flicker
flip-flop phenomenon
floating
>f. kidney
>f. spleen

"floating tooth" sign
flocculating
flocculent
flocculonodular
flood source
floppy disk
florid
flow
>blood f. measurement
>cerebral blood f.
>collateral f.
>effective renal plasma f.
>electron f.
>f. graph
>f. imaging

flow *(continued)*
    f. potential
    pulmonary f.
    f. study
FLS – fibrous long-spacing
   (collagen)
fluctuation
    intensity f.
    noise f's
fluffy margins
fluid
    bland f.
    cerebrospinal f.
    extraperitoneal f.
    free peritoneal f.
    intraperitoneal f.
    mediastinal f.
    pleural f.
    synovial f.
    toxic f.
fluid-fluid level
fluorescence
fluorescent
    f. phosphor
    f. ray
    f. scan
    f. screen
fluoride
    f. poisoning
fluorine 19
fluorine F 18
fluorochloride
fluorography
fluorometer
fluorometric
fluorometry
fluoronephelometer
fluororoentgenography

fluoroscope
    Edison's f.
fluoroscopic
    f. image
    f. image intensifier
    f. timer
fluoroscopical
fluoroscopy
    computerized f.
    digital f.
    image-amplified f.
fluorosis
flutter
    atrial f.
    auricular f.
    diaphragmatic f.
    mediastinal f.
    ventricular f.
flutter-fibrillation
flux
    electric f.
    f. jumping
    f. line
    magnetic f.
    photon f.
focal
    f. dermal dysplasia
    f. disease
    f. film distance
    f. length
    f. plane level
    f. plane tomography
    f. pyelonephritis
    f. spot
    f. thyroiditis
    f. zone
foci *(see* focus)

focus (foci)
    conjugate f.
    f. film distance
    grid f.
    line f.
    linear f.
    f. object distance
    f. size
    virtual f.
focused grid
focusing cup
FOD – focus object distance
fogging
fold
    aryepiglottic f.
    axillary f's
    bulboventricular f.
    gastric f's
    lacrimal f.
    medullary f.
    pharyngoepiglottic f.
    rugal f.
    semilunar f.
    vestibular f.
folic acid
follicle
    graafian f.
    lymphoid f's
follicular
folliculitis
folliculoma
    f. lipidique
FONAR – focused nuclear
   magnetic resonance
fontanelle
Food and Drug Administration
foot
    Madura f.

"football" sign
foramen (foramina)
    anterior sacral f.
    basal f.
    emissary f.
    hypoglossal f.
    infraorbital f.
    interventricular f.
    intervertebral f.
    jugular f.
    f. lacerum
    f. of Luschka
    f. of Magendie
    f. magnum
    mental f.
    f. of Monro
    neural f.
    nutrient f.
    obturator f.
    optic f.
    f. ovale
    palatine f.
    parietal f.
    f. rotundum
    sacral f.
    f. spinosum
    stylomastoid f.
    supraorbital f.
    f. transversa-
      rium
    transverse f.
    vascular f.
    venous f.
    vertebral f.
    f. of Vesalius
    f. of Winslow
    zygomaticofacial f.
foraminal

foraminous spiral tract
force
    centrifugal f.
    centripetal f.
    Coulomb's f.
    electric lines of f.
    electrical f.
    electromotive f.
    electrostatic f.
    field of f.
    gravitational f.
    Lorentz's f.
    molecular f.
    nuclear f.
forearm
forebrain
forefoot
foreign body
formation
    "ruffled border"
        bone f.
formatter
formula
    autotransformer f.
    power f.
    projection f.
fornix (fornices)
fossa (fossae)
    cerebral f.
    condyloid f.
    coronoid f.
    cubital f.
    gallbladder f.
    glenoid f.
    Gruber's f.
    hepatorenal f.
    hypophyseal f.
    iliac f.

fossa (fossae) *(continued)*
    infraspinatus f.
    intercondylar f.
    interpeduncular f.
    Jobert's f.
    jugular f.
    malleolar f.
    mandibular f.
    nasal f.
    olecranon f.
    paraduodenal f.
    paravesical f.
    parietal f.
    patellar f.
    pituitary f.
    popliteal f.
    posterior f.
    pterygoid f.
    pterygopalatine f.
    radial f.
    renal f.
    semilunar f.
    supraclavicular f.
    supraspinatus f.
    temporal f.
    temporomandibular f.
    tibiofemoral f.
    trochanteric f.
    ulnar f.
    zygomatic f.
Fourier
    direct transformation
      imaging
    discrete transformation
    multislice modified
      KWE direct imaging
    transformation recon-
      struction

Fourier *(continued)*
  transformation zeugma-
    tography
  two-dimensional imag-
    ing
  two-dimensional projec-
    tion reconstruction
four-valve-tube rectification
four-vessel angiography
fovea (foveae)
foveola
Fowler's position
fps – feet per second
fraction
  branching f.
  ejection f.
  penetration f.
  scatter f.
fractional
fractionation
fracture
  acetabular f.
  acromial f.
  articular f.
  avulsion f.
  Barton's f.
  basal neck f.
  Bennett's f.
  bimalleolar f.
  "blow-out" f.
  "boxer's" f.
  buckle handle f.
  bumper f.
  "burst" f.
  calcaneal f.
  carpal f.
  carpometacarpal f.
  Chance's f.

fracture *(continued)*
  Chauffeur's f.
  chisel f.
  chondral f.
  Chopart's f.
  clavicular f.
  "clay-shoveler's" f.
  closed f.
  Colles' f.
  comminuted f.
  compound f.
  compression f.
  condylar f.
  "contrecoup" f.
  convulsive f.
  coracoid process f.
  Cotton's f.
  cough f.
  dashboard f.
  dens f.
  depressed f.
  diacondylar f.
  dislocation f.
  displaced f.
  distraction f.
  Dupuytren's f.
  Duverney's f.
  epiphyseal f.
  Essex-Lopresti's f.
  extra-articular f.
  extracapsular f.
  fatigue f.
  femoral neck f.
  femoral shaft f.
  fibular shaft f.
  flexion f.
  Galeazzi's f.
  Gosselin's f.

fracture *(continued)*
> greenstick f.
> "growing" f.
> hangman's f.
> humeral condyle f.
> Hutchison's f.
> iliopubic ramus f.
> impaction f.
> intercondylar f.
> internal f.
> interperiosteal f.
> intertrochanteric f.
> intra-articular f.
> intracapsular f.
> intraperiosteal f.
> ischial f.
> Jefferson's f.
> Jones' f.
> Lefort's f.
> Lisfranc's f.-dislocation
> long bone f.
> lumbar f.
> Maissoneuf's f.
> Malgaigne's f.
> malleolus f.
> malunion f.
> march f.
> metacarpal f.
> metacarpal head f.
> metacarpal neck f.
> metaphyseal corner f.
> metatarsal f.
> Monteggia's f.-disloca-
>   tion
> Moore's f.
> navicular f.
> nightstick f.
> nonarticular f.

fracture *(continued)*
> oblique f.
> olecranon f.
> open f.
> osteochondral f.
> patellar f.
> pelvic ring f.
> peritrochanteric f.
> phalangeal f.
> Piedmont's f.
> Pott's f.
> pubic rami f.
> Quervain's f.
> rim f.
> Rolando's f.
> scaphoid f.
> Shepherd's f.
> Skillern's f.
> Smith's f.
> spiral f.
> splintered f.
> Stieda's f.
> stress f.
> subcapital f.
> subperiosteal f.
> subtrochanteric f.
> supracondylar f.
> T-f.
> teardrop f.
> thoracolumbar f.
> Thurston-Holland f.
> tibial condylar f.
> tibial plafond f.
> tibial shaft f.
> Tillaux's f.
> toddler's f.
> torsion f.
> torus f.

fracture *(continued)*
    transcervical f.
    transcondylar f.
    transverse f.
    trimalleolar f.
    "tripod" f.
    ulnar styloid f.
    vertebral f.
    volar plate f.
    wagonwheel f.
    Wagstaffe's f.
    Walther's f.
    Y-f.
fragile X syndrome
fragmentation
Francisella
    F. tularenis
francium
Frankfort
    line
    plane
Franseen needle
"frayed string" appearance
free
    f. air
    f. air ionization chamber
    f. electron
    f. induction decay
    f. isolated spin
    f. peritoneal air
    f. tissue water
Freiberger's method
Freiberg's infarction
fremitus
French polyethylene catheter
frenulum (frenula)

frequency
    energy f.
    Larmor's f.
    Larmor's precession f.
    f. waves
Fresnel's zone plate
Freund's adjuvant
friction marks
Friedländer's
    bacillus
    pneumobacillus
    pneumonia
Friedman's
    method
    position
Friend's erythroleukemia
frilling
frog-leg view
frontal
frontalis
frontodigital
frontoethmoidal
frontolacrimal
frontomalar
frontomaxillary
frontometaphyseal
    f. dysplasia
frontonasal
    f. dysplasia
fronto-occipital
frontoparietal
frontopontine
frontosphenoid
frontozygomatic
frostbite
fructose
FS – focal spot

FSH – follicle stimulating hormone
^{18}F sodium fluoride
Fuchs'
    method
    position
fucose
fucosidosis
fulcrum
full
    f. line scanning
    f.-wave rectification
    f.-wave rectifier
    f.-width at half-maximum
function
    line spread f.
    modulation transfer f.
    point spread f.
    renal f.
    Shepp-Logan filter f.
    Zeeman's hamiltonian f.
"functional asplenia"
fundal
fundament
fundi
fundiform
fundoplication
    Nissen's f.
fundus (fundi)
fungal

fungus (fungi)
funicular
funiculitis
funiculoepididymitis
funiculus (funiculi)
funnel
    f. breast
    mitral f.
    pial f.
    vascular f.
furosemide
furuncle
fused
fusiform
fusion
    atlantoaxial f.
    capitate-hamate f.
    capitate-trapezoid f.
    lunate-scaphoid f.
    lunate-triquetrum f.
    nuclear f.
    pisiform-hamate f.
    scaphoid-trapezium f.
    sutural f.
    trapezium-trapezoid f.
    triquetrum-hamate f.
    triquetrum-lunate f.
    vertebral f.
F(v) – velocity distribution function
FWHM – full-width at half-maximum
FZ – focal zone

G g

G –
- conductance
- gauss
- generator
- grid

γ – gamma rays

Ga – gallium

gadolinium
- g. 159 hydroxycitrate
- g. oxysulfide

gait
- antalgic g.
- gluteus medius g.
- paralytic g.
- short leg g.
- Trendelenburg's g.

galactorrhea

galactose

galactosemia

galactosidase deficiency

Galeazzi's fracture

Galen's vein "aneurysm"

gallbladder
- "porcelain" g.

gallium
- g. citrate Ga 67
- g. scanning
- radioactive g.
  - Ga 67
- g. uptake

gallstones

galvanometer

gamekeeper's thumb

gamma
- g.-aminobutyrate
- g. camera
- g. cascade
- g. emitter
- g. film
- g. heating
- g. radiation
- g. radiography
- g. ray
- g.-ray counter
- g.-ray level indicator
- g.-ray scanner
- g.-ray spectra
- g.-ray spectrometer
- g. scanning
- g. well counter

gammaphoto

gammopathy
- monoclonal g.

ganglia (*see* ganglion)

ganglioglioma

ganglion (ganglia or ganglions)
- intraosseous g.

ganglioneuroblastoma

ganglioneuroma

ganglioneuromatosis

gangliosidosis

gangrene
- gas g.
- pulmonary g.

gangrenous

gantry
gargoyle syndrome
gargoylism
    Pfaundler-Hurler g.
Garn's method
Garré's sclerosing osteomyelitis
gas
    g. amplification
    extraluminal g.
    g. gangrene
    g. infarction
    intraluminal g.
    intramural g.
    intraperitoneal g.
    g. myelography
    radioactive g.
    g. recovery
    retroperitoneal g.
    ventilator-induced g.
gaseous
gastrectomy
gastric
    g. antrum
    g. artery
    g. bubble
    g. carcinoma
    g. contents
    g. dilatation
    g. duplication
    g. emptying
    g. folds
    g. lymph node
    g. perforation
    g. polyp
    g. resection
    g. ulcer
gastrin

gastrinoma
gastritides
gastritis
    antral g.
    atrophic g.
    catarrhal g.
    cystic g.
    emphysematous g.
    eosinophilic g.
    erosive g.
    exfoliative g.
    follicular g.
    hypertrophic g.
    phlegmonous g.
    polypous g.
    pseudomembranous g.
    radiation g.
    toxic g.
    zonal g.
gastrocamera
gastrocele
gastrocnemial
    g. ridge
gastrocolic
gastroduodenal
gastroduodenostomy
gastroduodenum
gastroenteritis
    eosinophilic g.
    g. typhosa
    viral g.
gastroenterocolitis
gastroenterology
gastroenteroptosis
gastroepiploic
gastroesophageal
    g. reflux

gastroesophagography
    radionuclide g.
gastrogenic
Gastrografin
gastrointestinal
    g. bleeding
    g. blood loss test
    g. edema
    g. hemorrhage
    g. perforation
    g. protein loss test
    g. series
    g. system
    g. tract
gastrojejunostomy
gastropathy
gastropulmonary
gastropyloric
gastroradiculitis
gastrosplenic
gated
    g. blood pool imaging
    g. CT scanner
gauss
gaussian distribution
gavage
Gaynor-Hart
    method
    position
Geiger counter
Geiger-Müller counter
gelatinous
General Electric CT/T7 800
    scanner
General Electric 8800 scanner
generator
    direct current g.
    electric g.

generator *(continued)*
    electrostatic g.
    molybdenum-
      technetium g.
    polyphase g.
    resonance g.
    6-pulse 3-phase g.
    supervoltage g.
    three-phase g.
    Triphasix g.
    12-pulse 3-
      phase g.
    Van de Graaff's g.
    x-ray g.
genetic
genetically
    g. significant dose
genial
geniculate
geniculum (genicula)
geniohyoid
genital
genitalia
genitography
genitourinary
genu (genua)
    g. recurvatum
    g. valgum
    g. varum
genucubital
genufacial
genupectoral
geographic
geometric
    g. artifact
    g. distortion
    g. factor
geometrical

geometry
  g. factor
  Golay g.
  slice g.
Gerlach's tendon
German horizontal plane
germanium
germicide
germinal
germinoma
  pineal g.
Gerota's
  capsule
  fascia
GE scan – gastroesophageal scan
gestation
gestational trophoblastic disease
GFR – glomerular filtration rate
GHA – glucoheptanoic acid/glucoheptonate
GI – gastrointestinal
giant cell
  g. c. arteritis
  g. c. chondrodysplasia
  g. c. pneumonitis
  g. c. tumor
  g. c. xanthoma
giantism
Gianturco coils
Giardia
  G. intestinalis
  G. lamblia
giardiasis
gibbus
gigantism

giggle incontinence
Gill's method
gingiva (gingivae)
gingival
gingivitis
ginglymoarthrodial
ginglymoid
ginglymus
girdle
  pelvic g.
  shoulder g.
Girout's method
glabella
glabelloalveolar line
glabellomeatal line
glabrous
glacial acetic acid
gladiolus
gladiomanubrial
gland
  adrenal g.
  Brunner's g.
  bulbourethral g.
  endocrine g.
  exocrine g.
  lacrimal g.
  mammary g.
  mucous g.
  parathyroid g.
  parotid g.
  pineal g.
  pituitary g.
  prostate g.
  salivary g.
  sublingual g.
  submandibular g.
  submaxillary g.
  suprarenal g.

gland *(continued)*
    thymus g.
    thyroid g. uptake
glandular
glandulography
Glass
    hepatic test of G.
glass
    g. blower's emphysema
    g. envelope
glenohumeral
glenoid
glenoidal
glia
glial
glioblastoma
    g. multiforme
glioma
    brainstem g.
    optic chiasm g.
    pontine g.
global
globoid
globus (globi)
    g. pallidus
glomangioma
glomera (*see* glomus)
glomerular
glomerulitis
glomerulonephritis
glomerulonephropathy
glomerulopathy
glomerulosa
glomerulosclerosis
glomerulus (glomeruli)
glomus (glomera)
glomus (glomera)
    g. jugulare tumor

glomus (glomera) *(continued)*
    g. tympanicum tumor
glossa
glossal
glossoepiglottic
glossopalatine
glossopharyngeal
glottic
glottides
glottis (glottides)
glow modular tube
glucagon
glucocerebrosidase deficiency
glucocorticoid
glucoheptonate
gluconate
gluconeogenesis
glucosaminidase
glucose-6-phosphate dehydro-
    genase deficiency
β – glucuronidase deficiency
glucuronide
    g. conjugate
glutamate
glutaraldehyde
gluteal
gluten
gluteus medius gait
glycerol
glycerolphosphorylcholine
glycogen storage disease
glycolysis
glycosaminoglycan
gm – gram
G-M counter – Geiger-Müeller
    counter
goiter
    colloid g.

goiter *(continued)*
    diffuse g.
    intrathoracic g.
    mediastinal g.
    multinodular g.
    nontoxic g.
    retrosternal g.
    substernal g.
goitrogen
Golay
    coils
    geometry
gold Au 198
Golden's "S" sign
gompholic
gomphosis
gonad
    g. shielding
    mean g. dose
gonadal shield
gonadoblastoma
gonion
gonococcal
Goodpasture's syndrome
Gosselin's fracture
gout
gouty
GPC – glycerolphosphorylcho-
    line
graafian
    g. follicle
    g. vesicle
gradient
    g. coil
    edge g.
    field g.
    potential g.
    g. power amplifier

gradient *(continued)*
    g. system
    g. waveform generation
graft
    aortocoronary artery
      bypass g.
    aortoiliac g.
    coronary artery by-
      pass g.
    intra-abdominal g.
    saphenous vein aortoco-
      ronary bypass g.
graininess
gram
    g.-negative cocci
    g.-negative rods
    g.-positive cocci
    g.-stain
Grandy's method
granular
    g. pits
granularity
granulation
granuloma
    calcified g.
    eosinophilic g.
    g. inguinale venereum
    midline g.
    optic g.
    periapical g.
    plasma cell g.
    pulmonary g.
    Wegener's g.
granulomatosis
    eosinophilic g.
    lymphomatoid g.
    Wegener's g.
granulomatous

graphite
Grashey's
    method
    position
gravel
Graves' scapula
gravid
gravida
Gravigards intrauterine device
gravitational
    g. force
    g. potential energy
gravity
    specific g.
Grawitz's tumor
gray-scale ultrasonography
Grebe's chondrodysplasia
Green needle
greenstick fracture
Greig's cephalopolydactyly
grenz ray
Greulich-Pyle atlas
grid
    Bucky's g.
    g. cassette
    electronic g.
    g. film
    g. focus
    focused g.
    g. line
    linear g.
    Lysholm's g.
    moving g.
    oscillating g.
    parallel g.
    Potter-Bucky g.
    radiographic g.
    g. radius

grid *(continued)*
    g. ratio
    reciprocating g.
    rhombic g.
    stationary g.
groin
Grollman pigtail catheter
groove
    bicipital g.
    costal g.
    optic g.
    supraorbital g.
    ulnar g.
    vascular g.
Grossman's principle
"ground-glass" appearance
grounding
"growing" fracture
Gruber's fossa
Grüntzig balloon-tip catheter
GSD – genetically significant
    dose
gumma (gummas or gummata)
    miliary g.
    tuberculous g.
Gunson's method
gutter
    paracolonic g.
gynecography
gynecoid
gynecologic
gynecology
gynecomastia
gynogram
gynography
Gyratome
gyri *(see* gyrus)
gyromagnetic ratio

106 GYRUS – HAMILTONIAN

gyrus (gyri)
    cingulate g.
    frontal g.
    hippocampal g.
    lingual g.

gyrus (gyri) *(continued)*
    occipitotemporal g.
    parahippocampal g.
    rectal g.
    temporal g.

H h

H –
    henries
    Hounsfield unit
    hydrogen
$^2_1$H – deuterium
H_2 breath test
Haas'
    method
    position
habenula
habenular
habitus
hafnium
"hair brush" pattern
"hairpin" loop
"hair-standing-on-end" appearance
halation
half-cycle
half-life
    biological h-l.
    effective h-l.
    physical h-l.
    h-l layer
    radioactive h-l.

half-thickness
half-time of exchange
half-value layer
half-wave rectification
halide
hallux (halluces)
    h. dolorosa
    h. malleus
    h. rigidus
    h. valgus
    h. varus
halogenated
"halo" sign
HAM – human albumin microspheres
hamartoblastoma
hamartochondroma
hamartoma
    chondromatous h.
hamartomatosis
hamartomatous
hamate
hamiltonian
    h. equation
    Zeeman's h. function

Hamman's sign
"hammered brass" appearance
hammer toe
"hammocking"
Hampton's
        hump
        view
hamstring
hamulus (hamuli)
HAN – hyperplastic alveolar
    nodules
H & D curve – Hurter and Drif-
    field photographic curve
hand
        "rosebud" h.
        "windswept" h.
hand-foot-genital syndrome
hand-foot syndrome
hand-foot-uterus syn-
        drome
"hanging fruit" pattern
hangman's fracture
Harrison-Stubbs method
Hartmann's pouch
Hashimoto's thyroiditis
Hatt's method
haustral
        h. churning
        h. pattern
        h. sacculations
haustration
haustrum (haustra)
haversian
Hawkin's needle
Haygarth's node
hCG – human chorionic gonad-
    otropin
Hct_b – whole-body hematocrit

Hct_v – venous hematocrit
HDP – hydroxydiphosphonate
Health Maintenance Organiza-
    tion
Health Systems Agency
heart
        h. block
        h. failure
        "snowman" h.
heartworm
heat
        h. dissipation
        h. exchanger
        h. shield
        h. sink
        h. unit
heavy-chain disease
heavy ion imaging
"heavy markings"
heavy particle therapy
Heberden's node
Hector's tendon
heel effect
Heister's valve
helium atom
helix
Helmholtz's pair
hemangiectatic
        h. hypertrophy
hemangioblastoma
hemangioblastomatosis
hemangioendothelioblas-
        toma
hemangioendothelioma
hemangioendotheliosarcoma
hemangiofibroma
hemangioma
        cavernous h.

hemangioma *(continued)*
  h. lymphangioma
  orbital h.
  subglottic h.
  vertebral h.
hemangiomata
hemangiomatosis
  intraosseous h.
hemangiopericytoma
hemangiosarcoma
hemarthrosis
hematemesis
hematencephalon
hematocele
hematochezia
hematocolpos
hematocrit
  elevated venous h.
  mean circulatory h.
hematogenous
hematologic system
hematoma
  cerebral h.
  epidural h.
  extrapleural h.
  hepatic h.
  iliacus h.
  intracapsular h.
  intracerebral h.
  intracranial h.
  intramural h.
  intrarenal h.
  intrasplenic h.
  paraspinal h.
  perianal h.
  perinephric h.
  pulmonary h.
  retrouterine h.

hematoma *(continued)*
  splenic h.
  subcapsular h.
  subdural h.
  subungual h.
hematomyelia
hematomyelitis
hematopoiesis
hematopoietic
hematuria
  microscopic h.
  renal h.
  urethral h.
  vesical h.
hemianesthesia
hemiangiectatic
hemianopia
  h. homonymous
hemiataxia
hemiatrophy
hemiazygos
hemicranium
hemidiaphragm
hemifacial
  h. microsomia
hemigigantism
hemihepatectomy
hemihypertrophy
hemimelia
hemiparesis
hemiplegia
hemiscrotum
hemisphere
  cerebellar h.
  cerebral h.
  dominant h.
  vegetal h.
hemispherium

hemithorax
hemivertebra
hemochromatosis
hemocoelom
hemocytoblastoma
hemocytoma
hemodialysis
hemodilution
hemodynamic
hemoglobin S-S disease
hemolysis
hemolytic
    h. anemia
    h. icterus
    h.-uremic syndrome
hemopericardium
hemophilia
hemophiliac
hemophilic
Hemophilus
    H. influenzae
hemoptysis
hemorrhage
    cerebellar h.
    gastrointestinal h.
    intracerebral h.
    intracranial h.
    intraperitoneal h.
    mediastinal h.
    parenchymal h.
    perirenal h.
    pulmonary h.
    retroperitoneal h.
    subarachnoid h.
    subdural h.
    tracheobronchial h.
    variceal h.
hemorrhagic shock

hemorrhoid
hemosiderin
hemosiderosis
    idiopathic pulmonary h.
hemostasis
hemothorax
Henle's loop
Henoch-Schönlein purpura
Henschen's method
HEPA – high efficiency partic-
    ulate arrestance
heparan sulfate
heparin
hepatic
    h. angiography
    h. angle
    h. arteriography
    h. artery
    h. cord
    h. cyst
    h. duct
    h. flexure
    h. laceration
    h. lobe
    h. lymph node
    h. sphincter
    h. test of Glass
hepaticopulmonary
hepatitis
    neonatal h.
    radiation h.
hepatoadenoma
hepatobiliary
    h. scan
hepatoblastoma
hepatobronchial
hepatocarcinogenesis
hepatocarcinoma

hepatocellular
hepatocholangitis
hepatocirrhosis
hepatocolic
hepatocystic
hepatocyte
hepatodiaphragmatic
hepatoenteric
hepatofugal
hepatogastric
hepatogenic
hepatogenous
hepatoglycemia
hepatogram
hepatography
hepatojugular
    h. reflux
hepatolenticular
hepatolienal
hepatolienography
hepatolith
hepatoma
    diffuse h.
    infarcted h.
    multifocal h.
    pedunculated h.
    solitary h.
hepatomalacia
hepatomegaly
hepatomelanosis
hepatomphalocele
hepatomphalos
hepatonephric
hepatonephritic
hepatonephritis
hepatonephromegaly
hepatopancreas
hepatoperitonitis

hepatophlebitis
hepatophlebography
hepatopleural
hepatoportal
hepatopulmonary
hepatorenal
hepatorrhagia
hepatorrhea
hepatoscan
hepatoscopy
hepatosplenic
hepatosplenography
hepatosplenomegaly
hepatosplenopathy
hepatotoxemia
hepatotoxic
hepatotoxicity
hereditary
heredofamilial
Herellea
    H. vaginicola
hernia
    Bochdalek's h.
    cervical h.
    diaphragmatic h.
    hepatic h.
    hiatal h.
    inguinal h.
    intercostal h.
    Morgagni's h.
    omental h.
    paraesopha-
      geal h.
    pericardial h.
    spigelian h.
    umbilical h.
hernial
herniated

herniation
    transtentorial h.
herniogram
herniography
Herophili
    torcular H.
herpes
    h. encephalitis
    genital h.
    h. simplex
    h. zoster
herpesvirus
"herring-bone" pattern
hertz
heterogeneity
heterogeneous
heterogenous
heterotopia
heterotopic
Heublein's method
HEW – Department of Health,
    Education and Welfare
Hexabrix
hexamethonium
^{203}Hg chlormerodrin
^{203}Hg fluorescein
Hg meralluride
^{197}Hg mercurihydroxpro-
    pane
HGA – homogentisic acid
hiatal
hiatus
    h. semilunaris
Hickey's
    method
    position
HIDA – acetanilidoiminodi-
    acetic acid

high
    h.-contrast film
    h. efficiency particulate
        arrestance
    h.-lying patella
    h.-powered liquid chro-
        matography
    h. resolution images
    h. vacuum
    h. voltage transformer
Highmore's antrum
hila (*see* hilum)
hilar
Hill-Sachs deformity
hilum (hila)
    h. convergence sign
    h. overlay sign
    "pruned h."
hilus (hili)
hindbrain
hindfoot
HIPDM – ^{123}I hydroxyiodoben-
    zyl-propane-diamine
    method
hippocampal
hippocampus
Hippuran
hippurate
Hirtz's method
histamine
histiocytic
histiocytoma
histiocytomatosis
histiocytosis
    lipid h.
    sinus h.
    h. X
histogram

HIDA scan

histography
histologic
histology
histopathologic
histopathology
Histoplasma
      H. capsulatum
      H. duboisii
histoplasmic
histoplasmin
histoplasmoma
histoplasmosis
historadiography
"hitchhiker's" thumb
Hittorf's tube
HL – half-life
HLA – human leukocyte antigen
HMD — hyaline membrane disease
HMDP – hydroxymethylene diphosphonate
HMO – Health Maintenance Organization
hobnail liver
HOCM – hypertrophic obstructive cardiomyopathy
Hodgkin's lymphoma
Holmblad's method
holmium
holography
holoprosencephaly
holosystolic
Homer-Spaulding sign
homocystinuria
homogeneity
homogeneous
homogeneously

homogentisic acid oxidase deficiency
homologous
homonymous
homotypical
homozygous
honeycomb
    h. lung
    h. pattern
honeycombing
horizontal
    h. beam study
hormone
    luteinizing h.
    parathyroid h.
hormonopoietic
horn
    anterior h.
    frontal h.
    inferior h.
    occipital h.
    temporal h.
horsepower
horseshoe
    h. configuration
    h. kidney
hot
    h. cathode x-ray tube
    h. lesion
    "h. spot"
    h. wire
"hot-cross-bun" appearance
Hough's method
Hounsfield
    scale
    unit
hourglass chest
Howell-Jolly bodies

Howship's lacuna
HPLC – high powered liquid
   chromatography
HSA –
   Health Systems Agency
   human serum albumin
Hsieh's method
HU – Hounsfield unit
H.U. – heat unit
Hughston's method
humeral
humeri (*see* humerus)
humeroradial
humeroscapular
humeroulnar
humerus (humeri)
   h. varus
humidification
humidifier
humor
   aqueous h.
   crystalline h.
   plasmoid h.
   vitreous h.
hump
   ''dromedary h.''
   Hampton's h.
hunchback
Hurler-Scheie compound
Hurter and Driffield photographic curve
''Hutch'' diverticula
Hutchison's fracture
''H'' vertebra
HVL – half-value layer
hyalase
hyaline
   h. arteriosclerosis

hyaline *(continued)*
   h. cartilage
   h. membrane disease
hyalinosis cutis et mucosae
hybrid
hydantoin syndrome
hydatid
hydatidiform
hydatiduria
hydralazine
hydramnios
hydranencephaly
hydrarthritis
hydrarthrosis
hydrated
hydration
hydrocarbon
hydrocele
   cervical h.
   communicating h.
   diffused h.
   encysted h.
   funicular h.
   hernial h.
   h. renalis
   scrotal h.
   h. spinalis
hydrocephalus
   adult h.
   atrophic h.
   communicating h.
   intermediate h.
   h. internus
   noncommunicating h.
   obstructive h.
   h. occlusus
hydrocolpos
hydrocortisone

hydrocystadenoma
hydrodynamics
hydrogen
    h. atom
    h. density
    h. off-resonance beat
        pattern
hydrogen(¦H, atomic
    number 1)
hydrometer
hydrometrocolpos-polydactyly
    syndrome
hydromyelia
hydronephrosis
hydronephrotic
hydrophilic
hydropneumothorax
hydrops
    h. fetalis
    h. folliculi
hydroquinone
hydrothorax
hydroxide
hydroxyapatite
25-hydroxycholecalci-
    ferol
hydroxycitrate
hydroxy corticosteroid
25-hydroxyergocalciferol
hydroxymethylene diphosphon-
    ate
hygroma
hyoid
Hypaque
    H.-Cysto
    H. M.
    H. meglumine
    H. sodium

hyparterial
hypaxial
hyperaeration
    compensatory h.
    nonobstructive h.
    obstructive h.
    pulmonary h.
hyperaldosteronism
hyperalimentation
hyperamylasemia
hyperamylasuria
hyperandrogenism
hypercalcemia
hypercalciuria
hypercapnia
hypercementosis
hypercontraction
hypercortisonism
hypercycloidal
hyperdense
hyperechoic
hyperemia
hyperesthesia
hyperextension
hypergonadism
hyperimmunoglobulin E
hyperinflation
hyperkinetic
hyperlipidemia
hyperlucency
hyperlucent
hypermobility
hypermotility
hypernephroma
hyperosmolar
hyperosmotic
hyperostosis
    cortical h.

hyperostosis *(continued)*
    h. corticalis generali-
      sata
    diffuse idiopathic skele-
      tal h.
    h. frontalis interna
    infantile cortical h.
    van Buchem's endo-
      steal h.
hyperostotic
hyperoxaluria
hyperparathyroidism
hyperphalangia
hyperphalangism
hyperphosphatasia
hyperphosphatemia
hyperpituitarism
hyperplasia
    adrenal h.
    adrenocortical h.
    lymphoid h.
    nodular h.
    pituitary h.
hyperplastic
hyperpnea
hyperprolactinemia
hyperreactivity
hypersecretion
hypersecretory
hypersensitivity
hyperspasticity
hypersplenism
hypersthenic
hypertelorism
hypertension
    adrenal h.
    hyperkinetic h.
    portal h.

hypertension *(continued)*
    pulmonary h.
    renal h.
    renovascular h.
    splenoportal h.
    vascular h.
    vaso-occlusive h.
    venous h.
hypertensive
hyperthyroid
hyperthyroidism
hypertonic
hypertonicity
hypertriglyceridemia
hypertrophic
    h. arthritis
    h. gastritis
    h. obstructive cardiomy-
      opathy
    h. pulmonary osteoar-
      thropathy
    h. spurring
hypertrophy
    hemiangiecta-
      tic h.
    left ventricular h.
    prostatic h.
hypertubulation
hyperuricemia
hyperuricosuria
hypervascularity
hypervitaminosis
    h. A
    h. D
hypoadrenalism
hypoaeration
hypocalcemia
hypocalciuria

hypochondriac
hypochondrium
hypochondroplasia
hypochromic
hypocitraturia
hypocomplementemic
hypocycloidal
hypodactyly
hypodense
hypoechoic
hypofunction
hypogammaglobuline-
    mia
hypogastric
hypogenesis
hypogenetic
hypoglossal
hypoglycemia
hypogonadism
hypohepatia
hypokalemia
hypokinetic
hypolarynx
hypolipoproteinemia
hypomegakaryocytic
        h. thrombocytopenia
hyponatremia
hypoparathyroidism
hypophalangism
hypopharyngeal
hypopharynx
hypophosphatasia
hypophosphatemia
hypophosphatemic
hypophyseal
hypophyseoportal
hypophysis

hypopituitarism
hypoplasia
    campomelic h.
    central h.
    focal dermal h.
    spondylohumerofe-
        moral h.
hypoplastic
hypoproteinemia
hypospadias
hyposthenic
hypotension
    orthostatic h.
hypothalamic hamartoblastoma
    syndrome
hypothalamicohypophyseal
hypothalamic-pituitary function
hypothalamus
hypothenar hammer syndrome
hypothermia
hypothyroid
hypothyroidism
hypotonic
hypotonicity
hypovascularity
hypovegetative
hypoventilation
    alveolar h.
hypovitaminosis
    h. C
    h. D
hypovolemia
hypoxanthine-guanine phos-
    phoribosyltransferase defi-
    ciency
hypoxemia
hypoxia

Hyrtl's sphincter
hysterectomy
hysteresis
hysterography

hysterosalpingogram
hysterosalpingography
Hytrast
Hz – hertz

I
i

I –
  electric current
  intensity
  iodine
^{123}I, ^{125}I, ^{131}I – iodine radio-
  pharmaceuticals
IACB – intra-aortic counterpulsation balloon
iatrogenic
"iceberg"
    "i" sign
    "i" tumor
I-cell disease
ichthyosis
ICRP – International Commission on Radiological Pro-
  tection
ICRU – International Commission on Radiation Units
  and Measurements
icterus
ictus
ICW – intracellular
  water
ID – internal diameter
IDA – iminodiacetic acid

IDE – Investigational Device
  Exemption
idiopathic
    i. capsulitis
    i. familial acro-
      osteolysis
    i. hypercalcemia
    i. inflammatory bowel
      disease
    i. juvenile osteoporosis
    i. megacolon
    i. osteoarthropathy
    i. pulmonary fibrosis
    i. pulmonary hemoside-
      rosis
    i. scoliosis
iduronidase
IF –
  screen intensifying factor
  intrinsic factor
^{125}I-fibrinogen uptake test
IgA deficiency
^{123}I hexadecenoic acid
IHF – interhemispheric fissure
IHSS – idiopathic hypertrophic
  subaortic stenosis

¹²³I hippuran
¹³¹I hippuran
¹³¹I iodocholesterol
¹³¹I-labelled cholesterol
¹³¹I-labelled macroaggregated
    albumin
¹³¹I-labelled rose bengal
ileac
ileal
ileitis
    "backwash i."
    Crohn's i.
ileocecal
ileocecum
ileocolic
ileocolitis
    tuberculous i.
    i. ulcerosa chronica
ileorectal
ileosigmoid
ileostomy
ileotransverse
ileum
ileus
    adynamic i.
    colonic i.
    dynamic i.
    gallstone i.
    mechanical i.
    meconium i.
    paralytic i.
    spastic i.
ilia
iliac
    i. angle
    i. colon
    i. crest
    i. fossa

iliac *(continued)*
    i. lymph node
    i. osteomyelitis
    i. region
    i. spine
    i. spur
iliacus
iliocostal
iliofemoral
ilioinguinal
ilioischial
iliolumbar
iliolumbocostoabdominal
iliopelvic
iliopsoas
iliopubic
iliosacral
iliotibial
ilium (ilia)
ill-defined
IMA – inferior mesenteric ar-
    tery
image
    i. aliasing
    i. amplifier
    i. analysis
    calculated i.
    i. chains
    i. contrast
    i. converter
    fluoroscopic i.
    i.-forming system
    gated i.
    i. intensification
    i. intensifier system
    i. intensifier tube
    inversion recovery i.
    i. noise

image *(continued)*
>   nuclear magnetic reso-
>   nance i's
>   i. orthicon tube
>   phantom i.
>   i. quality
>   radiographic i.
>   i. reconstruction
>   i. reformation
>   renal i.
>   i. resolution
>   saturation recovery i.
>   scout i.
>   i. sharpness
>   i. slice thickness
>   spin echo i.
>   static renal i.
>   x-ray i.

imaging
>   adrenal i.
>   blood pool i.
>   cardiac blood pool i.
>   coded-aperture i.
>   diagnostic i.
>   digital vascular i.
>   direct Fourier transfor-
>   mation i.
>   dynamic volume i.
>   echo-planar i.
>   electrostatic i.
>   flow i.
>   gated blood pool i.
>   gray-scale i.
>   heavy ion i.
>   infarct-avid i.
>   isotope colloid i.
>   isotope hepatobiliary i.
>   longitudinal section i.

imaging *(continued)*
>   lymph node i.
>   magnetic resonance i.
>   microwave i.
>   multigated i.
>   multiplanar i.
>   multiple-gated blood
>   pool i.
>   multiple spin echo total
>   volume i.
>   multislice modified
>   KWE direct Four-
>   ier i.
>   myocardial infarct i.
>   myocardial perfusion i.
>   nuclear i.
>   nuclear magnetic reso-
>   nance i.
>   planar i.
>   projection reconstruc-
>   tion i.
>   pyrophosphate i.
>   quantitative brain i.
>   radionuclide i.
>   reconstructive i.
>   reticuloendothelial i.
>   rotating frame i.
>   selective excitation pro-
>   jection reconstruc-
>   tion i.
>   sensitive plane projec-
>   tion reconstruction i.
>   sequential first pass i.
>   sequential plane i.
>   single slice modified
>   KWE direct Fourier i.
>   spin-warp i.
>   thallium-201 i.

imaging *(continued)*
    three-dimensional echo planar i.
    three-dimensional Fourier i.
    three-dimensional i.
    three-dimensional KWE direct Fourier i.
    three-dimensional projection reconstruction i.
    transverse section i.
    two-dimensional Fourier i.
    two-dimensional Fourier transformation i.
    two-dimensional KWE direct Fourier i.
    two-dimensional modified KWE direct Fourier i.
    ultrasound i.
    ventilation perfusion i.
imidodiphosphonate
iminodiacetic acid
immobilization
immobilization device
    Pigg-O-Stat i. d.
immotile cilia syndrome
immovable
immunity
immunoadsorbent
immunoassay
immunoblastic
immunodeficiency
immunoelectrophoresis
immunofiltration
immunofluorescence

immunogenetics
immunoglobulin
immunosuppression
immunosuppressive
impacted
impaction
    i. fracture
    mucoid i.
impalpable
impedance
imperforate
IMPH – 1-iodomercuri-2-hydroxypropane
impinge
impingement
implant
    augmentation mammoplasty i.
    therapeutic radiology i.
    water density i.
implantation
impotence
impression
    basilar i.
impulse
    electrical i.
    i. timer
I_n chelate
^{111}In chloride
incipient
incisura (incisurae)
    i. angularis
    i. cardiaca
incisure
indium
    i. 111 leukocyte scanning
    i. nuclides

indium *(continued)*
    i. 111 oxine
incontinence
    giggle i.
    overflow i.
    paradoxical i.
    stress i.
    urge i.
incrementation
incudomalleal
incudomalleolar
incudostapedial
incus
IND – Investigational New
    Drug
indentation
    "ring-like" i.
    "wasp-waist" i.
index
    Cronqvist's cranial i.
    sesamoid i.
indirect volume image recon-
    struction
indium-111
indolent
"Indomitable" scanner
inductance
induction
inductive reactance
inductor generator
induration
industrial
    i. monitoring
    i. radiography
indwelling
    i. T-tube
inert
inertia

infantile
infarct
    i.-avid image
    i. scanning
infarcted
infarction
    anteroseptal i.
    atrial i.
    bone i.
    cerebral i.
    Freiberg's i.
    gas i.
    global renal i.
    lacunar i.
    mesenteric i.
    myocardial i.
    pulmonary i.
    renal i.
    splenic i.
    subendocardial i.
    thrombotic i.
    transmural i.
infection
infectious
infective
    i. endocarditis
    i. mononucleosis
inferior
    i. horn
    i. ramus
    i. vena cava occlusion
inferosuperior
^{113}m In ferric hydroxide
infestation
infiltrate
infiltration
infiltrative
inflammation

inflammatory
inflation
influenza
    i. A viral pneumonia
infradiaphragmatic
inframammary
inframesocolic
infraorbital
infraorbitomeatal
infraperitoneal
infrared
    i. radiation
    i. ray
infrasellar
infraspinatus
infratentorial
infratragal
infundibular
infundibulum (infundibula)
infusion
ingest
ingestion
Ingram's trocar catheter
inguinal
inhalation
inherent
    i. density
    i. filtration
    i. resistance
inheritance
inhibition
inhibitor
inhomogeneity
inhomogeneous
iniencephaly
inion
injection
    cisternal i.

injection *(continued)*
    opaque i.
    perinephric air i.
    transduodenal fiber-
        scopic duct i.
    i. urethrogram
[111] In-labelled autologous leu-
    kocytes
inlet
    pelvic i.
    thoracic i.
innominate
inorganic
inoscultation
[111] In-oxine-labelled autologous
    leukocytes
[111] In-oxine-labelled plate-
    lets
insoluble
inspiration
inspiratory
inspissated
instability
instillation
insufficiency
insufflation
    air i.
    intraperitoneal gas i.
    perirenal i.
    retroperitoneal gas i.
insula (insulae)
insular
insulator
insulinase
insulin-iodine
insulinoma
integral
integumentary

integumentum
    i. commune
intensification
    i. factor
    image i.
intensifier
intensifying
intensity
    electrical i.
    field i.
    i. fluctuation
    radiation
interaction
interarticular
    i. ridge
interatrial
intercalary
intercarpal
intercartilaginous
interceptive nervous system
interchondral
intercompartmental
intercondylar
    i. notch line
intercondyle
intercondyloid
intercostal
intercostohumeral
intercrural
intercuneiform
interdigital
interendognathic
interface
    acoustic i.
interfacet
interference
interhemispheric
interlace

interlobar
interlobular
interlock
intermalleolar
intermaxillary
intermediate
intermetacarpal
intermetatarsal
intermittent positive pressure
    breathing
internal
    i. auditory meatus
    i. conversion
    i. fracture
    i. radiation hazard
    i. resistance
internasal
International Commission on
    Radiation Units and Meas-
    urements
International Commission on
    Radiological Protection
interorbital
interosseous
interparietal
interpediculate
interpeduncular
interperiosteal
interphalangeal
interposition
    hepatodiaphragmatic i.
interpupillary
interrenal
intersegmental
interseptal
intersexual
interspace
interspinous

intersternal
interstice
interstitial
    i. infiltrates
    i. pneumonitis
    i. radiation
    i. radiotherapy
interstitium
intertarsal
interthalamic
intertrabecular
intertrochanteric
    i. ridge
intertubercular
interventricular
intervertebral
intestinal
    i. atresia
    i. duplication
    i. knot syndrome
    i. malrotation
    i. obstruction
    i. tract
intestine
    blind i.
    empty i.
    iced i.
    jejunoileal i.
    large i.
    mesenterial i.
    segmented i.
    straight i.
intestinum (intestina)
intima
intimal
intoxication
intra-abdominal
intra-alveolar

intra-aortic counterpulsation
    balloon
intra-articular
intrabronchial
intracapsular
intracardiac
    i. shunt
intracartilaginous
intracavitary
    i. radiotherapy
intracellular
intracerebral
intracolonic
intraconal
intracranial
intraductal
intradural
intraglottic
intrahepatic
intralobar
intraluminal
intramammary
intramedullary
intramembranous
intramural
intranodal
^{113}m In transferrin
intraoccipital
intraoperative
intraoral
intraosseous
    i. ganglia
    i. hemangiomatosis
intrapericardial
intraperiosteal
intraperitoneal
intrapleural
intrapulmonary

intraradial
intrarenal
    i. reflux
intrasellar
intrasplenic
    i. hematoma
    i. lymphangioma
intrathecal
intrathoracic
intratracheal
intrauterine
intrauterine device
    copper-7 i. d.
    copper T i. d.
    Dalkon shield i. d.
    double coil i. d.
    Gravigards i. d.
    Lippes loop i. d.
    Progestasert i. d.
    safety coils i. d.
intravascular
intravenous
    i. cholangiography
    i. cholecystography
    i. hyperalimentation
    i. pyelography
    i. urography
intraventricular
intrinsic
    i. factor
    i. nuclear spin
introducer
Intropaque
intubation
    endotracheal
    intratracheal i.
    nasal i.
    nasotracheal i.

intubation *(continued)*
    oral i.
    orotracheal i.
    tracheal i.
intussuscepting
intussusception
in utero [L] – in uterus
invaginated
invagination
    basilar i.
invasive
inverse
    "i.-comma" appearance
    i. square law of radiation
    i. voltage
inversely proportional
inversion
    i. recovery image
    i. recovery sequence
invert
Investigational Device Exemption
Investigational New Drug
in vitro [L] – in glass
in vivo [L] – in something alive
in-vivo crossmatch
involucrum
involuntary nervous system
iobenzamic acid
iobutoic acid
iocarmate meglumine
iocarmic acid
iocetamate
iocetamic acid
iodamic acid
iodamide

iodatol
iodecol
iodide
        potassium i.
        silver i.
        sodium i.
        i. transport
iodinated
        i. albumin
        i. contrast media
        i. I 125 fibrinogen
        i. I 125 serum albumin
        i. I 131 aggregated al-
          bumin (human)
        i. I 131 serum albumin
          (human)
iodination
iodine
        i. polyvinylpyrrolidone
          (PVP) bond
        radioactive i.
iodine$(^{126}_{53}$I, atomic number 53)
iodine 131
iodipamide
        i. meglumine
        i. sodium
iodized oil
iodoalphionic acid
iodocholesterol
iodohippurate
iodolipid
1-iodomercuri-2-hydroxypro-
    pane
iodomethamate
iodomethyl-19-norcholes-5-
    (10)-en-3B-o1 (NP-59)
iodophendylate
iodophthalein

iodopyracet
iodoxamate
iodoxamic acid
iodoxyl
ioglicate
ioglicic acid
ioglucol
ioglucomide
ioglunide
ioglycamic acid
ioglycamide
iogulamide
iohexol
IOM – infraorbital margin
iomide
IOML – infraorbitomeatal line
ion
        amphoteric dipolar i.
        i. chamber
        negative i.
        i. pair
        pertechnetate i.
        positive i.
ionic
        i. binding
        i. dimers
        i. monomers
        i. polar valence
        i. solution
ionization
        i. chamber
        i. counter
        i. current
        i. density
        i. instrument
        i. potential
        i. radiation
ionized

ionizing
ionograph
ionography
ionophore
iopamidol
iopanoate
iopanoic acid
iophendylate
iophenoxic acid
ioprocemic acid
iopromide
iopronic acid
iopydol
iopydone
iosefamate
iosefamic acid
ioseric acid
iosulamide
iosumetic acid
iotasul
ioteric acid
iothalamate
      i. meglumine
      i. sodium
iothalamic acid
iotrol
iotroxamide
iotroxic acid
IOV – inferior ophthalmic
    vein
ioxaglate
ioxaglic acid
ioxithalamate
ioxithalamic acid
iozomic acid
IPC – interpeduncular cistern
IPF – idiopathic pulmonary fi-
    brosis

IPH – idiopathic pulmonary
    hemosiderosis
ipodate
      i. calcium
      i. sodium
ipodic acid
IPPB – intermittent positive
    pressure breathing
ipsilateral
IRA-400 resin
iridium
^{191}m iridium
IRM – inferior rectus muscle
iron
      i. absorption
      i. core
      i.-core transformer
      i. deficiency anemia
      i./dextran
      i. hydroxide
      i./indium
      radioactive i.
      i. storage disease
irradiated
irradiation
irregularity
irritable
ischemia
      global i.
      mesenteric i.
      myocardial i.
      renal i.
      i. retinae
      transient myocardial i.
ischemic
ischial
      i. varus sign
ischioacetabular

ischioanal
ischiobulbar
ischiocapsular
ischiocele
ischiococcygeal
ischiococcygeus
ischiofemoral
ischiofibular
ischiopubic
ischiorectal
ischiosacral
ischiovaginal
ischiovertebral
ischium
Isherwood's
    method
    position
islet cell tumor
isobar
isobaric transition
isocenter
isocentric mounting
Isocon camera
isodense
isodose
    i. curve
    i. chart
isoelectric
isointense
isokinetic monitoring
isomer
isomeric
    i. decay
    i. transition

iso-osmotic
Isopaque
isosthenuria
isotone
isotope
    i. bone scan
    i. colloid imaging
    i. effect
    i. hepatobiliary imaging
    radioactive i.
    i. study
    i. voiding cystoureth-
        rography
isotopic
isotopism
isotopy
Isovue
isthmus (isthmi)
ITU – intensive therapy
    unit
IUD – intrauterine device
IUGR –intrauterine growth re-
    tardation
i.v. –intravenous pyelography
IVC –
    inferior vena cava
    intravenous cholangio-
        gram
IVCU –isotope voiding cys-
    tourethrography
"ivory" vertebrae
IVP –intravenous pyelogram
IVS –interventricular septum
IVU –intravenous urography

j

Jaccoud's
- arthritis
- arthropathy

"jail bars" appearance

Jamshide needle

jaundice
- cholestatic j.
- hemorrhagic j.
- infectious j.
- leptospiral j.
- obstructive j.
- spirochetal j.

JCAH – Joint Commission on Accreditation of Hospitals

Jefferson's fracture

jejunal
- j. carcinoma
- j. diverticulum
- j. intussusception
- j. ulcer

jejunalization

jejunitis
- Crohn's j.

jejunoileal

jejunum

Jewett-Marshall system

JGA – juxtaglomerular apparatus

JM – juxtamedullary

Jobert's fossa

Johnson's
- method
- position

joint
- acromioclavicular j.
- amphiarthrodial j.
- ankle j.
- anterior intraoccipital j.
- apophyseal j.
- arthrodial j.
- atlanto-occipital j.
- ball-and-socket j.
- biaxial j.
- bicondylar j.
- bilocular j.
- bleeder's j.
- Brodie's j.
- Budin's j.
- calcaneocuboid j.
- j. calcification
- capitular j.
- carpal j's
- carpometacarpal j's
- cartilaginous j.
- Charcot's j.
- Chopart's j.
- Clutton's j's
- coccygeal j.
- cochlear j.
- composite j.
- compound j.
- condylar j.
- condyloid j's
- j. contracture
- costochondral j.
- costotransverse j.

joint *(continued)*
    costovertebral j's
    cotyloid j.
    cricoarytenoid j.
    cricothyroid j.
    Cruveilhier's j.
    cubital j.
    cuboideonavicular j.
    cuneocuboid j.
    cuneometatarsal j's
    cuneonavicular j.
    dentoalveolar j.
    diarthrodial j's
    digital j's
    distal interphalangeal
      (DIP) j's
    dry j.
    j. effusion
    elbow j.
    ellipsoidal j.
    enarthrodial j.
    facet j's
    false j.
    femoropatellar j.
    fibrocartilaginous j.
    fibrous j.
    flail j.
    freely movable j.
    fringe j.
    ginglymoid j.
    glenohumeral j.
    gliding j's
    gompholic j.
    hemophilic j.
    hinge j's
    hip j.
    humeroradial j.
    humeroulnar j.

joint *(continued)*
    hysteric j.
    immovable j.
    incudomalleolar j.
    incudostapedial j.
    inferior radiolunar j.
    inferior tibiofibular j.
    interarticular j's
    intercarpal j's
    interchondral j's
    intercuneiform j's
    intermetacarpal j's
    intermetatarsal j's
    interphalangeal j's
    intersternebral j's
    intertarsal j's
    intervertebral j.
    irritable j.
    jaw j.
    knee j.
    lateral atlantoaxial j.
    lateral atlantoepistro-
      phic j.
    ligamentous j.
    Lisfranc's j's
    lumbosacral j.
    Luschka's j's
    mandibular j.
    manubriosternal j.
    median atlantoaxial j.
    metacarpophalangeal j's
    metatarsocuneiform j's
    metatarsophalangeal j's
    midcarpal j.
    midtarsal j.
    mixed j.
    mortise j.
    movable j.

joint *(continued)*
>   multiaxial j.
>   navicular j's
>   neurocentral j.
>   neuropathic j.
>   peg-and-socket j.
>   petro-occipital j.
>   phalangeal j's
>   pisotriquetral j.
>   pivot j's
>   plane j.
>   polyaxial j.
>   posterior intraoccipital j.
>   proximal interphalan-
>   geal (PIP) j's
>   radiocarpal j.
>   radioulnar j.
>   rotary j.
>   sacrococcygeal j.
>   sacroiliac j's
>   saddle j's
>   scapuloclavicular j.
>   schindyletic j.
>   screw j.
>   sellar j.
>   shoulder j.
>   simple j.
>   socket j.
>   spheno-occipital j.
>   spheroidal j.
>   spiral j.
>   sternal j's
>   sternoclavicular j.
>   sternocostal j's
>   stifle j.
>   subtalar j.
>   superior radioulnar j.
>   suture j.

joint *(continued)*
>   synarthrodial j.
>   synchondrodial j.
>   syndesmodial j.
>   synovial j.
>   talocalcaneal j.
>   talocalcaneonavicular j.
>   talonavicular j.
>   tarsal j's
>   tarsometatarsal j's
>   temporomandibular j's
>   thigh j.
>   through j.
>   tibiofibular j's
>   tibiotalar j's
>   trochoid j.
>   uncovertebral j's
>   uniaxial j.
>   unilocular j.
>   wedge-and-groove j.
>   wrist j.
>   xiphisternal j.
>   zygapophyseal j's

Joint Commission on Accredi-
>   tation of Hospitals

"joint mice"

Joint Review Committee

Joint Review Committee on
>   Education in Radiologic
>   Technology

Jones' fracture

joule

JRA – juvenile rheumatoid ar-
>   thritis

JRC – Joint Review Committee

JRCERT – Joint Review Com-
>   mittee on Education in
>   Radiologic Technology

Judd's method
jugal
jugular
    j. bulb
    j. foramen
    j. fossa
    j. lymph sac
    j. notch
    j. reflux
    j. vein
jugum (juga)
junction
    bulbomedullary j.
    cervico-occipital j.
    corticomedullary j.
    craniovertebral j.
    esophagogastric j.
    ischiopubic j.
    myoneural j.
    rectosigmoid j.
    sclerocorneal j.
    ureteropelvic j.
    ureterovesical j.
juncture
    duodenojejunal j.

Junghans' pseudospondylolis-
    thesis
juvenile
    j. angiofibroma
    j. chronic polyarthropa-
      thy
    j. hyaline fibromatosis
    j. idiopathic osteopo-
      rosis
    j. kyphosis dorsalis
    j. rheumatoid arthritis
    j. tertiary syphilis
juxta-articular
juxtacortical
juxtaepiphyseal
juxtaglomerular apparatus
juxtamediastinal
juxtamedullary
juxtangina
juxtaphrenic
juxtaposition
juxtapyloric
juxtaspinal
juxtavertebral
juxtavesical

K –
    cathode
    kilo
Ka – kiloampere
Kandel's method

Kaposi's
    sarcoma
    varicelliform eruption
karyotypic
Karplus relationship

Kasabach's method
KBG syndrome
Kc –
    kilocycle
    kilocurie
K-capture
K-characteristic x-ray
K electron
keloid
Kemp Harper method
Kenotron tube
kerasin
keratan sulfate
keratinizing
keratoacanthoma
        subungual k.
Kerley's
        A line
        B line
"kernel of popcorn" appear-
    ance
kernicterus
ketamine
ketone bodies
ketogenic steroid
kev. – kilo-electron-volt
kg – kilogram
kidney
        abdominal k.
        arteriosclerotic k.
        atrophic k.
        cicatricial k.
        contracted k.
        cyanotic k.
        cystic k.
        "doughnut" k.
        duplex k.
        dysplastic k.

kidney *(continued)*
        ectopic k.
        floating k.
        fused k.
        horseshoe k.
        lardaceous k.
        medullary sponge k.
        multicystic k.
        myelin k.
        Page's k.
        parenchymal k.
        pelvic k.
        perirenal k.
        pyelonephritic k.
        sacciform k.
        sigmoid k.
        sponge k.
        supernumerary k.
        thoracic k.
        wandering k.
        k. washout
kilocalorie
kilocurie
kilocycle
kilo-electron-volt
kilogram
kilohm
kilomegacycle
kilometer
kilosecond
kilovolt
        k. -ampere
        k. meter
        k. peak
kilovoltage
        k. peak
        k. selector
kilovoltmeter

kilowatt
Kimberlin's method
kineradiography
kinescope radiography
kinetic energy
kinetics
    radionuclide k.
Kinevac
kinking
kinky hair syndrome
    Menkes' k. h. s.
Kirchhoff's law
Kirchner's wire
Kirdani's method
Kirner's deformity
"kissing ulcers"
Kistner tracheal "button"
Kite's method
Klatzkin's tumor
Klebsiella
    K. *aerobacter*
    K. *pneumoniae*
    K. *rhinoscleromatis*
"kleeblattschödel"
Klein's technique
K line
Klippel-Feil deformity
km - kilometer
Kniest's dysplasia
knob
    aortic k.
KO - kilo-
Kock's pouch
Köhler's
    bone disease
    "teardrop" sign
Kohm - kilohm

Kohn's pore
Kopan's needle
Kovacs' method
^{42}K potassium chloride
K radiation
^{81m}KR ventilation study
Krebs' cycle
Krukenberg's tumor
krypton 81m
KS - ketogenic steroid
K-shell
KUB - kidney, ureter
    and bladder
Kuchendorf's method
Kumar, Welti and Ernst
    method
Kupffer's cell
Kurzbauer's
    method
    position
kv - kilovolt
kv.A - kilovolt-ampere
kv.P - kilovolt peak
kw - kilowatt
kwashiorkor
KWE method - Kumar,
    Welti and Ernst
    method
kymograph
kymography
kymoscope
kymoscopy
kyphoscoliosis
kyphosis
    basal k.
    k. dorsalis
kyphotic

L l

L –
    coil
    inductance
λ – decay constant
LA – left atrium
labelled ligand
labial
labium (labia)
labrum (labra)
labyrinth
    acoustic l.
    bony l.
    cortical l.
    endolympha-
      tic l.
    ethmoidal l.
    membranous l.
    olfactory l.
    osseous l.
    perilymphatic l.
    statokinetic l.
labyrinthine
labyrinthitis
    l. obliterans
labyrinthus (labyrinthi)
"lace-like"
    "l." appearance
    l. periostitis
lacerated
laceration
    aortic l.
    hepatic l.
    pulmonary l.

lacrimal
    l. apparatus
    l. canal
    l. canaliculi
    l. caruncle
    l. gland
    l. lake
    l. papilla
    l. process
    l. punctum
    l. sac
    l. scanning
    l. system
lacrimo-auriculo-dento-digital
    syndrome
lacrimoconchal
lacrimoethmoidal
lacrimomaxillary
lacrimoturbinal
lactiferous
lactobezoar
lactose-barium
lacuna (lacunae)
    Howship's l.
lacunar
    l. infarction
    l. skull
Ladd's bands
Laennec's cirrhosis
LAL – limulus lysate
lambda
lambdoid
lambdoidal

135

Lambert's channel
lamina (laminae)
      l. dura
      l. papyracea
      l. terminalis
laminagram
laminagraph
laminagraphy
laminar
laminated
      l. core
      l. silicon steel plates
lamination
laminectomy
laminogram
laminography
lamp
      Wood's l.
lanthanum oxybromide
LAO – left anterior oblique
Laquerrière-Pierquin
      method
      position
lardaceous
Larkin's position
Larmor's
      equation
      frequency
      precession frequency
Laron's dwarfism
laryngeal
laryngectomy
laryngismus
      l. paralyticus
      l. stridulus
laryngocele
laryngogram
laryngography

laryngohypopharynx
laryngomalacia
laryngopharyngeal
laryngopharyngography
laryngopharynx
laryngoscleroma
laryngospasm
laryngotracheitis
laryngotracheobronchitis
laryngotracheoesophageal
      l. cleft
larynx
laser beam
Lasix test
latent
laterad
lateral
laterality
lateroconal
lateromedial
latitude
      density l.
      radiographic l.
lattice
      l. relaxation time
      l. vibrations
Lauenstein and Hickey
      method
      projection
lavage
law
      conservation of
        energy l.
      Coulomb's l.
      Curie's l.
      Doerner-Hoskins distri-
        bution l.
      electrostatic l.

law *(continued)*
>
> Faraday's l.
> Fick's l.
> l. of inertia
> inverse-square l.
> Kirchhoff's l.
> l. of magnetism
> Newton's l. of action-reaction
> Newton's l. of motion
> Ohm's l.
> l. of reciprocity
> l. of thermodynamics
> transformer l.

Lawrence's
>
> method
> position

lawrencium

Law's
>
> method
> position
> view

laxative

"lazy leukocyte syndrome"

LC – inductance-capacitance

LD – lethal dose

LD_{50} – median lethal dose

lead
>
> l. apron
> l. equivalent
> l. glass
> l. gloves
> l. protective chair
> l. rubber

lead ($^{207}_{82}$Pb, atomic number 82)

"lead pipe" colon

"leafless tree" appearance

leaflet
>
> aortic l.
> mitral l.

least-squares analysis

Lee & Westcott needle

Lee needle

Lefort's fracture

left-hand thumb rule

leiomyoblastoma

leiomyofibroma

leiomyoma

leiomyomata

leiomyosarcoma

Lenard's ray tube

lens
>
> objective l.
> Thorpe's plastic l.
> "zoom" l.

lenticular

lenticulostriate

lenticulothalamic

lentiform

lentigo (lentigines)

Leonard-George
>
> method
> position

leontiasis
>
> l. ossium

leopard syndrome

leprosy

leptomeningeal

leptomeninges

leptomeningioma

leptomeningitis

leptomyelolipoma

lepton

leptospiral

leptospirosis

Leri's pleonosteosis
lesion
    annular l.
    "apple core" l.
    "butterfly" l.
    cold l.
    "doughnut" l.
    "dumbbell" l.
    ellipsoid l.
    hot l.
    "napkin ring" l.
    "ring-like" l.
    sessile l.
    space occupying l.
    wedge-shaped l.
LET – linear energy transfer
lethal dose
leukemia
    chronic myelocytic l.
    myelogenous l.
    myelomonocytic l.
leukemic
leukocytosis
leukopenic
leukoplakia
levoangiocardiogram
levocardiogram
levoclination
levogram
Lewis'
    method
    position
LH – luteinizing hor-
   mone
licorice powder
lidocaine hydrochloride
lidofenin
Lieberkühn's crypts

lien
lienal
lienitis
lienography
ligament (*see* Part II, Table of
    Ligaments)
ligamentous
ligamentum (ligamenta)
    l. flavum
ligand
    antibody bound l.
    bound l.
    free l.
    labelled l.
    radiolabelled l.
    unlabelled l.
"light bulb" appearance
light photons
light-to-video conversion
Lilienfelds
    method
    position
lily pad sign
limbi (*see* limbus)
limbic
limbus (limbi)
    l. sphenoidalis
limen (limina)
    l. insulae
    l. nasi
limulus lysate test
Lindblom's
    method
    position
line
    absorption l.
    acanthiomeatal l.
    anterior junction l.

line *(continued)*

    anthropologic base l.
    anthropomorphic
      base l.
    auricular l.
    Blumensaat's l.
    calcaneal l.
    Camper's l.
    canthomeatal l.
    Chamberlain's l.
    epiphyseal plate l.
    field l.
    Fischgold's bimastoid l.
    Fischgold's biventer l.
    Fleischner's l.
    l. focus
    Frankfort l.
    glabelloalveolar l.
    glabellomeatal l.
    gluteal l.
    grid l.
    infraorbital l.
    infraorbitomeatal l.
    intercondylar
      notch l.
    intermalleolar l.
    interorbital l.
    interpupillary l.
    Kerley's A l.
    Kerley's B l.
    mammillary l.
    McGregor's l.
    mentomeatal l.
    metaphyseal l.
    midtalar l.
    nuchal l.
    obturator l.
    occlusal l.

line *(continued)*

    orbitomeatal base l.
    para-aortic l.
    paraesophageal l.
    paraspinal l.
    paratracheal l.
    paravertebral l.
    pericardial l.
    posterior junction l.
    psoas l.
    pubococcygeal l.
    radiographic base l.
    Reid's base l.
    l. saturation
    l. scanning
    Shenton's l.
    spigelian l.
    l. spread function
    subcostal l.
    transpyloric l.
    transtubercular l.
    transverse l.
    tuberculo-occipital pro-
      tuberance l.
    l. voltage compensator

linea
linear

    l. absorption coefficient
    l. accelerator
    l. array
    l. attenuation coefficient
    l. compartmental system
    l. energy transfer
    l. focus
    l. grid
    l. phased arrays
    l. photon
    l. resolution

linear *(continued)*
    l. scanning
    l. sequenced arrays
    l. system approach
    l. tomography
lingua (linguae)
lingual
lingula
lingular
linitis
    l. plastica
LIP – lymphocytic interstitial
   pneumonitis
lipid
lipidosis
Lipiodol
lipoatrophic
lipochondrodystrophy
lipodystrophy
lipogenesis
lipogenic
lipogranulomatosis
lipohyperplasia
lipoid
lipoma
lipomatosis
lipomatous
lipomeningocele
lipopolysaccharide
lipoproteinemia
    A-beta l.
liposarcoma
liposkeletogenic
Lippes loop intrauterine device
lipping
LIQ – lower inner quadrant
Liquipake

Lisfranc's
    fracture-dislocation
    joint
lissencephalic
lissencephaly
Listeria
liter
lithiasis
lithium
lithogenic
lithotomy
"Little Leaguer's elbow"
liver
    amyloid l.
    biliary cirrhotic l.
    brimstone l.
    bronze l.
    hobnail l.
    lardaceous l.
    pigmented l.
    polycystic l.
    sago l.
    stasis l.
    sugar-icing l.
    waxy l.
"Liverpool silicosis"
LL – left lateral
LLL – left lower lobe
LLQ – left lower quad-
   rant
Loa
    L. loa
lobar
    l. agenesis
    l. collapse
    l. consolidation
    l. emphysema

lobar *(continued)*
  "l. nephronia"
  l. pneumonia
  l. torsion
lobe
  accessory l.
  appendicular l.
  azygos l.
  caudate l.
  central l.
  cuneate l.
  flocculonodular l.
  frontal l.
  hepatic l.
  occipital l.
  parietal l.
  piriform l.
  polyalveolar l.
  quadrate l.
  Riedel's l.
  temporal l.
lobectomy
lobster claw deformity
lobular
lobulated
lobulation
lobule
lobus (lobi)
localization
localized
locular
loculated
loculus (loculi)
lodestone
Loepp's projection
Löffler's
  endocarditis

Löffler's *(continued)*
  eosinophilia
  pneumonia
log – logarithm
logarithm
long bone fracture
longitudinal
  l.arch
  l. axis
  l. relaxation
   time
  l. relaxation time con-
   stant
  l. section imaging
  l. section tomography
  l. suture
  l. time constant
  l. tomography
loop
  duodenal l.
  Henle's l.
  Lippes l.
loopogram
loose bodies
"Looser's transformation
  zones"
lopamidol
LOQ – lower outer quad-
  rant
lordosis
lordotic
Lorentz's force
Lorenz's
  method
  position
Löw-Beer
  method

Löw-Beer *(continued)*
    position
low-contrast film
LPO – left posterior oblique
LRM – lateral rectus muscle
LSF – line-spread function
lucency
lucent
lückenschädel
Ludwig's angina
luetic
    l. gumma
LUL – left upper lobe
lumbar
    l. aortography
    l. arch
    l. curve
    l. disc
    l. flexion and extension
        study
    l. lymph node
    l. myelography
    l. puncture
    l. region
    l. spine
    l. vertebra
lumbarization
lumboabdominal
lumbocostal
lumbocrural
lumbodorsal
lumboiliac
lumboinguinal
lumbosacral
    l. angle
    l. joint
    l. plexus
lumbrical

lumen
luminal
lunate
    bipartite l.
    l. scaphoid fusion
    l.-triquetrum fusion
lung
    l. agenesis
    "drowned l."
    esophageal l.
    farmer's l.
    honeycomb l.
    hyperlucent l.
    l. markings
    pigeon breeder's l.
    "respirator l."
    l. root
    "shock l."
    "stiff l."
lupus erythematosus
    discoid l. e.
    systemic l. e.
LUQ – left upper quadrant
Luschka's
    foramen
    joints
lutetium
luxated
luxation
"luxury perfusion" syndrome
LV –
    left ventricle
    left ventricular
LVH – left ventricular hyper-
    trophy
lymph
    l. node *(see* under node)
    l. sac

lymphadenectasis
lymphadenectomy
lymphadenitis
    caseous l.
    enteric l.
    histoplasmic l.
    mesenteric l.
    tuberculoid l.
    tuberculous l.
lymphadenogram
lymphadenography
lymphadenoma
lymphadenomatosis
lymphadenopathy
    axillary l.
    hilar l.
    immunoblastic l.
    mediastinal l.
    mesenteric l.
    tuberculous l.
lymphadenosis
lymphangiectasia
lymphangiectatic
lymphangiogram
lymphangiography
lymphangioma
    colonic l.
    cystic l.
    hemangioma l.
    intrasplenic l.
    mediastinal l.
lymphangiomatosis
lymphangiomyomatosis
lymphangiophlebitis
lymphangiosarcoma
lymphangitic
lymphangitis
    l. carcinomatosis

lymphatic
lymphedema
lymphenteritis
lymphoblastic
lymphoblastoma
lymphocele
lymphocyst
lymphocytic
lymphocytoma
lymphocytosis
lymphoendothelioma
lymphoepithelioma
lymphoepitheliomata
lymphogram
lymphogranuloma
    l. inguinale
    l. malignum
    l. venereum
lymphogranulomatosis
lymphography
lymphoid
    l. adenohypophysitis
    l. follicles
    l. hyperplasia
lymphoma
    alveolar l.
    Burkitt's l.
    clasmocytic l.
    disseminated l.
    giant follicular l.
    granulomatous l.
    histiocytic l.
    Hodgkin's l.
    lymphoblastic l.
    lymphocytic l.
    non-Hodgkin's l.
    retroperitoneal l.
    stem cell l.

lymphoma *(continued)*
    undifferenti-
      ated l.
lymphomatoid
lymphomatosum
lymphomatous
lymphomyxoma
lymphoproliferative
lymphoreticular
lymphosarcoma
    fascicular l.
    lymphoblastic l.

lymphosarcoma *(continued)*
    lymphocytic l.
    sclerosing l.
lymphosarcomatosis
lyophilized sulfur colloid
Lysholm's
    grid
    method
lysis
lysozyme
    l. inhibition
lytic

m

M –
    mega-
    meter
    micro-
    micron
    mutual inductance
m –
    micro-
    micron
    milli-
mA – milliam-
    pere
MAA – macroaggregated albu-
    min
macerate
maceration
Mach effect
Mackenzie Davidson method
macrencephaly

macroaggregated
    m. albumin
macroaggregates
macroangiography
macrocrania
macrodactyly
macrodystrophia
    m. lipomatosa
macroglobulinemia
    Waldenström's m.
macroglossia
macrogragh
macromolecular
macromolecule
macronodular
macrophage
macroradiography
macroscopic magnetization
    vector

Madayag needle
Madelung's deformity
Madura foot
maduromycosis
magenblase
Magendie
    foramen of M.
magenstrasse
magic numbers
magnesium
magnet
    beam-bending m.
    cryostable m.
    Eindhoven's m.
    permanent m.
    resistive m.
    superconductive m.
    Walker's m.
magnetic
    artificial permanent m.
    m. circuit
    m. disc
    m. domain
    m. field
    m. field strength
    m. flux
    m. focal plane
    m. force
    m. induction
    m. lines of force
    m. material
    m. moment
    m. nuclei
    m. permeability
    m. pole
    m. recording
    m. resonance imaging
    m. retentivity

magnetic (continued)
    superconducting m.
magnetism
magnetization
    m. transfer
magnetogyric
    m. ratio
magnification
    m. angiography
    m. factor
    m. percentage
    radiographic m.
    m. radiography
    vertebrobasilar m.
magnitude of ripple
main gain control
Maissoneuf's fracture
mal
    m. de mer
    grand m.
    petit m.
malabsorption
malacia
    "segmental m."
malaise
malakoplakia or malacoplakia
malalignment
maldevelopmental
malformation
    Arnold-Chiari m.
    arteriovenous m.
    Chiari's m.
    congenital m.
    Ebstein's m.
    Mondini's
    pulmonary arteriove-
        nous m.
    Scheibe's m.

malfunction
Malgaigne's fracture
malignancy
malignant
malleolar
malleolus (malleoli)
    fibular m.
    m. fracture
    lateral m.
    medial m.
    radial m.
    tibial m.
    ulnar m.
mallet finger
malleus
malnutrition
malocclusion
malomaxillary
malpighian
malposition
malrotation
malum
    m. coxae senilis
malunion
mamilla (mamillae)
mamillary system
mamillotegmental
mammary
    m. dysplasia
mammillary system
mammogram
mammography
Mammomat
mammoplasty
Mammorex
mandible
mandibular

mandibuloacral
    m. dysplasia
mandibulofacial
mandibulopharyngeal
maneuver
    Müller's m.
    toe-touch m.
    Valsalva's m.
manganese chloride
manifest image
Mankin's method
mannitol
mannosidosis
manometer
manubrial
manubriosternal
manubriosternoclavicular
manubrium (manubria)
manus
maple syrup urine disease
"maplike"
marble bone disease
Marchand's adrenals
march fracture
margin
    costal m.
    infraorbital m.
    midlateral orbital m.
    supraorbital m.
    synovial m.
marginal
margination
Martz's method
mAs – milliampere-second
Maslin's method
mass
    m. absorption coefficient

mass *(continued)*
- m. acceleration
- atomic m.
- m. energy equivalence
- intraluminal m.
- m. number
- relativistic m.
- m. spectrometer
- subcarinal m.
- m. units

massa (massae)
- m. intermedia

masseter
masseteric
Massiot's polytome
mastectomy
mastocarcinoma
mastochondroma
mastochondrosis
mastocytoma
mastocytosis
mastogram
mastography
mastoid
- m. air cells
- m. antrum
- m. portion
- m. process
- m. suture
- m. tip

mastoiditis
- "catarrhal" m.
- sclerotic m.
- suppurative m.

matrix
maturation
- delayed skeletal m.
- dysharmonic m.

maturation *(continued)*
- skeletal m.
- "maturity indicators"

maxicamera
maxilla (maxillae)
maxillary
- m. antra
- m. sinus

maximum permissible dose equivalent
maxwellian distribution
Maxwell's theory of radiation
Mayer's
- method
- position
- view

May's method
mc. or mCi – millicurie
μc. or μCi – microcurie
MCA – multichannel analyzer
McGregor's line
MCTD – mixed connective tissue disease
MDAC – multiplying digital-to-analog converter
MDP – methylene diphosphonate
MEA – multiple endocrine adenomatosis (syndrome)
mean
- m. deviation
- m. free path
- m. gonad dose
- m. life

measles
measurement
- Cobb's m.
- Ferguson's m.

meatus
Mecholyl
Meckel's
    cave
    cavity
    diverticulum
    stone
meconium
    m. aspiration syndrome
    m. ileus
    m. peritonitis
    m. plug syndrome
media (*see* medium)
    contrast m.
    opaque m.
mediad
medial
median
mediastinal
"mediastinal crunch"
mediastinitis
mediastinoscopy
mediastinum
Medical Research Council
mediolateral
Mediterranean
    anemia
    fever
medium (media)
    contrast m.
    culture m.
    radiopaque m.
medulla (medullae)
    m. oblongata
    m. spinalis
medullary
    m. canal
    m. conus

medullary *(continued)*
    m. cord
    m. space
    m. sponge kidney
    m. stenosis
medulloblastoma
Medx
    camera
    scanner
Meese's position
megabladder
megacalyces
megacalycosis
megacardia
megacephalic
megacholedochus
megacolon
    idiopathic m.
    psychogenic m.
megadontism
megaduodenum
mega-electron-volts
megaesophagus
megahertz
megalencephalon
megaloblastic
megalobulbus
megalocephaly
megalocheiria
megalocystis
megalodactyly
megaloureter
megavolt
megavoltage
megepiphyseal
meglumine
    m. diatrizoate
    m. iodipamide

meglumine *(continued)*
    m. iothalamate
megohm
Meiboom-Gill sequence
melanoameloblastoma
melanoma
melanotic
melatonin
melioidosis
melorheostosis
    m. leri
membranaceous
membrane
    periodontal m.
    m. phosphate
    synovial m.
    thyrohyoid m.
    tympanic m.
membranocartilaginous
membranous
mendelevium
mendosal
Menghini needle
meningeal
meninges
meningioma
    angioblastic m.
    en plaque m.
    falcine m.
    parasagittal m.
    sphenoid wing m.
    suprasellar m.
meningitis
meningoarteritis
meningoblastoma
meningocele
    sacral m.
    spurious m.

meningococcemia
meningococcus
meningocortical
meningoencephalitis
    amebic m.
    eosinophilic m.
    syphilitic m.
meningoencephalocele
meningoencephalomyelitis
meningomyelitis
meningomyelocele
meningomyeloencephalitis
meningomyeloradiculitis
meningoradicular
meningoradiculitis
meninx (meninges)
meniscal
meniscosynovial
meniscus (menisci)
    m. sign
Menkes' kinky hair syndrome
menopausal
menopause
menorrhagia
menstrual
menstruation
mental
    m. foramen
    m. point
    m. protuberance
    m. tubercle
mentomeatal
mento-occipital
mentum
"Mercedes-Benz" sign
Mercuhydrin
1-mercuri-2-hydroxypropane
mercury

meromelia
mesaticephalic
mesencephalon
mesenchyma
mesenchymal
mesenchymomatosis
mesenterial
mesenteric
    m. adenopathy
    m. arteriography
    m. fibrofatty prolifera-
      tion
    m. infarction
    m. ischemia
    m. lymphadenitis
    m. lymphadenopathy
    m. node
mesenteritis
    retractile m.
mesentery
mesial
mesiodistal
mesion
mesoazygos
mesoblastic
mesocephalic
mesocolon
mesodermal
mesomelic
meson
mesonephric
    m. ridge
mesothelioma
metabolic pathways
metabolism
metabolites
metacarpal

metacarpophalangeal
metacarpotalar syndrome
metacarpus
metachondromatosis
metallic
metaphyseal
    m. chondrodysplasia
    m. chondroplasia
    m. corner fracture
    m. dysostosis
    m. dysplasia
    m. irregularity
    m. line
    m. sclerosis
    m. transverse bands
    m. vessel
metaphysis (metaphyses)
metaphysitis
metaplasia
    agnogenic myeloid m.
    osseous m.
metaplastic
metastable
metastasis (metastases)
    mural m.
metastasize
metastatic
metatarsal
metatarsalgia
metatarsocuneiform
metatarsophalangeal
metatarsus
    m. adductus
    m. atavicus
    m. brevis
    m. latus
    m. primus varus

metatarsus *(continued)*
>   m. varus

metatropic
>   m. dysplasia

metencephalon

metencephalospinal

meteorism

meter
>   milliampere-second
>   (mAs) m.
>   m.-kilogram-second
>   (MKS) system

methacholine

methacrylate bone interface

methiodal
>   m. sodium

method
>   Albers-Schönberg m.
>   Alexander's m.
>   Anderson's m.
>   Andrén's m.
>   Arcelin's m.
>   Ball's m.
>   Bayler-Pinneau m.
>   Béclère's m.
>   Benassi's m.
>   Bertel's m.
>   Blackett-Healy m.
>   border detection m.
>   Broden's m.
>   Cahoon's m.
>   Caldwell-Moloy m.
>   Caldwell's m.
>   Cameron's m.
>   Camp-Gianturco m.
>   Causton's m.
>   Chamberlain's m.

method *(continued)*
>   Chassard-Lapiné m.
>   Chaussé's m.
>   Cleaves' m.
>   Cobb's m.
>   Colbert's m.
>   Colcher-Sussman m.
>   Davis' m.
>   Dooley, Caldwell and
>   Glass m.
>   Duncan-Hoen m.
>   Dunlap, Swanson and
>   Penner m.
>   dye-dilution m.
>   electrostatic m.
>   Erasmo's m.
>   Evan's m.
>   Feist's m.
>   Ferguson's m.
>   Fisk's m.
>   Fleischner's m.
>   Freiberger's m.
>   Friedman's m.
>   Fuchs' m.
>   Garn's m.
>   Gaynor-Hart m.
>   Gill's m.
>   Girout's m.
>   Grandy's m.
>   Grashey's m.
>   Gunson's m.
>   Haas' m.
>   Harrison-Stubbs m.
>   Hatt's m.
>   Henschen's m.
>   Heublein's m.
>   Hickey's m.

method *(continued)*

Hirtz's m.
Holmblad's m.
Hough's m.
Hsieh's m.
Hughston's m.
^{123}I hydroxyiodo-
  benzyl-propane-
  diamine m.
Isherwood's m.
Johnson's m.
Judd's m.
Kandel's m.
Kasabach's m.
Kemp Harper m.
Kimberlin's m.
Kirdani's m.
Kite's m.
Kovacs' m.
Kuchendorf's m.
Kumar, Welti and
  Ernst m.
Kurzbauer's m.
KWE m.
Laquerriere-Pierquin m.
Lauenstein and
  Hickey m.
Law's m.
Lawrence's m.
Leonard-George m.
Lewis' m.
Lilienfeld's m.
Lindblom's m.
Lorenz's m.
Löw-Beer m.
Lysholm's m.
Mackenzie Davidson m.
Mankin's m.

method *(continued)*

Martz's m.
Maslin's m.
May's m.
Mayer's m.
Miller's m.
Monte Carlo m.
multiple line
  scanning m.
multiple sensitive
  point m.
multisection m.
Nölke's m.
Ottonello's m.
Owen-Pendergrass m.
parallax m.
Parama's m.
Pawlow's m.
Pearson's m.
Pfeiffer-Comberg m.
Pirie's m.
Porcher's m.
QRS synchro m.
Quesada's m.
Rhese's m.
Sansregret's m.
Schüller's m.
sensitive line m.
sequential line m.
sequential point m.
Settegast's m.
Sommer-Foegella m.
Staunig's m.
Stecher's m.
Stenver's m.
Strickler's m.
surface coil m.
Sweet's m.

method *(continued)*
    Tanner-Whitehouse-
      Healy m.
    Tarrant's m.
    Taylor's m.
    Teufel's m.
    Thoms' m.
    Titterington's m.
    Twining's m.
    Valdini's m.
    Valvassori's m.
    Waters' m.
    Wehlin's m.
    Wigby-Taylor m.
    Williams' m.
    Wolf's m.
    Zanelli's m.
    Zimmer's m.
    Zizmor's m.
methodology
methotrexate
methylcellulose gel
methyl cholesterol
methylene diphospho-
    nate
methylglucamine
    m. iodipamide
    m. iodoxamate
    m. ioglycamide
    m. iothalamate
    m. iotroxamide
methyl methacrylate
methysergide
metoclopramide
metol
metopic
metra
metric system

metrizamide
    m. myelography
metrizamide-assisted computed
    tomography
metrizoate
metrizoic acid
metrosalpingography
metrotubography
Mev. – megaelectron volt
Meynet's node
MF – magnification factor
mf – microfarad
MHP – 1-mercuri-2-hydroxy-
    propane
MHz –
    megahertz
    270 m.
Michaelis' rhomboid
microadenoma
microangiogram
microatelectasis
microcephalic
microcephaly
microcolon
microcomputer
microcrania
microcurie
microcytic
microdosimetry
microembolization
microfarad
microfilm
microfocus
microfracture
microgeodic
micrognathia
microgram
microlithiasis

micromelia
micron
micronodular
Micropaque
microphthalmia
microradiogram
microradiography
microscopic
microsomia
microspheres
Microtrast
microtron
microwave imaging
micturition
midaxillary
midbrain
midcarpal
midcoronal
middle lobe syndrome
midfoot
midfrontal
midgut
midlateral
midoccipital
midplane
midriff
midsagittal
midsection
midtalar
midtarsal
midtegmentum
midthoracic
migraine
migration
miliary
milk-induced colitis
milk of calcium
    m. of c. bile

milk of calcium *(continued)*
    m. of c. calculi
Miller-Abbott tube
Miller's
    method
    position
milliammeter
milliamperage
milliampere
milliampere-minute
milliampere-second
millicurie
    m. -hour
milliequivalent
milligamma
milliliter
millimeter
millimicrocurie
millimicrogram
million-electron-volt
millirad
millirem
milliroentgen
millisecond
milliunit
millivolt
Mima
    M. polymorpha
"mimosa" pattern
mineralization
miniature radiography
minification
minometer
mirror image lung syndrome
miscibility
miscible
mithramycin
mitochondria

Mira luma
(one word)

mitochondrial
mitosis
mitotic
mitral
    m. atresia
    m. funnel
    m. leaflet
    m. murmur
    m. regurgitation
    m. stenosis
    m. valve prolapse
MKS – meter-kilogram-second
MLD – median lethal dose
MLS – multiple line scan
mm –
    micromicro-
    millimeter
MMFR – maximum midexpiratory flow rate
MMM syndrome
M-mode – time-motion mode
MMTV – mammary tumor viruses
Mo – molybdenum
mobile x-ray system
mobility
modulation
    amplitude m.
    brightness m.
    image m.
    object m.
    m. transfer function
mogul
    "third m."
Mohr-Wriedt's brachydactyly
molal
molality
molar volume

mole
    hydatidiform
molecular
    m. diffusion rate
    m. dynamics
    m. force
    m. structure
    m. vibration
molecule
Molnar disc
molybdenum
momentum
Mondini's pulmonary arteriovenous malformation
mongolism
mongoloidism
moniliasis
monitor
    air m.
    beam m.
    radiation m.
monitoring
    cardiovascular m.
    industrial m.
    television m.
monoarthritic
monochromatic
    m. radiation
monoclonal
monocular
monodactyly
monoenergetic
    m. radiation
monoglucuronide
monomers
    ionic m.
    nonionic m.
monomorphic

mononuclear
mononucleosis
    infectious m.
Monophen
monosodium
    m. urate monohydrate
monosomy
monostotic fibrous dysplasia
monoxide
Monro
    foramen of M.
Monte Carlo method
Monteggia's fracture-
    dislocation
Moore's fracture
morbid
morbus
    m. coxae senilis
Morgagni's hernia
moribund
morphea
morphine
morphologic
morphology
Morrison's pouch
mortification
mortise
mosaic
Mossbauer's spectrometer
''moth-eaten'' appearance
motility
    m. study
motoneuron
    multipolar m.
mottle
    photon m.
    quantum m.
    radiographic m.

mottle (continued)
    screen m.
mottled
movement
    arc to arc m.
    arc to line m.
    m. artifacts
    circular m.
    hypocycloidal m.
    linear m.
    line to line m.
    multidirectional m.
    symmetrical-unsym-
        metrical m.
moyamoya
MP – membrane phosphate
MPD – maximum permissible
    dose
mr – milliroentgen
mrad – millirad
MRC – Medical Research
    Council
mrem – millirem
MRI – magnetic resonance im-
    aging
MRM – medial rectus muscle
msec – millisecond
3M syndrome
MTF – modulation transfer
    function
mucin
mucinous
mucocele
mucocutaneous
mucoepidermoid
mucoid
mucolipidosis
Mucomyst

mucoperiosteum
mucopolysaccharidosis
      m. I-H
      m. I H/S
      m. I S
      m. II
      m. VI
Mucor
mucormycosis
mucosa
mucosal
mucous
mucoviscidosis
mucus
MUGA – multigated angio-
    gram
"mulberry-type" calcifica-
    tion
müllerian
Müller's maneuver
multangular
multiarticular
multiaxial
multicentric
multichannel
multicrystal camera
multicystic
multidirectional
multifocal
multiformat camera
multigated
      m. angiography
      m. imaging
multigravida
multilanigraph
multilobular
multilobulated
multilocular

multiloculated
multinodular
multipara
multiplanar
      m. imaging
      m. scanning
multiplane line integral projec-
    tion reconstruction
multiple
      m. endocrine adenoma-
        tosis syndrome
      m.-gated blood pool im-
        aging
      m.-gated blood pool
        scan
      m. infarct dementia
      m. line scanning
        method
      m. myeloma
      m. -nuclide
      m. plane integral recon-
        struction
      m. radiography
      m. sclerosis
      m. sensitive point
        method
      m. spin echo total vol-
        ume imaging
      m. synostoses syn-
        drome
      m. xanthomatosis
multiplex
multiplexing
multiscaler
multisection
      m. cassette
      m. method
      simultaneous m.

multislice
    m. full line scan
    m. modified KWE direct Fourier imaging
    m. scanner
multitomography
mummify
mural
murmur
    amphoric m.
    aneurysmal m.
    aortic m.
    apical diastolic m.
    arterial m.
    asymptomatic m.
    cardiac m.
    congenital m.
    crescendo m.
    diastolic m.
    ejection m.
    innocent m.
    mitral m.
    noninvasive m.
    pansystolic m.
    pleuropericardial m.
    prediastolic m.
    presystolic m.
    pulmonic m.
    regurgitant m.
    subclavicular m.
    systolic m.
    tricuspid m.
    vascular m.
    venous m.
muscle (*see* Part II, Table of Muscles)
muscular
musculature

musculomembranous
musculoskeletal
musculotendinous
mustache sign
mutation
myasthenia gravis
mycelium (mycelia)
mycetoma
mycobacteria
Mycobacterium
    M. kansasii
    M. leprae
mycologist
mycology
mycopathology
Mycoplasma
    M. pneumoniae
mycoplasma
mycoplasmal
mycoplasmosis
mycosis
mycotic
myelencephalitis
myelin
myelinoclasis
myelitis
myeloblastoma
myelocele
myelocisternoencephalography
myelocytic
myelocytoma
myelofibrosis
myelogenous
myelogram (*see* myelography)
myelographic
myelography
    cervical m.
    computed m.

myelography *(continued)*
    gas m.
    lumbar m.
    metrizamide m.
    opaque m.
    positive contrast m.
    thoracic m.
myeloid
myelolipoma
myeloma
    endothelial m.
    giant cell m.
    multiple m.
    osteosclerotic m.
    plasma cell m.
myelomeningitis
myelomeningocele
myelomonocytic
myelopathy
myeloperoxidase
myelophthisic
myeloproliferative
myeloradiculitis
myeloradiculodysplasia
myeloradiculopathy
myelosarcoma
myeloschisis
myelosclerosis
myelosclerotic
myelosis
Mylar
Myleran
myoblastoma
myocardial
    m. contusion
    m. failure
    m. infarct imaging
    m. infarction

myocardial *(continued)*
    m. ischemia
    m. necrosis
    m. perforation
    m. perfusion imaging
myocardium
Myodil
myoepithelial
myoepithelioma
myoglobinuria
myolipoma
myoma
myometrial
myonecrosis
myoneural
myopathy
myorelaxant
myositis
    interstitial m.
    m. ossificans progres-
      siva
    m. purulenta
    rheumatoid m.
    suppurative m.
myotonic
myxadenoma
myxedema
    circumscribed m.
    papular m.
    pituitary m.
    pretibial m.
myxedematoid
myxedematous
myxoadenoma
myxoblastoma
myxochondrofibrosar-
    coma
myxochondroma

myxochondrosarcoma
myxocystoma
myxoenchondroma
myxoendothelioma
myxofibroma
myxofibrosarcoma
myxoglioma
myxoid

myxoma (myxomas or myxo-
     mata)
myxomatosis
myxomatous
myxomyoma
myxopapilloma
myxosarcoma
myxosarcomatous

N –
     neutral number
     newton
NA – Nomina Anatomica
Na atoms
nail
          Plummer's n.
          Smith-Petersen n.
nail-patella syndrome
NaI – sodium iodide
nanocephaly
nanocurie
nanogram
nanosomia
"napkin ring"
          "n. r." defect
          "n. r." lesion
naris (nares)
narrow-beam half-
     thickness
nasal
nasion
nasoantral

nasoantritis
nasobronchial
nasociliary
nasofrontal
nasogastric
nasolabial
nasolacrimal
nasomaxillary
naso-oral
nasopalatine
nasopharyngeal
nasopharyngitis
nasopharyngography
nasopharynx
naso-pineal angle
nasorostral
nasoseptal
nasoseptitis
nasosinusitis
nasospinale
nasotracheal
nasoturbinal
nates

National Council on Radiation
    Protection and Measure-
    ments
National Health Service (UK)
National Radiological Commis-
    sion
National Radiological Protec-
    tion Board
nausea
navel
navicular
NC - no connection
nc. or nCi - nanocurie
NCRPM - National Council on
    Radiation Protection and
    Measurements
NDA - New Drug Application
nearthrosis
nebulization
necrobiotic
necropsy
necrosis
    acute tubular n.
    aseptic n.
    avascular n.
    carpal n.
    coagulation n.
    colliquative n.
    embolic n.
    epiphyseal ischemic n.
    exanthematous n.
    familial carpal n.
    fat n.
    gangrenous n.
    myocardial n.
    osseous n.
    peripheral n.
    radiation n.

necrosis *(continued)*
    scaphoid n.
    syphilitic n.
necrotic
necrotizing
needle
    anesthetic n.
    Chiba n.
    Craig n.
    flexible biopsy n.
    Franseen n.
    Green n.
    Hawkins n.
    Jamshide n.
    Kopan's n.
    Lee n.
    Lee & Westcott n.
    Madayag n.
    Menghini n.
    percutaneous n.
    Rotex n.
    sheathed n.
    skinny n.
    TruCut n.
    Turkel n.
    Turner's n.
    Vim-Silverman n.
    Westcott n.
negative
    n. charge
    n. direction
    n. electron
    n. ion
    n. potential
    n. terminal
negatron
    n. emission
neodymium

Neo-Iopax
neon
neonatal
neoplasia
neoplasm
    retroperitoneal n.
neoplastic
neostigmine
neovascularity
nephradenoma
nephrectomy
nephredema
nephrelcosis
nephremia
nephritic
nephritis
nephroabdominal
nephroblastoma
    cystic differenti-
      ated n.
    polycystic n.
nephrocalcino-
  sis
nephrocardiac
nephrocystitis
nephrogastric
nephrogenic
nephrogram
nephrography
nephrohypertrophy
nephrolith
nephrolithiasis
nephroma
    embryonal n.
    mesoblastic n.
    multicystic n.
    multilocular cystic n.
nephron

nephronia
    "lobar n."
nephronophthisis
nephropathy
nephropexy
nephroptosis
nephropyelography
nephrosclerosis
nephrosis
    Finnish type n.
nephrosonephritis
nephrosonography
nephrostogram
nephrostomy
    percutaneous n.
nephrotomogram
nephrotomography
    bolus injection n.
    infusion n.
nephrotuberculosis
nephrourography
neptunium
nerve (*see* Part II, Table of
    Nerves)
nervous system
neural
neuralgia
neurenteric
neurilemma
neurilemmitis
neurilemoma
neurinoma
neuroangiographic
neuroarthropathy
neuroastrocytoma
neuroblastoma
neurocanal
neurocentral

neurocranial
neurocranium
neurocutaneous
neurocytoma
neurodiagnostic
neuroectodermal
neurofibroma
neurofibromatosis
neurofibrosarcoma
neurogenic
neurogenous
neuroglia
neurogliocytoma
neuroglioma
neurohypophyseal
neurohypophysis
neurologic
neurolysis
neuroma
    acoustic n.
    mucosal n.
    trigeminal n.
neuromatosis
neuromatous
neuromeningeal
neuromotor
neuromuscular
    n. scoliosis
neuron
neuropathic
neuropathy
    radicular n.
neuroradiologist
neuroradiology
neuroroentgenography
neurosarcoma
neuroskeletal
neurotrophic

neurovasculotropic
neurovisceral
    n. lipidosis
    n. storage disease
neutral atom
neutrino
neutron
    n. absorption process
    n. activation analysis
    epithermal n.
    n. excess
    fast n.
    intermediate n.
    n. number
    slow n.
    thermal n.
neutrophil
    n. dysfunction syn-
      drome
    gram-positive n.
nevoid basal cell carcinoma
newton
Newton's
    law of action-reaction
    law of motion
NHS – National Health Service
    (UK)
niche
nickel
nidus
nightstick fracture
nigra
    substantia n.
nigral
niobium
Niopam
Nissen's fundoplication
nitrate

nitrofurantoin
nitrogen ($^{14}_{7}$N, atomic
    number 7)
nitrogen mustard
nitrogenous
nitrous oxide
NMR – nuclear magnetic reso-
    nance
nobelium
Noble's position
Nocardia
    N. brasiliensis
nocardial
nocardiosis
nodal
node
    aortic n.
    aortic-pulmonic
        lymph n.
    aortocaval n.
    atrioventricular n.
    axillary n.
    azygos lymph n.
    Bouchard's n.
    bronchopulmonary
        lymph n.
    buccal lymph n.
    carinal n.
    celiac lymph. n.
    cervical lymph n.
    circumcardiac lymph n.
    Cloquet's n.
    gastric lymph n.
    gastroepiploic lymph n.
    gouty n.
    Haygarth's n.
    Heberden's n.
    hepatic lymph n.

node *(continued)*
    hilar n.
    ileocolic lymph n.
    iliac lymph n.
    inguinal lymph n.
    lumbar lymph n.
    lymph n.
    mammary n.
    mandibular lymph n.
    mediastinal lymph n.
    mesenteric lymph n.
    Meynet's n.
    obturator n.
    Osler's n.
    pancreatic lymph n.
    pancreaticosplenic
        lymph n.
    para-aortic n.
    parasternal lymph n.
    paratracheal n.
    parotid lymph n.
    periaortic n.
    phrenic lymph n.
    popliteal lymph n.
    prelaryngeal n.
    pretracheal n.
    prevascular lymph n.
    pulmonary lymph n.
    pyloric lymph n.
    retroauricular lymph n.
    retrocrural n.
    retroperitoneal lymph n.
    retropharyngeal lymph n.
    Rotter's n.
    sacral lymph n.
    Schmorl's n.
    sentinel n.
    sinoatrial n.

node *(continued)*
    sinus n.
    subcarinal n.
    submandibular lymph n.
    submental lymph n.
    syphilitic n.
    tracheal lymph n.
    tracheobronchial
        lymph n.
nodular
nodulation
nodule
    acinar n.
    acinus n.
    air-containing n.
    alveolar n.
    autonomous n.
    cold n.
    hot n.
    interstitial n.
    miliary n.
    pulmonary n.
    solitary n.
    thyroid n.
noise
    n. averaging behavior
    n. fluctuation
    Poisson's n. fluctua-
        tions
    quantum n.
Nölke's
    method
    position
Nomina Anatomica
nomogram
nonarticular
nonbullous
noncalcified

noncommunicating
nonconductor
nonfiberoptic
nonflocculating
nongated CT scan
nongoiterous
nongummatous
non-Hodgkin's lymphoma
nonhomogeneity
nonhomogeneous
noninvasive
nonionic
    n. dimers
    n. monomers
nonischemic
nonlinear
nonlinearity
nonmagnetic
non-neoplastic
nonobstructive
nonodontogenic
non-ohmic resistor
nonopacification
nonopacified
nonopaque
nonossifying
nonosteogenic
nonparasitic
nonpyogenic
nonradiopaque
nonresectable
nonrotation
non-screen film
nonseminomatous
nonsequestrating
nonspecific
nonsuppurative
nontoxic

nonuniformity
nonunion
nonventricular
    n. cerebrospinal
      fluid space disease
nonviscous
nonvisualization
nonvisualized
norepinephrine
normalized plateau slope
normal salt solution
normoxic/hypoxic spectra
"nose-chin" position
"nose-forehead" position
notch
    angular n.
    capitate n.
    cardiac n.
    cerebellar n.
    ethmoidal n.
    infratragal n.
    intercondylar n.
    jugular n.
    mandibular n.
    manubrial n.
    radial n.
    scapular n.
    sciatic n.
    n. sign
    spinoglenoid n.
    sternal n.
    suprascapular n.
    suprasternal n.
    supratragal n.
    tentorial n.
    trochlear n.
    vertebral n.
notching

Novopaque
NRC –
    National Radiological
      Commission
    Nuclear Regulatory Com-
      mission
NRPB – National Radiological
    Protection Board
NSD – nominal single dose
n-type semiconductors
nuchal line
nuchofrontal
nuclear
    n. angiography
    n. cardiology
    n. decay
    n. disintegration
    n. emulsion
    n. energy
    n. fission
    n. force
    n. fusion
    n. magnetic moments
    n. medicine
    n. imaging
    n. particle
    n. probe
    n. radiation
    n. reaction
    n. reactor
    n. relaxation
    n. scanner
    n. scanning
    n. scintigraphy
    n. spin
    n. structure
nuclear magnetic resonance
    n. m. r. images

nuclear magnetic resonance
   (continued)
      n. m. r. imaging
      n. m. r. Fourier trans-
        formation
      n. m. r. phantoms
      pulsed n. m. r.
      n. m. r. relaxation rate
        enhancement
      n. m. r. scanning se-
        quences
      n. m. r. signal intensity
      n. m. r. spectra
      n. m. r. spectral param-
        eters
      n. m. r. spectrometer
      n. m. r. spectroscopy
      n. m. r. spin-warp
        method
      n. m. r. tomography
Nuclear Regulatory Commission
nuclease
nuclei
nucleic acid
nucleide
nucleiform
nucleography
nucleoid
nucleoliform
nucleon
nucleonics
nucleoprotein

nucleoreticulum
nucleoside
nucleotherapy
nucleotide
nucleus
      amygdaloid n.
      atomic n.
      caudate n.
      daughter n.
      lentiform n.
      parent n.
      n. pulposus
      red n.
nuclide
nullipara
number
      atomic n.
      Avogadro's n.
      body atomic n.
      effective atomic n.
      Euler's n.
      mass n.
      nucleon n.
      n. profile
numerical
      n. dissection
      n. projection display
      n. projection/dissolu-
        tion display
nutrient
nutrition
Nyegaard
nystagmus

O

O –
Ω – ohm
oat cell carcinoma
obesity
obex
object-film distance
objective
    o. lens
    o. plane
oblique
obliquity
obliterative
obscuration
obstetrics
obstruction
    airway o.
    atrial o.
    biliary o.
    bronchial o.
    cystic duct o.
    esophageal o.
    intestinal o.
    intraductal o.
    mechanical o.
    renal o.
    small bowel o.
    transhepatic o.
    ureteral o.
    ureteropelvic junc-
       tion o.
    ureterovesical junc-
       tion o.
    urinary tract o.

obstructive
    o. carcinoma
    o. cardiomyopathy
    o. collapse
    o. hydrocephalus
    o. hyperaeration
    o. jaundice
    o. nephropathy
    o. uropathy
obturator
    o. line
    o. sign
OC – outer canthus
occipital
    o. horn
    o. lobe
    o. plane
    o. protuberance
    o. sulcus
    o. vertebra
occipitalization
occipitoanterior
occipitoatloid
occipitoaxoid
occipitobasilar
occipitobregmatic
occipitocalcarine
occipitocervical
occipitofacial
occipitofrontal
occipitomastoid
occipitomental
occipitoparietal

occipitoposterior
occipitosphenoidal
occipitotemporal
occipitothalamic
occipitovertical
occiput
occlusal line
occlusion
occult
occupational radiation
OCG – oral cholecystogram
ochronosis
OCR – optical character recognition
octapeptide
octet rule
ocular
oculo-auricular-vertebral dysplasia
oculo-cerebro-renal syndrome
oculo-dento-digital syndrome
oculo-dento-osseous dysplasia
oculomotor
Odelca camera unit
Oddi's sphincter
odontogenic
odontoid
odontoma
OER – oxygen extraction rate
OFD – object-film distance
off-resonance proton
OHCS – hydroxy corticosteroid
Ohio Nuclear Delta 50 FS scanner
Ohio Nuclear Delta 50 scanner
Ohio Nuclear Delta 2000 scanner
ohm

ohmic
   o. resistance
   o. resistor
ohmmeter
Ohm's law
OIH – orthoiodohippurate
oil
   brominized o.
   iodized o.
olecranon
   o. fossa
   o. fracture
   o. process
oleic acid I 125
oleothorax
olfactory
oligemia
oligoarthritis
oligoarticular
oligodactylia
oligodactyly
oligodendrocyte
oligodendroglioma
oligomenorrhea
oliguria
olivocerebellar
olivopontocerebellar
olivospinal
OMBL – orbitomeatal base line
omental
omentoportography
omentum
OML – orbitomeatal line
Omnipaque
omphalocele
omphalomesenteric
omphalophlebitis

oncocytoma
oncologist
oncology
"onion skin" appearance
onychodystrophy
onycholysis
onycho-osteo-arthro dysplasia
opacification
opacified
opacity
opaque
    o. arthrography
    o. enema
    o. injection
    o. media
    o. myelography
OPD syndrome – oto-palato-
    digital syndrome
open bronchus sign
operating voltage
operculum (opercula)
ophthalmic
ophthalmology
ophthalmoplegia
opisthocranion
opisthotonos
OPLL – ossification of the pos-
    terior longitudinal ligament
opportunistic
    o. pneumonia
optic
    o. canal
    o. chiasma
    o. foramen
    o. granuloma
    o. groove
    o. nerve
    o. radiation

optic *(continued)*
    o. tract
optical amplifying system
opticochiasmatic
optimum
Optiplanimat automated unit
Orabilex
Oragrafin
oral
    o. cholangiography
    o. cholecystogram
    o. cholecystography
    o. intubation
Oravue
orbicular
orbit
    atomic o.
    electron o.
orbital
    o. base
    o. cavity
    o. electron
    o. fat
    o. fissure
    o. hemangioma
    o. plane
    o. plate
orbitography
orbitomeatal
Orbitome tomographic system
orbitoparietal
Orbix x-ray unit
ordography
organic
organoaxial
    o. rotation
organophosphate
orifice

oro-digito-facial syndrome
oro-facio-digital syndrome
orolingual
oromaxillary
oronasal
oropharynx
orotracheal
Orthicon television camera
orthodiagram
orthodiagraph
orthodiagraphy
orthodiascope
orthodiascopy
orthoiodohippurate
orthopantomography
orthopedics
orthoroentgenography
orthoscopic
orthoskiagraph
orthostatic
orthovoltage
os (ora)
    o. uteri
os (ossa)
    o. calcis
    o. centrale
    o. coxae
    o. innominatum
    o. magnum
    o. odontoideum
    o. styloideum
    o. trapezium secundar-
      ium
    o. triangulare
Osbil
oscillating
    o. electron
    o. grid

oscilloscope
Osler's node
OSMED – oto-spondylo-me-
    gaepiphyseal dysplasia
osmium
osmolality
osseous
    o. metaplasia
    o. necrosis
    o. spicule
    o. synostosis
ossicle
ossiculum
ossification
    cartilaginous o.
    dichotomous o.
    ectopic o.
    endochondral o.
    intracartilaginous o.
    intramembranous o.
    metaplastic o.
    perichondral o.
    periosteal o.
    pulmonary o.
    vertebral o.
ossifying
osteitis
    o. condensans ilii
    o. deformans
    o. fibrosa cystica
    o. pubis
    radiation o.
    rubella o.
osteoarthritis
osteoarthropathy
osteoarthrosis
    intervertebral o.
osteoblast

osteoblastic
osteoblastoma
osteochondral
osteochondritides
osteochondritis
    o. dissecans
    o. necroticans
osteochondrodystrophy
osteochondroma
osteochondromatosis
osteochondromyxoma
osteochondropathia
    o. cretinoidea
osteochondropathy
osteochondrosarcoma
osteochondrosis
    o. dissecans
    intervertebral o.
osteoclast
osteoclastoma
osteocystoma
osteocyte
osteodysplasty
osteodystrophia
    o. cystica
    o. fibrosa
osteodystrophy
    Albright's o.
    renal o.
osteoectasia
osteofibroma
osteofibromatosis
osteogenesis
    o. imperfecta
    o. imperfecta cystica
osteogenic
osteoglophonic

osteohypertrophic-varicose
    nevus syndrome
osteoid
    o. osteoma
osteolipoma
osteoliposarcoma
osteology
osteolysis
osteolytic
osteoma
    o. cutis
    o. eburneum
    o. medullare
    osteoid o.
    o. sarcomatosum
    o. spongiosum
    "tropical ulcer" o.
osteomalacia
osteomyelitis
    Brucella o.
    calvarial o.
    Candida o.
    fungal o.
    Garré's sclerosing o.
    hematologic o.
    Hemophilus influenzae o.
    iliac o.
    Klebsiella o.
    luetic o.
    multifocal o.
    neonatal o.
    nocardial o.
    nonsequestrating o.
    pyogenic o.
    Salmonella o.
    tuberculous o.

osteomyelitis *(continued)*
 o. variolosa
osteomyelodysplasia
osteomyelography
osteomyxochondroma
osteonecrosis
osteo-onycho-dysostosis
osteopathia
 o. striata
osteopathy
osteopenia
osteopetrosis
osteophyte
osteophytic
osteophytosis
osteopoikilosis
osteoporosis
 o. circumscripta
 congenital o.
 endocrine o.
 hyperparathyroid o.
 iatrogenic o.
 idiopathic juvenile o.
 neurovasculotropic o.
 nutritional deficiency o.
 senile o.
 spinal o.
 subchondral o.
osteoprogenitor cell
osteosarcoma
osteosclerosis
 autosomal dominant o.
osteosclerotic
osteoscope
osteosynovitis
ostium
OTD – organ tolerance dose

otic
otitis externa
otitis media
 chronic adhesive o. m.
 fibro-osseous o. m.
oto-palato-digital
 syndrome
otorrhea
otosclerosis
 cochlear o.
 fenestral o.
oto-spondylo-megaepiphyseal
 dysplasia
''otospongiosis''
Otto-Krobak pelvis
Ottonello's method
outlet
 pelvic o.
 thoracic o.
out-of-phase
outpouching
output
 cardiac o.
 o. phosphor
 o. side
ovarian
ovary
overaeration
overcouch
 o. exposure
 o. tube
 o. view
overdevelopmental
overdistention
overexposure
overflow incontinence
Overhauser's effect

overinflation
"overlap shadow"
overpenetrated film
overriding
overvoltage
"over writing"
oviduct
Owen-Pendergrass method

oxalosis
oxidation
oxycephalic
oxycephaly
oxygen($^{16}_{8}$O, atomic number 8)
oxygenated
oxyphil
oxysulfide

p

P –
 phosphorus
 posterior
 primary winding
^{32}P – radioactive phosphorus
PA –
 posteroanterior
 thyroxine-binding prealbu-
  min
pacchionian
  p. villi
pacemaker
  diaphragmatic p.
  transvenous p.
pachycephalic
pachydermoperiostitis
pachydermoperiostosis
pachygyria
pachyonychia
  p. congenita
packing fraction
Page's kidney

PAH – para-aminohippurate
pair
  p. annihilation
  electron-positron p.
  Helmholtz's p.
  ion p.
  p. production
palate
palatine tonsil
palatoethmoidal
palatograph
palatography
palatomyograph
palatopharyngeal
palindromic
  p. rheumatism
palladium
palliative
palmar
palmitate
palmitic acid
palsy

panacinar
panagraphy
"pancake"
      p. appearance
      p. compression
Pancoast's tumor
pancreas
pancreatic
pancreaticoduodenal
pancreaticosplenic
pancreatitis
pancreatogram
pancreatography
pancytopenia
      congenital p.
      p.-dysmelia syndrome
      Fanconi's p.
"panda" appearance
pangynecography
panlobular
panmural
panniculitis
pannus
pan-oral
panoramic
      p. radiography
      p. tomography
      p. view
panoramix
Panorex
pansinusitis
pansystolic
pantomographic view
pantomography
      concentric p.
      eccentric p.
Pantopaque
pantothenic acid

papaverine
papilla
      duodenal p.
      lacrimal p.
      p. of Vater
papillary
papillitis
papilloma
      choroid plexus p.
      squamous cell p.
papillomata
papillomatosis
papular
papule
papulosis
papulosquamous
papulovesicular
para-aminohippurate
para-aminohippuric acid
para-aminosalicylic
      acid
para-aortic
paracentesis
"parachute string"
paracicatricial
paracolic
paracolonic
paracondyloid
paradoxical
      p. incontinence
paraduodenal
paraesophageal
paraffinoma
paraganglioma
paragonimiasis
Paragonimus
parahilar
parahippocampal

parainfluenza
    p. viral pneumonia
parallax method
parallel
    p. circuit
    p. grid
    p. ray
paralysis
    p. agitans
paralytic
    p. gait
paralyze
paramagnetic
    p. ion
    p. relaxation
    p. shift
paramagnetism
Parama's method
paramedian
parameter
paranasal
paranasopharyngeal
paraneoplastic
parapelvic
parapharyngeal
paraplegia
pararenal
parasagittal
parasellar
paraseptal
parasinoidal
parasite
parasitic
paraspinal
paraspinous
parasternal
parastremmatic
    p. dysplasia

parasutural
    p. sclerosis
parasympathetic
parathormone
parathyroid
paratracheal
paratyphoid
paraureteral
paraventricular
paravertebral
paravesical
paravirus
parenchyma
parenchymal
    p. kidney
    p. transit time index
parent
    p. element
    p. nucleus
    p. nuclide
parenteral
"parentheses-like" calcification
paresis
    pharyngeal p.
    Todd's p.
paries (parietes)
parietal
    p. fenestra
    p. foramina
    p. lobe
    p. peritoneum
    "p. star"
    p. stellate
parietoacanthial
parietography
parietomastoid
parieto-occipital

parieto-orbital
parietotemporal
paronychia
parosteal
parotid
parotitis
pars (partes)
    p. distalis
    p. interarticularis
    p. intermedia
    p. nervosa
    p. petrosa
    p. tuberalis
partial volume
particle
    alpha p.
    beta p.
    nuclear p.
    viral p.
    p. waves
partition
    p. coefficient
part-thickness
parturition
PAS – para-aminosalicylic acid
Pasteurella
    P. multocida
pastille radiometer
patch
    lymphoid p's
    Peyer's p's
patella
    p. alta
    p. baja
    high-lying p.
patellar
patelliform
patellofemoral

patency
patent ductus arteriosus
pathoanatomy
pathogenesis
pathogenetic
pathognomonic
pathologic
    p. diagnosis
    p. discrimination
    p. tissue
pathology
pathophysiology
pathway
    Embden-Meyerhof gly-
      colytic p.
    visual p.
pattern
    alveolar p.
    "broken bough" p.
    "butterfly" p.
    convolutional p.
    corkscrew p.
    cystic p.
    "fingerprint" p.
    "hair brush" p.
    "hanging fruit" p.
    haustral p.
    "herring-bone" p.
    honeycomb p.
    "mimosa" p.
    rugal p.
    solid p.
    start test p.
    three-dimensional physi-
      ologic flow p.
patulous
pauciarthritic
pauciarticular

Pauli's exclusion principle
Pawlow's
        method
        position
Pb – lead
PBI – protein-bound iodine
PC – pentose cycle
p.c. – post cibum
pc. or pCi – picocurie
PCr – phosphocreatine
PCW – pulmonary capillary
    wedge pressure
PDA – patent ductus arterio-
    sus
PE – photographic effect
peak
        Bragg's p.
        characteristic p.
        p. kilovoltage
        p.-to-peak
        p. value
Pearson's
        method
        position
pectineal
pectiniform
pectoral aplasia-dysdactyly
    syndrome
pectoralis
pectus
        p. carinatum
        p. excavatum
        p. gallinatum
        p. recurvatum
pediatric
pedicle
pedicular

pediculate
peduncle
peduncular
pedunculated
PEEP – positive end-expiratory
    pressure
PEG –
        pneumoencephalography
        polyethyleneglycol
peizoelectric
pelvic
        p. abscess
        p. cavity
        p. colon
        p. girdle
        p. inflammatory disease
        p. inlet
        p. kidney
        p. outlet
        p. pneumography
        p. portion
        p. ring fracture
pelvicalyceal
pelvicephalography
pelvicephalometer
pelvicephalometry
pelvimetry
pelviography
pelvioradiography
pelvioscopy
pelviradiography
pelviroentgenography
pelvis (pelves)
        Otto-Krobak p.
        renal p.
pelviureteric
pelvocalyceal

pemphigus
"pencil-in-cup" defor-
    mity
"penciling" deformity
"pencil-like" deformity
pendelluft
pendulum
penetration
        radiographic p.
penetrology
penetrometer
        Benoist's p.
penicillin
pentagastrin
pentose cycle
penumbra
"pepper-pot" pitting
peptic ulcer
percent depth dose
perception
        depth p.
perchlorate
        p. discharge test
        potassium p.
percussion
percutaneous
        p. antegrade pyelogra-
            phy
        p. antegrade urography
        p. biopsy
        p. carotid arteriography
        p. drainage
        p. hepatobiliary cholan-
            giography
        p. liver biopsy
        p. needle
        p. nephrostomy

percutaneous *(continued)*
        p. transhepatic cholan-
            giography
        p. transhepatic puncture
        p. transtracheal bron-
            chography
perforated
perforating ulcer
perforation
        colonic p.
        duodenal p.
        gastric p.
        gastrointestinal p.
        hypopharyngeal p.
        myocardial p.
        pharyngeal p.
        pulmonary p.
        retroperitoneal p.
        tracheal p.
perfusion
        p. lung scan
        luxury p.
        myocardial p.
        peripheral p.
        p. scanning
        p. study
periacetabular
perianal
perianeurysmal
periaortic
periapical
periappendiceal
periaqueductal
periarticular
periaxial
peribiliary
peribronchial

peribronchiolar
peribronchiolitis
peribronchitis
pericallosal
pericardiac
pericardial
    p. adhesions
    p. calcification
    p. cavity
    p. cyst
    p. disease
    p. effusion
    p. fat pad
    p. hernia
    p. line
    p. sac
pericardiectomy
pericardiocentesis
pericarditis
    bacterial p.
    carcinomatous p.
    mediastinal p.
    suppurative p.
    tuberculous p.
    uremic p.
pericardium
pericholangitis
pericholecystic
perichondral
perichondrium
pericolonic
perigastric
perigraft
perihepatic
perihilar
perilunate
perilymphatic

perimesencephalic
perimeter
    p. ratio
perineal
perineosacral
perinephric
perineuronal
perinodal
perinuclear
periodontal
periodontitis
    p. complex
    p. simplex
periorbital
periosteal
    p. apposition
    p. chondroma
    p. cloaking
    p. desmoid
    p. elevation
    p. reaction
    p. resorption
    p. thickening
periosteum
periostitis
    florid reactive p.
    "lace-like" p.
    sesamoid p.
peripancreatic
peripelvic
peripheral
    p. angiography
    p. arteriography
    p. arteriosclerosis
    p. entrapment
    p. necrosis
    p. nervous system
    p. perfusion

peripheral *(continued)*
- p. vascular disease
- p. venography

periphery
perirectal
perirenal
- p. air study

perisellar
perisigmoidal
perisplenic
peristalsis
peristaltic
peritendinitis
- p. calcarea

peritoneal
peritoneography
peritoneum
- parietal p.
- visceral p.

peritonitis
peritonoscopy
peritonsillar
peritrochanteric
peritumoral
periureteric
periventricular
perivesical
Perlmann's tumor
permeability
- p. constant
- magnetic p.

permeative
permissible dose
pernicious
perodactyly
peromelia
peronarthrosis
peroneal

peroneotibial
perpendicular
persistent
- p. fetal circulation syndrome
- p. mode
- p. switch

pertechnetate
- sodium p.

pes
- p. abductus
- p. adductus
- p. anserinus
- p. cavus
- p. planus
- p. pronatus
- p. supinatus
- p. valgus
- p. varus

PET – positron emission tomography
petrobasilar
petroclinoid
petromastoid
petro-occipital
petropharyngeus
petrosal
petrosphenobasilar
petrospheno-occipital
petrosquamous
petrotympanic
petrous
- p. apex
- p. portion
- p. pyramid
- p. ridge
- p. temporal
- p. tip

PETT – positron emission transverse tomography
Peyer's patches
Pfaundler-Hurler gargoylism
PFC – persistent fetal circulation
Pfeiffer-Comberg method
Pfeiffer's acrocephalosyndactyly
PFFD syndrome – proximal femoral focal deficiency syndrome
Pfizer 200 FS scanner
Pfizer 0450 scanner
PGA – pyridoxilene glutamate
pH – hydrogen ion concentration
phagocyte
phagocytose
phagocytosis
phalangeal
    p. microgeodic syndrome
    p. tufts
phalanges (see phalanx)
phalangophalangeal
phalanx (phalanges)
    delta p.
    distal p.
    proximal p.
phantom
    p. chest
    p. image
    p. resolving power
    ultrasound p's
pharmacodynamics
pharmacologic
pharmacoradiology

pharyngeal tonsil
pharyngocele
pharyngoepiglottic
pharyngoesophageal
pharyngoesophagraphy
pharyngography
pharyngolaryngeal
pharyngomaxillary
pharynx
phase
    arterial p.
    capillary p.
    p. coherence
    p. distortion
    electrical p.
    exudative p.
    pneumonic p.
    reparative p.
    venous p.
phenidone
phenobarbital
phenobutiodyl
phenolphthalein
phenolsulfonphthalein
phenoltetrachlorophthalein
phenomenon
    flip-flop p.
    interference p.
    pulmonary vascular autoregulatory p.
    "vacuum p."
phenotype
    Turner's p.
phentetiothalein
phenylalanine
phenyldiphenyloxadiazole
phenylketonuria
phenyloxazolyl

pheochromocytoma
phlebitis
phlebogram
phlebography
phlebolith
phlegmon
phlegmonous
phocomelia
phonate
phonation
    expiratory p.
    inspiratory p.
    p. study
phosphatase
phosphate
    sodium p.
phosphene
phosphocreatine
phospholipid
phosphor
    fluorescent p.
    output p.
    scintillating p.
phosphorated
phosphorescence
phosphorescent
phosphorus ($^{31}_{15}$P, atomic number 15)
phosphorus 32 diisofluorophosphate
Phospho-soda
photocathode
photochemical
photoconductive
photodisintegration
photodisplay unit
photoelectric
    p. absorption

photoelectric *(continued)*
    p. circuit
    p. effect
    p. emission
    p. interaction
    p. timer
photoelectron
photoflow
photofluorographic
photofluorography
photographic
    p. effect
    p. radiometer
    p. subtraction
photomicrograph
photomultiplier tube
photon
    Compton's scattering p.
    degraded p.
    dual p.
    p. energy
    p. flux
    linear p.
    p. mottle
    p. theory of radiation
photoneutron
photonuclear
photorecording
photoroentgenography
photoscanner
photosensitivity
photosensitization
phototimer
phototiming
phototube output circuit
photovolt pH meter
PHP – pseudohypoparathyroidism

phrygian cap deformity (gallbladder)

phrenic
phrenicocolic
phrenicoesophageal
phrenicovertebral
phrenocostal
phrenopyloric
phrenovertebral
physical half-life
physicist
physics
physiological
physiology
physiotherapy
physis
phytate
pi
>p. lines
>p. mesons

pial
pia mater
Picker Synerview 600 scanner
picocurie
"picture frame" appearance
PID – pelvic inflammatory disease
PIE – pulmonary interstitial emphysema
Piedmont's fracture
piezoelectric
>p. crystals
>p. effect

pig (a lead container used to store radioisotopes and radioactive materials)
pigeon breast
pigeon breeder's lung
Pigg-O-Stat
>immobilization device

Pigg-O-Stat *(continued)*
>pneumonias

pigmentary
pigmented
pigtail catheter
pile
pillar
pillion
pilocytic
pin
>Smith-Petersen p.

pin-cushion distortion
pineal
pinealoblastoma
pinealoma
>ectopic p.

pinealopathy
pinhole collimator
piniform
"pink eye"
"pink puffer"
pinna
pion beam
PIP – proximal interphalangeal (joint)
PIPIDA – *p*-isopropylacetanilido-iminodiacetic acid
Pirie's
>method
>transoral projection

piriform
pisiform
p-isopropylacetanilido-iminodiacetic acid
pisotriquetral
PIT – plasma iron turnover
pitchblende
Pitressin

pitting
    "pepper-pot" p.
pituitary
    p. adenoma
    p. apoplexy
    p. fossa
    p. gland
pivot
    p. joints
    p. plane
pixel – picture element
PKU – phenylketonuria
placenta (placentas or placen-
    tae)
    p. previa
placental
placentography
plagiocephalic
plagiocephaly
plana (*see* planum)
planar imaging
Planck's
    constant
    quantum theory
plane
    Addison's p.
    auricular p.
    auriculoinfraorbital p.
    axial p.
    axiopetrosal p.
    coronal p.
    cross-sectional p.
    datum p.
    dextrosinistral p.
    p. encoding
    Frankfort p.
    frontal p.
    German horizontal p.

plane *(continued)*
    horizontal p.
    p. integral projection re-
        construction
    interparietal p.
    intertubercular p.
    median-raphe p.
    median sagittal p.
    midcoronal p.
    midfrontal p.
    midsagittal p.
    nasion-postcondylare p.
    occipital p.
    orbital p.
    parasagittal p.
    pivot p.
    popliteal p.
    Pöschl's p.
    sagittal p.
    semicircular p.
    semilongitudinal p.
    spinous p.
    sternal p.
    sternoxiphoid p.
    subcostal p.
    suprasternal p.
    temporal p.
    thoracic p.
    transpyloric p.
    transtubercular p.
    transverse p.
    umbilical p.
    vertical p.
    Virchow's p.
planigram
planigraphic
planigraphy
plantar

plantarflexion
plantodorsal
planum (plana)
    Calvé's vertebra p.
    p. sphenoidale
planus
plaque
plasma cell
    p. c. granuloma
    p. c. myeloma
plasmacytoma
plasma iron turnover
plasmapheresis
plasmatofibrous
plasmocytoma
plasmoid
plate
    atretic p.
    cribriform p.
    epiphyseal p.
    orbital p.
    perpendicular p.
    pterygoid p.
plateau
platelets
platelike
platinocyanide
platinum
platybasia
pleiotropism
pleiotropy
plenum
pleomorphic
pleonosteosis
    Leri's p.
plesiosectional tomography
plesiosette
plethora

plethysmography
    electrical impedance p.
pleura (pleurae)
    apical p.
    cervical p.
    costal p.
    diaphragmatic p.
    mediastinal p.
    parietal p.
    pericardiac p.
    pulmonary p.
    visceral p.
pleural
    p. cavity
    p. drainage tube
    p. effusion
    p. fluid
    p. meniscus
    p. plaque
    p. space
    p. thickening
pleurisy
pleuritic
pleurobronchitis
pleurocarditis
pleurocele
pleurocentrum
pleurocholecystitis
pleurocutaneous
pleurodynia
pleurography
pleurohepatitis
pleurolith
pleuropericardial
pleuroperitoneal
pleuropneumonia
pleuropulmonary
pleurovisceral

plexus (plexus or plexuses)
    Batson's p.
    brachial p.
    choroid p.
    lumbosacral p.
    venous p.
plica (plicae)
    p. colliculi
    p. sublingualis
plombage
plumbicon tube
Plummer's nail
pluridirectional tomography
Plurigraph
plutonium
PM – photomultiplier
pneumarthrogram
pneumarthrography
pneumatization
pneumatocele
pneumatogram
pneumatograph
pneumatosis
    p. cystoides coli
    p. intestinalis
    p. pulmonum
pneumencephalography
pneumoalveolography
pneumoangiogram
pneumoangiography
pneumoarthrogram
pneumoarthrography
pneumobacillus
    Friedländer's p.
pneumobilia
pneumocardiograph
pneumocardiography
pneumocephalus

pneumococcal
pneumococcus
pneumoconiosis
pneumocranium
pneumocystic
Pneumocystis
    P. carinii
pneumocystography
pneumocystotomography
pneumocyte
pneumoencephalogram
pneumoencephalography
pneumoencephalomyelogram
pneumoencephalomyelography
pneumofasciogram
pneumogastrography
pneumogastroscopy
pneumogram
pneumography
    cerebral p.
    pelvic p.
    retroperitoneal p.
pneumogynogram
pneumomediastinogram
pneumomediastinography
pneumomediastinum
pneumomyelography
pneumonectomy
pneumonia
    adenovirus p.
    aspiration p.
    asthmatic p.
    bacterial p.
    bronchial p.
    chickenpox p.
    Chlamydia p.
    cytomegaloviral p.
    desquamative p.

pneumonia *(continued)*
    diffuse p.
    eosinophilic p.
    Escherichia coli p.
    Friedländer's p.
    gram-positive p.
    granulomatous p.
    hair spray p.
    Hemophilus influenzae p.
    hospital acquired p.
    hydrocarbon p.
    influenza A viral p.
    interstitial p.
    Klebsiella p.
    lingular p.
    lipoid p.
    lobar p.
    Löffler's p.
    mineral oil p.
    mycoplasmal p.
    Mycoplasma pneumoniae p.
    neonatal p.
    opportunistic p.
    parainfluenza viral p.
    Pigg-O-Stat p's
    pneumococcal p.
    Pseudomonas aeruginosa p.
    radiation p.
    resolving p.
    respiratory syncytial viral p.
    ''round'' p.
    staphylococcal p.
    Staphylococcus aureus p.

pneumonia *(continued)*
    streptococcal p.
    Streptococcus pneumoniae p.
    Streptococcus pyogenes p.
    toxoplasmosis p.
    viral p.
pneumonic
pneumonitis
    aspiration p.
    chemical p.
    desquamative interstitial p.
    giant cell p.
    granulomatous p.
    lipoid p.
    lymphocytic interstitial p.
    ossifying p.
    Pneumocystis p.
    radiation p.
    uremic p.
pneumonograph
pneumonography
pneumopericardium
    ventilator-induced p.
pneumoperitoneography
pneumoperitoneum
    diagnostic p.
    spontaneous p.
    ventilator-induced p.
pneumopyelogram
pneumopyelography
pneumoradiography
    retroperitoneal p.

pneumoretroperitoneum
pneumoroentgenogram
pneumoroentgenography
pneumothorax
    diagnostic p.
    subpulmonary p.
    tension p.
    ventilator-induced p.
pneumotomography
pneumoventriculogram
pneumoventriculography
p-n junctions
pocket
    p. chamber
    p. dosimeter
poikiloderma
    p. congenitale
point
    auricular p.
    branching p.
    concentric p.
    mental p.
    saturation p.
    p. scanning
    p. spread function
poisoning
    radium p.
Poisson's
    distribution
    noise fluctuations
"poker" spine
polar
polarity
polarization
poliomyelitis
polonium
polyalveolar

polyarcuate
polyarthritic
polyarteritis
    p. nodosa
polyarthritis
polyarthropathy
polyarticular
polyaxial
polychondritis
polychromatic
polychromaticity
polycycloidal tomography
polycystic
polycystoma
polycythemia
    spurious p.
    p. vera
polydactyly
    postaxial p.
    preaxial p.
polydystrophic
polydystrophy
    pseudo-Hurler p.
polyenergetic
polyester
polyethylene
polyethyleneglycol
polygonal
polyhydramnios
polyhyperphalangism
polymer
    plastic p.
polymerization
polymyalgia
    p. rheumatica
polymyositis
polyostotic fibrous dysplasia

polyp
- adenomatous p.
- colonic p.
- dermoid p.
- duodenal p.
- epithelial p.
- fibroangiomatous p.
- fibrous p.
- gastric p.
- hyperplastic p.
- intussuscepting p.
- juvenile p.
- lymphoid p.
- nasal p.
- neoplastic p.
- sessile p.

polypeptide
polyperiostitis
- p. hyperesthetica

polyphase
polyphosphate
polyplastic
polypoid
polyposis
polypous
polyradiculitis
polyradiculoneuritis
polyradiculoneuropathy
polysplenia
polysyndactyly
polysynostosis
polysynovitis
polytendinitis
polytendinobursitis
polytenosynovitis
polytome
- Massiot's p.
- multidirectional p.

polytomogram
polytomography
- hypocycloidal p.

polyvinylchloride
polyvinylpyrrolidone
pons (pontes)
- p. cerebelli
- p. hepatis
- p.-oblongata

pontine
"popcorn" calcification
"popcorn-like" appearance
popliteal-pterygium syndrome
POPOP – 1,4-bis-a-(5-phenyl-
oxazolyl)-benzene
"porcelain" gallbladder
Porcher's method
pore
- Kohn's p.

porencephalic
porencephaly
pork insulin
porous
porphyria
porphyry
porta (portae)
- p. hepatis
- p. lienis
- p. omenti
- p. pulmonis

portacamera
portal
- p. canal
- p. hypertension
- p. vein
- p. venography

portion
- abdominal p.

portion *(continued)*
    cranial p.
    mastoid p.
    pelvic p.
    petrous p.
    pleural p.
    squamous p.
    vertebral p.
portocaval
    p. shunt
portography
portophlebography
portosplenography
portovenography
portwine marks
porus (pori)
    p. acusticus internus
    p. sudoriferus
Pöschl's plane
position
    Albers-Schönberg p.
    Albert's p.
    anatomic p.
    anterior p.
    anteroposterior (AP) p.
    axial p.
    axiolateral p.
    basilar p.
    Béclère's p.
    Benassi's p.
    Blackett-Healy p.
    Broden's p.
    brow-down p.
    brow-up p.
    butterfly p.
    Caldwell's p.
    Camp-Coventry p.
    Chassard-Lapiné p.

position *(continued)*
    Cleaves' p.
    Clements-Nakayama p.
    Coyle's trauma p.
    cross-table lateral p.
    decubitus p.
    dorsal p.
    dorsoplantar p.
    dorsosacral p.
    erect p.
    eversion p.
    extension p.
    Feist-Mankin p.
    Fick's p.
    Fleischner's p.
    flexion p.
    Fowler's p.
    Friedman's p.
    frog-leg p.
    fronto-occipital p.
    Fuchs' p.
    Gaynor-Hart p.
    Grashey's p.
    genucubital p.
    genufacial p.
    genupectoral p.
    Haas' p.
    half-axial p.
    hanging-head p.
    Hickey's p.
    hinge p.
    horizontal p.
    hyperextension p.
    inferosuperior p.
    inlet p.
    inversion p.
    Isherwood's p.
    Johnson's p.

position *(continued)*
    knee-chest p.
    Kurzbauer's p.
    Laquerrière-Pierquin p.
    Larkin's p.
    lateral p.
    lateral autotomogram p.
    lateromedial p.
    Lawrence's p.
    Law's p.
    left anterior oblique
        (LAO) p.
    left posterior oblique
        (LPO) p.
    Leonard-George p.
    Lewis' p.
    Lilienfeld's p.
    Lindblom's p.
    lithotomy p.
    lordotic p.
    Lorenz's p.
    Löw-Beer p.
    Mayer's p.
    medial oblique p.
    Meese's p.
    mento-occipital p.
    Miller's p.
    Noble's p.
    Nölke's p.
    "nose-chin" p.
    "nose-forehead" p.
    oblique p.
    oblique axial p.
    occipitofrontal p.
    occipitomental p.
    occipitovertical p.
    Pawlow's p.
    Pearson's p.

position *(continued)*
    posterior p.
    posteroanterior (PA) p.
    postvoid p.
    profile p.
    prone p.
    reclining p.
    recumbent p.
    retrosternal p.
    right anterior oblique
        (RAO) p.
    right posterior oblique
        (RPO) p.
    Schüller's p.
    semiaxial transoral p.
    semierect p.
    semiprone p.
    semirecumbent p.
    semisupine p.
    Settegast's p.
    Sims' p.
    Staunig's p.
    Stecher's p.
    Stenver's p.
    submentovertical p.
    superoinferior p.
    supine p.
    supraorbital p.
    swimmer's p.
    Tarrant's p.
    Taylor's p.
    Titterington's p.
    Towne's p.
    transabdominal p.
    transaxillary p.
    transorbital p.
    transthoracic p.
    Trendelenburg's p.

position *(continued)*
- "tripod" p.
- Twining's p.
- ulnar flexion p.
- upright p.
- upside-down p.
- ventral p.
- vertical p.
- verticomental p.
- verticosubmental p.
- Waters' p.
- Wigby-Taylor p.
- Zanelli's p.

positive
- p. charge
- p. direction
- p. electron
- p. end-expiratory pressure
- p. ion
- p. mask
- p. terminal

positrocephalogram

positron
- p.-coincidence
- p. decay
- p. emission tomography
- p. emission transverse tomography
- p. scintillation camera

positronium

postaxial

postcalcarine

postcaval

postcholecystectomy syndrome

post cibum

postcondylare

postcricoid

posterior
- p. arch
- p. fossa
- p. junction line
- p. view

posteroanterior

posterolateral

posteromedial

postevacuation

postfibrinous

postgastrectomy

postictal

posticus

postirradiation

postischemia

postmenopausal

postmyocardial

postnephrectomy

postoperative

postpericardiotomy
- p. syndrome

postpneumonectomy

postpubertal

postradiation

post release radiography

post-traumatic

postural

postvagotomy

postvoid radiography

potassium
- p. atom
- p. bromide
- p. iodide
- p. perchlorate

potential
- accelerating p.
- chemical p.
- p. difference

potential *(continued)*
    electrical p.
    p. energy
    flow p.
    p. gradient
    gravitational p.
    ionization p.
    mechanical p.
    negative p.
Potter-Bucky
    diaphragm
    grid
Potter's thumb
Pott's
    aneurysm
    fracture
pouch
    Douglas' p.
    Hartmann's p.
    Kock's p.
    Morrison's p.
power
    p. consumed formula
    electrical p.
    p. factor
    p. formula
    p. loss
    phantom resolving p.
    p. rule
    p. supply
PPD – phenyldiphenyloxadi-
    azole
PPHP – pseudopseudohypopar-
    athyroidism
PPO – 2,5-diphenyloxazole
PPS – posterior pararenal space
PR – projection reconstruction
Praestholm

praseodymium
preamplifier
preaxial
precession (gyro)
precocious
precocity
    sexual p.
predetector
prediastolic
prednisone
pre-epiglottic
pregnancy
    ectopic p.
    extrauterine p.
    intrauterine p.,
prelaryngeal
premalignant
premature
prematurity
premaxillary
prenatal
preneoplastic
prepubertal
prepyloric
presacral
presbyesophagus
presenile
presystolic
preternatural
pretibial
pretracheal
prevascular
primary
    p. beam
    p. radiation
    p. x-ray circuit
primigravida
primipara

primordial
princeps
    p. pollicis
principle
    air-gap p.
    Dodge's p.
    Fick's p.
    Grossman's p.
    Pauli's exclusion p.
    planigraphic p.
Prinzmetal's angina
Priodax
Pro-Banthine
probe
    fiberoptic p.
    p. matching
    nuclear p.
    p. renography
    scintillation p.
process (processes)
    acromion p.
    alveolar p.
    articular p.
    articulated p.
    basilar p's
    bremsstrahlung p.
    clinoid p.
    condyloid p.
    coracoid p.
    coronoid p.
    costal p.
    ensiform p.
    epitransverse p.
    frontal p.
    glenoid p.
    inflammatory p.
    lacrimal p.
    mastoid p.

process (processes) *(continued)*
    neutron absorption p.
    odontoid p.
    olecranon p.
    palatine p.
    paracondyloid p.
    pterygoid p.
    spinous p.
    styloid p.
    superior articulating p.
    supracondyloid p.
    transverse p.
    uncinate p.
    vermiform p.
    xiphoid p.
    zygomatic p.
processor
proctitis
profile ray view
progeria
Progestasert intrauterine device
prognathism
prognosis
progressive
    p. epiphyseal development
    p. portal fibrosis
projection
    abduction p.
    acanthiomental p.
    acanthioparietal p.
    adduction p.
    angled anteroposterior p.
    anterior p.
    anteroposterior p.
    apical lordotic p.
    axial p.

projection *(continued)*
- axillary p.
- axiolateral p.
- ball-catcher's p.
- basic p.
- basilar p.
- basovertical p.
- Berteil's p.
- biplane p.
- Blineau's p.
- blowout view p.
- Caldwell's p.
- caudal p.
- cephalad angled p.
- cephalic p.
- cephalic angula-
  tion p.
- Chassard-Lapiné p.
- Chaussé's p.
- chewing p.
- "Cleopatra" p.
- cone-down p.
- craniocaudad p.
- cross-sectional trans-
  verse p.
- decubitus p.
- distal p.
- dorsoplantar p.
- erect anteroposterior p.
- erect fluoro spot p.
- extraoral p.
- flexion, extension p.
- p. formula
- frontal p.
- geometrical p.
- half-axial p.
- inferior p.
- inferior-superior p.

projection *(continued)*
- inferosuperior p.
- intraoral p.
- L-5, S-1 p.
- lateral p.
- lateromedial p.
- Lauenstein and
  Hickey p.
- Loepp's p.
- lordotic p.
- lumbosacral p.
- medial p.
- medial oblique axial p.
- mediolateral p.
- navicular p.
- nuchofrontal p.
- oblique p.
- occipital p.
- odontoid p.
- open mouth p.
- orbitoparietal p.
- palmar p.
- parietal p.
- parietoacanthial p.
- parieto-orbital p.
- parietotemporal p.
- perineosacral p.
- pillar p.
- Pirie's transoral p.
- plantodorsal p.
- posteroanterior p.
- posterolateral p.
- posteromedial p.
- profile p.
- proximal p.
- p. reconstruction imag-
  ing
- recumbent p.

projection *(continued)*
    Runström's p.
    scaphoid p.
    semiaxial p.
    semierect p.
    skyline p.
    stereo right lateral p.
    stereoscopic p.
    submentovertex p.
    submentovertical p.
    "sunrise" p.
    superimposition p.
    superior p.
    superoinferior p.
    supine p.
    supraorbital p.
    swimmer's lateral p.
    tangential p.
    Templeton and Zim carpal tunnel p.
    transcranial p.
    transfacial p.
    translateral p.
    transoral p.
    transorbital p.
    transtabular p.
    transthoracic p.
    tunnel p.
    vertex p.
    verticosubmental p.
    Vogt's bone free p.
    volar p.
    Waters' p.
    weight-bearing p.
project reconstruction imaging
prolapse
    holosystolic p.
    mitral valve p.

prolapse *(continued)*
    systolic p.
proliferation
proliferative
prolongation
promethium
prominence
promontory
PROMs – programmable read-only memories
pronate
pronated
pronation
pronator
prone
Pronestyl
propagation
propantheline bromide
properitoneal
prophylactic
prophylaxis
proportional
    p. counter
    directly p.
    inversely p.
    p. region
proportionality
proprioception
proprioceptive
proprioceptor
proptosis
propyliodone
prosencephalon
prostaglandin E
prostate
prostatectomy
prostatic
prostatography

prosthesis (prostheses)
    Swanson's p.
prosthetic
Prostigmin
protactinium
protein
    p. binding
    p.-bound iodine
    p.-losing enteropathy
proteinosis
proteolytic
Proteus
    P. inconstans
    P. mirabilis
    P. morgani
    P. vulgaris
protocols
proton
    p. relaxation time
    p. spin-lattice relaxation
      time
    p. tunneling
    water p.
protoplasmic
protraction
protrusio
    p. acetabuli
protrusion
protuberance
    mental p.
    occipital p.
proximal
    p. femoral focal defi-
      ciency syndrome
    p. phalanx
    p. tibial
prune belly syndrome
"pruned hilum"

"pruned-tree"
    "p.-t." appearance
    "p.-t." arteriography
PS – pulmonic stenosis
psammoma
psammomatous
psammosarcoma
pseudarthrosis
pseudoachondroplasia
pseudoachondroplastic
    p. dysplasia
pseudoaneurysm
pseudoarthrosis
pseudobrachydactyly
pseudobronchiectasis
pseudobulbar
pseudocamptodactyly
pseudocapsule
pseudocleft hand
pseudocoarctation
pseudocyesis
pseudocyst
pseudocystic
pseudodiverticula
pseudoepiphysis
pseudofracture
pseudogout
pseudo-Hurler polydystrophy
pseudohydrocephalus
pseudohyperparathy-
    roidism
pseudohypoparathyroidism
pseudoleprechaunism
pseudolymphoma
pseudomembranous
Pseudomonas aeruginosa
pseudomyxoma
    p. peritonei

pseudo-obstruction
pseudopneumonia
pseudopodal
pseudopolyp
pseudopolypoid
pseudopseudohypoparathy-
    roidism
pseudosarcoma
pseudosarcomatous
pseudoscopic
pseudospicule
pseudospondylolisthesis
    p. of Junghans
pseudothalidomide
pseudothrombosis
pseudotruncus
    p. arteriosus
pseudotumor
pseudovalve
pseudovolvulus
pseudoxanthoma
    p. elasticum
PSF – point-spread function
PSIS – posterior superior iliac
    spine
psoas
    p. abscess
    p. line
    p. muscle
    p. shadow
psoriasis
psoriatic
PSP – phenolsulfonphthalein
^{31}P spectra
psychiatry
psychogenic
    p. constipation
    p. megacolon

psychogenic *(continued)*
    p. rheumatism
psychology
psychomotor
psychosocial
4p syndrome (Wolf-Hirschhorn
    syndrome)
5p syndrome (cri du chat syn-
    drome)
PT – pluridirectional tomogra-
    phy
PTA – percutaneous translu-
    minal angioplasty
PTAB – pterygoalar bar
PTC – percutaneous transhe-
    patic cholangiography
PTCA – percutaneous translu-
    minal coronary angio-
    plasty
pterygium
pterygoalar
pterygoid
    p. apophysis
    p. canal
    p. fossa
    p. hamulus
    p. plate
    p. process
pterygopalatine
pterygospinous
PTH – parathyroid hormone
ptosis
PTSB – pterygospinous bar
PTT – parenchymal transit
    time
p-type semiconductors
puberty
    precocious p.

pubic
- p. arch
- p. rami
- "p." sign

pubis (pubes)
pubococcygeal
Puck cutfilm changer
pudendal
"puddled"
"puddling"
puerile
puerperal
pulmonary
- p. airway
- p. amyloidosis
- p. angiography
- p. aplasia
- p. arteriography
- p. arteriovenous malformation
- p. arteritis
- p. artery
- p. aspergillosis
- p. aspiration
- p. atresia
- p. barotrauma
- p. blood volume
- p. capillary wedge pressure
- p. collapse
- p. contusion
- p. cyst
- p. edema
- p. embolism
- p. embolus
- p. emphysema
- p. extravascular lung water

pulmonary *(continued)*
- p. fibrosis
- p. flow
- p. gangrene
- p. granuloma
- p. hamartoma
- p. hematoma
- p. hemorrhage
- p. hemosiderosis
- p. hyperaeration
- p. hypertension
- p. hypoplasia
- p. infarction
- p. infiltrate
- p. insufficiency
- p. interstitial emphysema
- p. laceration
- p. lymph node
- p. nodule
- p. oat cell carcinoma
- p. oligemia
- p. ossification
- p. osteoarthropathy
- p. osteopathia
- p. parenchymal trauma
- p. pedicle
- p. perforation
- p. plethora
- p. ridge
- p. sequestration
- p. sling
- p. stenosis
- p. support
- p. trunk
- p. tuberculosis
- p. valve

pulmonary *(continued)*
    p. venolumbar syndrome
    p. venous hypertension
    p. ventilation
pulmonic
    p. regurgitation
    p. stenosis
pulsating
pulsation
pulse
    p.-height spectrum
    p. length (width)
    selective radiofrequency p.
pulsed
    p. NMR
    p. radiofrequency field
    p. response resonance
"pulseless disease"
pulvinar
    p. thalami
"punched out" appearance
punctate
punctum (puncta)
    p. lacrimale
puncture
    arterial p.
    cervical p.
    cisternal p.
    lumbar p.
    percutaneous transhepatic p.
PUO – pyrexia of unknown origin
purgative
purine nucleoside phosphorylase deficiency

purpura
    Henoch-Schönlein p.
purulent
pus (pura)
    burrowing p.
    sanious p.
putamen
putrefaction
putrescent
PVP – polyvinylpyrrolidone
PXE – pseudoxanthoma elasticum
pyelectasis
pyelitis
pyelocaliectasis
pyelofluoroscopy
pyelogram (*see* pyelography)
pyelography
    antegrade p.
    ascending p.
    drip-infusion p.
    hydrated p.
    intravenous p.
    percutaneous antegrade p.
    retrograde p.
    washout p.
pyelonephritic
pyelonephritis
    atrophic p.
    emphysematous p.
    focal p.
    suppurative p.
    xanthogranulomatous p.
pyeloscopy
pyelosinus
pyeloureterectasis

PYG – pyridoxylideneglutamate
pyknodysostosis
pyloric
    p. antrum
    p. atresia
    p. canal
    p. lymph node
    p. orifice
    p. portion
    p. sphincter
    p. stenosis
    p. ulcer
    p. valve
    p. vestibule
pylorospasm
pylorus
pyogenic

pyometrium
pyopneumothorax
PYP – ^{99m}Tc stannous pyro-
    phosphate
pyramid
    renal p.
pyramidal
pyrexia
pyridoxilene glutamate
pyridoxylideneglutamate
pyrogen
pyrogenic
pyrophosphate
    p. dihydrate
pyrosis
pyruvate
    p. kinase deficiency

q

QA – quality assurance
QC – quality control
18q chromosomal abnormality
QCT – quantitative computed
    tomography
Q electron
QF – quality factor
Q factor
QPC – quadrigeminal plate cis-
    tern
QRS cycle
QRS signal
QRS synchro method
Q shell
13Q syndrome
quadrant

quadrate
quadrature detection scheme
quadratus
    q. lumborum
quadrigeminal
    q. plate cistern
    q. lamina
quadrupole coil
qualimeter
quality
    q. factor
    radiographic q.
    therapy q.
quanta (*see* quantum)
. quantification
    shunt q.

quantitation
quantitative
    q. analysis
    q. bone mineral analy-
        sis
    q. brain imaging
    q. cardiology
    q. CT densitometry
    q. regional lung func-
        tion study
    q. tracer study
quantity
    radiographic q.

quantum (quanta)
    q. energy
    q. mechanics
    q. mottle
    q. noise
    q. number
    q. theory
quaternary
quenching
Quervain's fracture
Quesada's method
quickening

R

R –
    resistance
    resistor
    roentgen
RA – right atrium
Ra – radium
rabbit
racemose
rachitic
rad – radiation absorbed dose
radial
    r. aplasia
    r. deviation
    r. hemimelia
    r. hypoplasia
    r. nerve
    r. ray deficiency
radialis indicis volaris

radiant energy
radiation
    r. absorbed dose
    alpha r.
    annihilation r.
    background r.
    beta r.
    "braking" r.
    bremsstrahlung r.
    r. burn
    characteristic r.
    r. colitis
    corpuscular r.
    cosmic r.
    r. counter
    cyclotron r.
    r. dermatitis
    r. detector

radiation *(continued)*
>   direct r.
>   dose equivalent r.
>   electromagnetic r.
>   r. energy
>   r. enteropathy
>   r. equivalent man
>   r. exposure
>   gamma r.
>   r. gastritis
>   r. hepatitis
>   infrared r.
>   r. injury
>   r. intensity
>   interstitial r.
>   ionization r.
>   r. leakage
>   man-made environmental r.
>   Maxwell's theory of r.
>   r. monitor
>   monochromatic r.
>   monoenergetic r.
>   natural r.
>   r. necrosis
>   nuclear r.
>   occupational r.
>   optic r.
>   r. osteitis
>   photon theory of r.
>   r. physics
>   r. pneumonia
>   r. pneumonitis
>   primary r.
>   r. protection
>   recoil r.
>   remnant r.
>   scattered r.

radiation *(continued)*
>   r. sickness
>   specific r.
>   spontaneous r.
>   r. syndrome
>   terrestrial r.
>   r. therapy
>   thermal r.
>   r. warning symbol
>   white r.
>   r. window

radiation production
>   Cerenkov's r. p.

radicular

radiculopathy

radioactive
>   r. decay
>   r. disintegration
>   r. effluents
>   r. element
>   r. equilibrium
>   r. fallout
>   r. gallium
>   r. gases
>   r. half-life
>   r. isotope
>   r. nuclide
>   r. series
>   r. source
>   r. thorium

radioactivity

radioactor

radioanaphylaxis

radioassay

radioautograph

radioautography

radiobe

radiobioassay

radiobiological
radiobiologist
radiobiology
radiocalcium
radiocarbon
radiocarcinogenesis
radiocardiogram
radiocardiography
radiocarpal
radiocesium
radiochemical
radiochemistry
radiochemotherapy
radiochemy
radiocholecystography
radiocholesterol
radiochroism
radiochromatography
radiocinematograph
radiocolloid
radiocurable
radiocystitis
radiode
radiodensity
radiodermatitis
radiodermatoglyphics
radiodermatography
radiodiagnosis
radiodiagnostics
radiodiaphane
radiodigital
radiodontia
radioelectrocardiogram
radioelectrocardiograph
radioelectrocardiography
radioelement
radioencephalogram
radioencephalography

radiofluorine
radiofrequency
    r. amplifier
    r. coil
    r. magnetic field
    r. pulse
    r. stimulation
radiogallium
radiogenic
radiogold
radiogram (*see* radiography)
radiograph
radiographer
radiographic
    r. base line
    r. contrast
    r. density
    r. distortion
    r. effect
    r. grid
    r. image
    r. latitude
    r. magnification
    r. mottle
    r. penetration
    r. quality
    r. quantity
    r. resolution
    r. sensitometry
radiography
    air contrast r.
    biomedical r.
    body section r.
    bone age r.
    "chalky" r.
    diagrammatic r.
    electron r.
    r. filter

radiography *(continued)*
    gamma r.
    industrial r.
    kinescope r.
    magnification r.
    miniature r.
    multiple r.
    pan-oral r.
    panoramic r.
    post release r.
    postvoid r.
    scanned projection r.
    scout r.
    spill r.
    "split film" r.
    stereoscopic r.
radiohepatographic
radiohumeral
radioimmunity
radioimmunoassay
radioimmunodiffusion
radioimmunoelectrophoresis
radioimmunoprecipitation
radioinduction
radioiodine
radioiodinated orthoiodohippu-
    rate
radioiron
    r. half-life
    r. incorporation rate
radioisotope scanner
radioisotopic
radiokymography
radiolabelled
radiolead
radiolesion
radiologic
    r. capsule

radiological
Radiological Society of North
    America
radiologist
radiology
radiolucency
radiolucent
radiolysis
radiometacarpal
radiometallography
radiometer
    pastille r.
    photographic r.
radiometric
radiomicrometer
radiomimetic
radiomuscular
radion
radionecrosis
radionitrogen
radionuclide
    r. angiocardiography
    r. angiography
    r. cholescintigraphy
    r. cisternography
    r. cystography
    r. emission tomography
    r. gastroesophagography
    r. imaging
    r. kinetics
    r. purity
    r. scanning
    r. venography
    r. ventriculography
    r. voiding cystoure-
    thrography
radiopacity
radiopaque

radioparency
radioparent
radiopathology
radiopelvimetry
radiopharmaceutical
radiophobia
radiophosphorus
radiophotography
radiophylaxis
radiophysics
radioplastic
radiopotassium
radiopotentiation
radiopulmonography
radioreaction
radioreceptor
radioresistant
radioresponsive
radiosclerosis
radioscope
radioscopy
radiosensitive
radiosensitivity
radiosodium
radiospirometry
radiostereoscopy
radiostrontium
radiosulfur
radiotechnetium
     r. polyphosphate
radiotelemetry
radiotellurium
radiotherapeutics
radiotherapy
    computerized r.
    interstitial r.
    intracavitary r.
radiothorium

radiotoxemia
radiotracer
radiotransparency
radiotransparent
radioulnar
    r. synostosis
radium
radius
    Bohr's r.
    grid r.
radon
"railroad track" appearance
rale
ramus (rami)
    inferior r.
    ipsilateral r.
    mandibular r.
    pubic r.
    superior r.
range
RAO - right anterior oblique
raphe
rapid drip study
Rapido
Rapido-mat
rarefaction
Rasmussen's aneurysm
raster
ratemeter
Rathke's pouch tumor
ratio
    branching r.
    grid r.
    gyromagnetic r.
    magnetogyric r.
    perimeter r.
    rectosigmoid r.
    signal-to-noise r.

ratio *(continued)*
  target-to-nontarget r.
  r. transformer
"rat tail" deformity
ray
  alpha r.
  beta r.
  cathode r.
  central r.
  cosmic r.
  delta r.
  fluorescent r.
  gamma r.
  grenz r.
  infrared r.
  parallel r.
  roentgen r.
  secondary r.
  vertical r.
Raybar 75
Rayopak
Rayvist
RBC – red blood cell
RBE – relative biologic effectiveness
RBL –
  radiographic base line
  Reid's base line
18r chromosomal abnormality
rd. – rutherford
reactance
reaction
  biomolecular r.
  endoergic r.
  nuclear r.
  periosteal r.
  thermonuclear r.

reactive
reactor
real-time
  r.-t. scanning
  r.-t. ultrasonography
  r.-t. ultrasound
recanalization
receptor
recess
  azygoesophageal r.
  epitympanic r.
reciprocating grid
reciprocity
recirculation system
reclining
recoil
  r. electron
  r. radiation
recombination
reconstruction
  Fourier transformation r.
  plane integral projection r.
  single slice line integral projection r.
  single slice projection r.
  "target" r.
  two-dimensional line integral projection r.
  two-dimensional projection r.
  "zoom" r.
reconstructive imaging
reconstructor
  dynamic planar r.
  dynamic spatial r.
recovery
  inversion r.

recovery *(continued)*
    inversion r. sequence
    saturation r.
    silver r.
    r. time
rectification
    full-wave r.
    self-r.
    solid-state r.
rectified current
rectifier
    full-wave r.
    self-r.
    silicon r.
    solid-state diode r.
    valve tube r.
rectifying
    r. circuit
    r. system
    r. tube
rectilinear scanner
rectosigmoid
rectum
recumbency
recumbent
reducing agent
redundancy
redundant
reduplication
reflex sympathetic dystrophy
   syndrome
reflux
    duodenogastric
      bile r.
    esophageal r.
    gastroesophageal r.
    hepatojugular r.
    intrarenal r.

reflux *(continued)*
    jugular r.
    r. nephropathy
    ureteric r.
    ureterovesical r.
    vaginal r.
    vesicoureteral r.
refractory
region
    hypochondriac r.
    iliac r.
    inguinal r.
    lumbar r.
    proportional r.
    saturation r.
regional
    r. enteritis
    r. extravascular lung
      water
    r. lung function test
    r. ventilation/perfusion
      study
regression
regurgitant
regurgitation
    aortic r.
    mitral r.
    pulmonic r.
    tricuspid r.
    valvular r.
    vesicoureteral r.
Reid's base line
reimplantation
reintussusception
Reiter's arthritis
rejection
relationship
    Karplus r.

210 RELATIVE BIOLOGIC EFFECTIVENESS – REPULSION

relative biologic effectiveness
"relative mutation risk"
relativistic
  r. mass
  r. mechanics
relaxation
  r. rates
  r. times
REM – roentgen equivalent
  man
remnant radiation
REMP – roentgen equivalent
  man period
renal
  r. angiography
  r. aortography
  r. arteriography
  r. calculus
  r. carbuncle
  r. cell carcinoma
  r. cholesteatoma
  r. cortex
  r. cyst
  r. duplication
  r. dysplasia
  r. echogram
  r. failure
  r. fossa
  r. function
  "r. halo" sign
  r. hematuria
  r. image
  r. infarction
  r. ischemia
  r. localization
  r. medullary contamina-
    tion

renal *(continued)*
  r. obstruction
  r. osteodystrophy
  r. outline
  r. pelvis
  r. plasma flow
  r. pyramid
  r. radionuclide stu-
    dies
  r. scan
  r. scanning
  r. scintigraphy
  r. transit time
  r. transplant
  r. transplantation
  r. tubular acidosis
  r. venography
reniform
renipelvic
reniportal
renocystogram
Renografin
renogram
renography
Reno-M-30
Reno-M-60
Reno-M-Dip
renovascular
Renovist
Renovue
REP – roentgen equivalent
  physical
reparative
replenisher
replenishment system
reproductive
repulsion
    electrostatic r.

RES – reticuloendothelial sys-
    tem
resection
resin
resistance
resistive
resistivity
resistor
    non-ohmic r.
    ohmic r.
    variable r.
resolution
    axial r.
    contrast r.
    density r.
    energy r.
    hole-pair limiting r.
    image r.
    linear r.
    plane-pair r.
    radiographic r.
    spatial r.
    spatiotemporal r.
    r. target
    temporal r.
    ultrasound r.
resolving power
resonance
    r. capture
    r. condition
    electron paramagnetic r.
    electron spin r.
    field focusing nuclear
      magnetic r.
    r. generator
    magnetic r.
    pulsed response r.
    topical magnetic r.

resonant frequency
resorption
    r. pits
respiration
    pendulum r.
"respirator lung"
respiratory
    r. distress syndrome
      (adult) (ARDS)
    r. excursion
    r. failure
    r. support
    r. syncytial virus
    r. system
    r. tract
restrictive
resuscitation
retained gastric antrum syn-
    drome
retardation
retention
retentivity
reticular
reticulation
reticulocyte count
reticulocytes
reticuloendothelial
    r. cell
    r. imaging
    r. system
reticuloendothelioses
reticulohistiocytoma
reticulohistiocytosis
    multicentric r.
reticulosarcoma
reticulosis
"reticulum cell" sarcoma
retina

retinoblastoma
retractile
retroauricular
retrobulbar
retrocaval
retrocecal
retrococcygeal
    r. air study
Retro-Conray
retrocrural
retroesophageal
retrograde
    r. aortography
    r. cardioangiography
    r. cholangiography
    r. cystography
    r. cystourethrography
    r. pyelography
    r. urethrography
    r. urography
retroiliac
retrolental
retrolisthesis
retromammary
retroperitoneal
    r. abscess
    r. air study
    r. echogram
    r. fibrosis
    r. gas
    r. lymph node
    r. lymphoma
    r. neoplasm
    r. perforation
    r. pneumography
    r. pneumoradiography
    r. space
retroperitoneum

retropharyngeal
retrorectal
retrosternal
retrothymic
retrotracheal
retrouterine
retroverted
revascularization
"reverse three" sign
reversible
RF – radiofrequency
RFC – radio frequency
    coil
RGAS – retained gastric
    antrum syndrome
rhabdoid
rhabdomyoma
rhabdomyosarcoma
rhenium
rheostat
Rhese's method
rheumatic
    r. fever
rheumatism
    palindromic r.
    psychogenic r.
rheumatoid
    r. arthritis
    r. factor
rhinal
rhinorrhea
rhinoscleroma
rhinovirus
rhizomelia
rhizomelic chondrodysplasia
    punctata
rhodium
rhombic grid

rhomboid
    Michaelis' r.
rhonchus (rhonchi)
rhythmic segmentation
RIA – radioimmunoassay
riboflavin
ribonucleic acid
ribose
ribosome
ribosyl
ribothymidine
ribulose
rickets
ridge
    alveolar r.
    epicondylic r.
    gastrocnemial r.
    interarticular r.
    interosseous r.
    intertrochanteric r.
    mesonephric r.
    petrous r.
    pulmonary r.
    sphenoid r.
    supracondylar r.
    tentorial r.
Riedel's lobe
right middle lobe syndrome
rima (rimae)
    r. glottidis
    r. vestibuli
rim fracture
"rim sign"
ring
    r. B chromosome
    "r. of bone" concept
    Cannon's r.
    commutator r.

ring *(continued)*
    cricoid r.
    "r.-like" indentation
    "r.-like" lesion
    "r." shadow
    r. sign
    slip r's
    tendinous r.
    vascular r.
Ring-McLean catheter
ripple
    electrical r.
    r. voltage
Rivinus' duct
RL – right lateral
RLL – right lower lobe
RLQ – right lower quadrant
R-meter
RML – right middle lobe
rmm – relative molecular mass
RMS – root mean square
RN – radionuclide
Rn – radon
RNA – ribonucleic acid
RNV – radionuclide venog-
    raphy
Robin's
    anomalad
    sequence
ROC – receiver-operating char-
    acteristic
roentgen
    r. equivalent man
    r. equivalent man pe-
        riod
    r. equivalent physical
    r. kymography
    r. ray

roentgenogram
roentgenography
roentgenologic
roentgenologist
roentgenology
ROI – region of interest
Rokitansky's diverticulum
Rolando's fracture
root
        aortic r.
        r. mean square (voltage)
        r. sleeve fibrosis
rose
        r. bengal
"rosebud" hand
rostrum (rostrums or rostra)
        r. of corpus callosum
        sphenoidal r.
rotary
rotate-rotate scanning
rotate-stationary scanning
rotating
        r. anode target
        r. anode tube
        r. frame imaging
rotation
        organoaxial r.
        scaphoid r.
rotational
rotator cuff tear
rotavirus
Rotex needle
rotography
rotor
roto-tomography
Rotter's node
"round" pneumonia
RP – retrograde pyelogram

RPF – renal plasma flow
RPM – rapid processing mode
    (par speed screens)
rpm – revolutions per minute
RPO – right posterior oblique
RSNA – Radiological Society
    of North America
RSV – respiratory syncytial vi-
    rus
rT3 – L-3, 3', 5',-triiodo-
    thyronine (reverse T3)
RT (N) –
    certified radiologic tech-
        nologist—
    nuclear medicine
RT (R) –
    certified radiologic tech-
        nologist—
    diagnostic medicine
RT (T) – certified radiol-
    ogic technologist—
    oncology
rubella
        r. osteitis
rubidium
rubor
rubroreticular
rudimentary
"ruffled border" bone forma-
    tion
ruga (rugae)
rugal
        r. fold
        r. pattern
"rugger jersey" appearance
RUL –
    right upper lobe
    right upper lung

rule
    octet r.
    Simpson's r.
Runström's
    projection
    view
rupture
    aortic r.
    bronchial r.
    esophageal r.
    splenic r.

rupture *(continued)*
    tracheobronchial r.
RUQ – right upper quadrant
ruthenium
rutherford
RV – right ventricle
RVG – radionuclide ventriculo-
    gram
RVOT – right ventricular out-
    flow tract

S

S – secondary winding
s – screen containing cassette
SA – specific activity
saber-sheath trachea
"saber shin" appearance
sac
    abdominal s.
    alveolar s.
    amniotic s.
    aortic s.
    chorionic s.
    conjunctival s.
    dental s.
    dural s.
    embryonic s.
    endolymphatic s.
    epiploic s.
    gestation s.
    hernial s.
    jugular lymph s.

sac *(continued)*
    lacrimal s.
    lymph s.
    omental s.
    pericardial s.
    peritoneal s.
    pleural s.
    splenic s.
    thecal s.
sacciform
saccular
sacculated
sacculation
saccule
sacral
    s. agenesis
    s. canal
    s. cornu
    s. curve
    s. hiatus

sacral *(continued)*
    s. lymph node
    s. meningocele
    s. promontory
    s. spine
    s. vertebra
sacralization
sacroanterior
sacrococcygeal
sacrocoxitis
sacroiliac
sacroiliitis
sacrolisthesis
sacrolumbar
sacroperineal
sacroposterior
sacropromontory
sacrosciatic
sacrospinal
sacrotransverse
sacrouterine
sacrovertebral
sacrum
Saethre-Chotzen acrocephalo-
    syndactyly
sagittal
sagittalis
sago
sail shadow
salicylates
saline solution
salivary
Salmonella
    S. typhi
salpingitis
    s. isthmica nodosa
salpingocele
salpingography

salpingolithiasis
salpingo-oophorectomy
salpingo-oophorocele
salpingoperitonitis
salpingopharyngeal
salpingostaphyline
salpinx (salpinges)
Salpix
Salter-Harris classification
Salyrgan
samarium
Sanchez-Perez cassette charger
"sandwich"
    "s." appearance
    "s." sign
    "s." vertebrae
"sandwichlike"
sanious
Sansregret's method
saphenous
sarcoidosis
sarcoma
    ameloblastic s.
    s. botryoides
    Ewing's s.
    Kaposi's s.
    neurogenic s.
    osteogenic s.
    parosteal s.
    "reticulum cell" s.
    synovial s.
    Walker's s.
sarcomatous
saturable reactor
saturation
    s. analysis
    s. current
    s. plateau

saturation *(continued)*
    s. point
    s. recovery
    s. region
    tube s.
    s. voltage
Satvioni's cryptoscope
"sawtooth" configuration
SBFT – small bowel follow-
    through
SBS – small bowel series
scale
    Hounsfield s.
scaler
scalloped
scalloping
scan
    adrenal s.
    blood pool s.
    bone s.
    brain s.
    capillary blockade per-
      fusion s.
    CT s.
    dynamic CT s.
    fluorescent s.
    hepatobiliary s.
    isotope bone s.
    liver/spleen s.
    multiple gated blood
      pool s.
    multislice full line s.
    nongated CT s.
    perfusion lung s.
    renal s.
    salivary gland s.
    selective excitation
      line s.

scan *(continued)*
    single line s.
    single pass sector s.
    spleen s.
    thallium myocardial s.
    thyroid s.
    ventilation s.
    whole body s.
scandium
scanner
    beam CT s.
    CT body s.
    Elscint Excel 905 s.
    EMI 7070 s.
    EMI CT 500 s.
    gamma-ray s.
    gated CT s.
    General Electric 8800 s.
    General Electric CT/T7
      800 s.
    "Indomitable" s.
    Medx s.
    millisecond s.
    multislice s.
    neurodiagnostic s.
    nongated CT s.
    nuclear s.
    Ohio Nuclear Delta
      50 s.
    Ohio Nuclear Delta 50
      FS s.
    Ohio Nuclear Delta
      2000 s.
    Pfizer 0450 s.
    Pfizer 200 FS s.
    Picker Synerview 600 s.
    radioisotope s.
    rectilinear s.

scanner *(continued)*
    Siemens Somatom 2 s.
    supercam scintillation s.
    Technicare Delta
       2020 s.
    tomographic multi-
       plane s.
    Varian CT s.
    whole body s.
scanning
    A-mode (amplitude
       modulation) s.
    B-mode (brightness
       modulation) s.
    bone marrow s.
    brain s.
    cine CT s.
    compound s.
    contiguous s.
    full line s.
    gallium s.
    gamma s.
    infarct s.
    lacrimal s.
    line s.
    linear s.
    M-mode (time-
       motion) s.
    multiplanar s.
    nuclear s.
    perfusion s.
    point s.
    radioisotope s.
    radionuclide s.
    real-time s.
    renal s.
    rotate-rotate s.
    rotate-stationary s.

scanning *(continued)*
    sector s.
    sensitive point s.
    s. sequence
    single pass s.
    s. spot
    three-phase bone s.
    transverse s.
    water path s.
    whole body s.
scanography
scaphocephalic
scaphocephaly
scaphoid
    s.-capitate fracture dis-
       location
    s.-lunate dislocation
    s. necrosis
    s. rotation
    s. scapula
    s.-trapezium fusion
scapho-lunate
    s.-l. angle
    s.-l. dissociation
scapula (scapulae)
    alar s.
    Graves' s.
    scaphoid s.
    winged s.
scapular
scapuloanterior
scapuloclavicular
scapulohumeral
scapuloposterior
scattered radiation
scattering
    Compton's s.
    self-s.

scattering *(continued)*
    Thomson's s.
    ultrasound s.
scatter radiation
    Compton's s. r.
Scheibe's malformation
Schilling test
schindylesis
schindyletic
schistosoma
Schistosoma japonicum
schistosomiasis
    s. japonica
    s. mansoni
Schmorl's node
Schonander film changer
Schroedinger's equation
Schüller's
    method
    position
schwannoma
sciatic
scientific notation
scimitar
    s. shadow
    "s. sign"
    s. syndrome
scintiangiography
scintigram *(see* scintigraphy)
scintigraphic
    s. "hot spot"
scintigraphy
    nuclear s.
    renal s.
    thallium perfusion s.
scintillating
scintillation
    s. camera

scintillation *(continued)*
    collimated s. detector
    s. counter
    s. probe
    s. spectrometer
scintiphotograph
scintiphotography
scintiphotosplenoportography
scintiscan
scintiscanner
scintiview
sclera (sclerae)
scleritis
sclerocorneal
scleroderma
sclerodermatous
scleroma
scleromalacia
scleromyxedema
sclerosarcoma
sclerosing
sclerosis
    amyotrophic lateral s.
    annular s.
    cortical s.
    diaphyseal s.
    endosteal s.
    metaphyseal s.
    multiple s.
    parasutural s.
    subchondral s.
    subendocardial s.
    tuberous s.
    vascular s.
    venous s.
    ventrolateral s.
sclerosteosis
sclerotic

scoliosis
   congenital s.
   idiopathic s.
   neuromuscular s.
scorbutic
   s. rosary
"scottie dog"
   "s. d." appearance
   "s. d." view
scout
   s. image
   s. radiography
   s. view
screen
   s.-film contact
   fluorescent s.
   intensifying s.
   s. lag
   s. mottle
   s. thickness
   s.-type film
screening
scrofula
scrotal
scrotum
scurvy
scutum
   s. pectoris
SD – phase sensitive detector
s.d. – standard deviation
"seat-belt" injury
sebaceous
sebaceum
sec. – seconds
secondary
   s. curve
   s. electron
secreta

secrete
secretion
section thickness
sectoring
secular
sedative
sedimentation rate
"segmental malacia"
segmented
Seidlitz powder test
seizure
   epileptiform s.
^{75}Se-labelled taurine conjugate
   of 23-selena-25-homo-
   cholic acid
Seldinger's
   catherization
   percutaneous technique
selective
   s. angiocardiography
   s. arteriography
   s. radiofrequency pulse
   s. venography
   s. visceral aortogra-
   phy
selective excitation
   s. e. irradiation technique
   s. e. line scan
   s. e. projection reconstruction imaging
selenium
selenomethionine
self
   s.-absorption
   s.-developing film
   s.-inductance
   s.-induction

self *(continued)*
    s.-quenched counter tube
    s.-rectification
    s.-rectified circuit
    s.-rectifier
    s.-scattering
sella (sellae)
    dorsum s.
    ''empty'' s.
    s. turcica
sellar
semiautomatic system
semiaxial
semicircular
semicoma
semiconductor
    s. chip
    s. detector
semierect
semiflexion
semilongitudinal
semilunar
seminal
seminiferous
seminoma
seminomatous
semiprone
semirecumbent
semispinalis
    s. capitis
semisupine
senescent
Sengstaken-Blakemore tube
senile
senograph
senography

sensitive
    s. line method
    s. plane
    s. plane projection re-construction imaging
    s. point scanning
sensitivity
sensitometer
    electroluminescent s.
sensitometry
sensory
sentinal
Sephadex
sepsis
septa (*see* septum)
septal
septation
septic
    s. shock
septicemia
septomarginal
septum (septa)
    s. canalis musculotuba-rii
    interatrial s.
    interventricular s.
    s. lucidum
    nasal s.
    s. pellucidum
    s. primum defect
sequela (sequelae)
sequence
    Carr-Purcell s.
    direct mapping s.
    inversion recovery s.
    Meiboom-Gill s.
    Robin's s.
    scanning s.

sestamibi scan

sequence *(continued)*
    spin-echo s.
sequential
    s. film
    s. first pass imaging
    s. line method
    s. plane imaging
    s. point method
sequestration
sequestrum (sequestra)
    "button" s.
sera
serendipitous
serialoangiocardiography
serialogram
serialograph
series
    s. circuit
    gastrointestinal s.
    radioactive s.
    small bowel s.
seroma
seronegative
seropositive
serous
serpentine
serpiginous
Serratia
    S. marcescens
sesamoid
    s. index
    s. periostitis
^{75}Se selenomethionine
^{75}Se selenomethyl cholesterol
sessile
Settegast's
    method
    position

SFP or SSFP – steady-state-
    free-precession
shadow
    acoustic s.
    "bat's-wing" s.
    "butterfly" s.
    calcific s's
    double-bubble s.
    "overlap" s.
    psoas s.
    "ring" s.
    sail s.
    scimitar s.
    s. shield
    "triple line" s's
shadowgram
shadowgraph
shadowgraphy
shaft
shaggy
shape
    "baseball bat" s.
    "cricket bat" s.
    "dumbbell" s.
Sharpey's fibers
sheath
    tendon s.
sheathed
shell
    atomic s.
    "s. of bone" appear-
      ance
    first or K-s.
    second or L-s.
    third or M-s.
    fourth or N-s.
    fifth or O-s.
    sixth or P-s.

shell *(continued)*
  seventh or Q-s.
  valence s.
"shell-like" demarcation
Shenton's line
"shepherd's crook" deformity
Shepherd's fracture
Shepp-Logan filter function
shield
  Dalkon s.
  lead gonad s.
  shadow s.
shielding
shigella *Chiatski ring*
shim coils
shimming
shock
  cardiogenic s.
  hemorrhagic s.
  "s. lung"
  septic s.
short leg gait
short scale contrast
shoulder
  s. girdle
  s. sign
shunt
  arteriovenous s.
  atrial septal defect s.
  cardiac s.
  cystoperitoneal s.
  extracardiac s.
  intracardiac s.
  portocaval s.
  s. quantification
  venous s.
  ventriculoperitoneal s.
sialaden

sialadenitis
sialadenography
sialectasia
sialectasis
sialoangiography
sialodochitis
sialogram
sialography
sialolithiasis
sicca syndrome
sickle cell anemia
SID – source-to-image receptor
  distance
SIDS – sudden infant death
  syndrome
Siemens Somatom 2 scanner
sigmoid
  s. colon
  s. elevator sign
  s. kidney
  s. sinus
  s. sulcus
  s. volvulus
sigmoidoscopy
sign
  air-bronchogram s.
  air cap s.
  air crescent s.
  air dome s.
  beak s.
  "bite s."
  black pleura s.
  border s.
  "bowing" s.
  "Carman-Kirklin me-
   niscus" s.
  cervicothoracic s.
  chest-abdomen s.

sign *(continued)*
   "crowfoot" s.
   cut-off s.
   "dagger" s.
   Deuel's halo s.
   "double bubble" s.
   double lesion s.
   double track s.
   "double wall" s.
   doughnut s.
   ellipse s.
   extrapleural s.
   fat pad s.
   "floating tooth" s.
   "football" s.
   Golden's S s.
   "halo" s.
   Hamman's s.
   high convergence s.
   high overlay s.
   hilum convergence s.
   hilum overlay s.
   Homer-Spaulding s.
   "iceberg" s.
   ischial varus s.
   Köhler's "teardrop" s.
   lily pad s.
   meniscus s.
   "Mercedes-Benz" s.
   mustache s.
   notch s.
   obturator s.
   open bronchus s.
   "pubic" s.
   "renal halo" s.
   "reverse three" s.
   "rim s."
   ring s.

sign *(continued)*
   "sandwich" s.
   "scimitar s."
   shoulder s.
   sigmoid elevator s.
   silhouette s.
   Spalding's s.
   "spine" s.
   Spinnaker sail s.
   stacked coin s.
   tring s.
   teat s.
   thoracoabdominal s.
   thymic wave s.
   Turner's s.
   vallecular s.
   Westmark's s.
   Wimberger's s.
signal-to-noise ratio
silhouette
   s. sign
silicate
silicon
silicone
   s. rectifier
silicoproteinosis
silicosis
   "Liverpool s."
silicotic
silver
   s. bromide
   s. halide
   s. iodide
   metallic s.
   s. nitrate
   s. recovery
simean crease
Simmons' catheter

simplex
Simpson's rule
Sims' position
simulation
simultaneous
    s. three-dimensional
        measurement
    s. multifilm tomography
sincalide
sinciput
sine wave
single
    s. contrast barium
        enema
    s. contrast study
    s. emulsion film
    s.-film automatic system
    s. line scan
    s. pass scanning
    s. pass sector scan
    s. phase system
    s. photon counting (sys-
        tem)
    s. photon emission test
    s. photon emission
        computed tomogra-
        phy
    s.-pole double-throw
    s. slice line integral
        projection reconstruc-
        tion
    s. slice modified KWE
        direct Fourier imag-
        ing
    s. slice projection re-
        construction
sinistrad
sinistral

sinoatrial
Sinografin
sinogram
sinography
sinospiral
sinus
    s. bradycardia
    cavernous s.
    confluence of s's
    costophrenic s.
    dural s.
    dura mater s.
    ethmoidal s's
    frontal s.
    s. histiocytosis
    maxillary s.
    s. node
    occipital s.
    paranasal s.
    s. pericranii
    petrosal s.
    phrenocostal s.
    piriform s.
    sagittal s.
    sigmoid s.
    sphenoid s.
    sphenoparietal s.
    straight s.
    transverse s.
    tympanic s.
    venous s.
sinusitis
sinusography
siphon
    carotid s.
Siregraph 2
Siremat
sirenomelia

situs (situs)
    s. inversus
    s. perversus
    s. transversus
six-pulse three-phase generator
skeletal
skeleton
    appendicular s.
    axial s.
skiagram
skiagraph
skiagraphy
Skillern's fracture
skin
    s. dose
    s. sparing
Skiodan
Skiodan Acacia
skip
    s. areas
    s. tomography
skull
    brachycephalic s.
    cloverleaf s.
    contracting s.
    dolichocephalic s.
    lacunar s.
    mesocephalic s.
skyline view
slice
    CT s.
    s. geometry
    s. selection
sling
    vascular s.
slip rings
SLS – segment long-spacing
    (collagen)

sludge
slug
SMA – superior mesenteric artery
small bowel series
smallpox
small rounded opacities
Smith-Petersen
    nail
    pin
Smith's fracture
SNM – Society of Nuclear Medicine
"snowman" heart
"soap bubble" appearance
Society of Nuclear Medicine
socket
sodium
    s. bicarbonate
    s. bromide
    s. carbonate
    s. chloride
    s. chromate
    diatrizoate s.
    s. hydroxide
    s. iodide
    iodipamide s.
    iodohippurate s.
    iodomethamate s.
    iodophthalein s.
    iothalamate s.
    ipodate s.
    methiodal s.
    Oragrafin s.
    s. pertechnetate
    s. phosphate
    s. radioiodine
    s. rose bengal

sodium *(continued)*
  s. sulfite
  s. thiosulfate
  s. thorium tartrate
  tyropanoate s.
  s. warfarin
software
soft x-ray
SOG – supraorbital groove
solarization
solenoid
solid
  s. pattern
  s.-state diode rectifier
  s.-state physics
  s.-state rectification
solitary
solubilize
Solu-Biloptin
soluble
solution
  Carnoy's s.
  hundredth-normal s.
  hypertonic s.
  ionic s.
  molal s.
Solutrast
SOM – supraorbital margin
somatic
somatomedin
somesthetic
Sommer-Foegella method
sonar
sonarography
sonics
sonofluoroscope
sonogram
sonographer

sonographic
sonography
sonolucent
sorbitol
sound waves
source-skin distance
source-to-image receptor distance
SP – sugar phosphate
space
  axillary s.
  capsular s.
  s.-charge
  s.-charge compensator
  complemental s.
  disc s.
  epicerebral s.
  epidural s.
  epitympanic s.
  extradural s.
  extrapleural s.
  iliocostal s.
  intercostal s.
  intercrural s.
  interosseous s.
  interseptal s.
  intertrabecular s.
  ischiorectal s.
  medullary s.
  meningeal s.
  s. occupying lesion
  pararenal s.
  parasinoidal s.
  periaxial s.
  perihepatic s.
  perineal s.
  perineuronal s.
  perinuclear s.

space *(continued)*
  pharyngomaxillary s.
  phrenocostal s.
  pleural s.
  popliteal s.
  pre-epiglottic s.
  presacral s.
  pretracheal s.
  prevascular s.
  retrobulbar s.
  retrocrural s.
  retromammary s.
  retroperitoneal s.
  retropharyngeal s.
  retrorectal s.
  retrosternal s.
  retrotracheal s.
  subacromial s.
  subarachnoid s.
  subcarinal s.
  subdural s.
  subepicranial s.
  subhepatic s.
  submaxillary s.
  subphrenic s.
  subtrapezial s.
  thenar s.
  thyrohyal s.
"spadelike" appearance
Spalding's sign
spallation
spasm
  coronary s.
  esophageal s.
spastic
spatial
  s. dose distribution
  s. filter

spatial *(continued)*
  s. information
  s. nonuniformity
  s. resolution
  s. uniformity
spatiotemporal
  s. resolution
SPC – single photon counting
    (system)
spdt – single-pole double-throw
specific
  s. activity
  s. gravity
  s. radiation
speckled
SPECT – single-photon emis-
    sion computed tomogra-
    phy
spectral
spectrograph
spectrometer
  beta-ray s.
  Bragg's s.
  gamma-ray s.
  mass s.
  Mossbauer's s.
  scintillation s.
  x-ray s.
spectrometry
  pulse height s.
spectrophotofluorome-
    ter
spectrophotometer
  absorption s.
spectrophotometry
spectroscope
spectroscopic
spectroscopy

spectrum (spectra)
    absorption x-ray s.
    atomic s.
    characteristic s.
    chromatic s.
    electromagnetic
      energy s.
    emission s. x-ray
    pulse-height s.
    thermal s.
    x-ray s.
spermatic
spermatocele
sphenobasilar
sphenoethmoid
sphenoethmoidal
sphenofrontal
sphenoid
    s. ridge
sphenoidal
    s. rostrum
sphenomalar
sphenomaxillary
spheno-occipital
spheno-orbital
sphenopalatine
sphenoparietal
sphenopetrosal
sphenopharyngeal
sphenorbital
sphenosquamosal
sphenosquamous
sphenotemporal
sphenoturbinal
sphenovomerine
sphenozygomatic
sphere
spherical

spherocytosis
spheroidal
spherophakia brachymorphia
sphincter
    s. ani
    cardiac s.
    cardioesophageal s.
    gastroesophageal s.
    hepatic s.
    Hyrtl's s.
    inguinal s.
    s. of Oddi
    palatopharyngeal s.
    pharyngoesophageal s.
    prepyloric s.
    pyloric s.
sphincteroplasty
sphingomyelin
spiculated
spiculation
spicule-like
spiculum (spicula)
"spiderweb-like"
spigelian
    s. hernia
    s. line
spin
    s. coupling
    s. density
    s. echo
    s. echo sequence
    s.-lattice relaxation time
    s.-lattice relaxation time
      constant
    s.-spin relaxation time
    s.-spin relaxation time
      constant
    s.-warp imaging

spina (spinae)
    s. bifida
    s. bifida occulta
    s. luetica
    s. ventosa
spinal
    s. canal
    s. cord
    s. dysraphism
    s. fusion
    s. osteoporosis
    s. stenosis
"spindle cell" carcinoma
spindling
spine
    anterior nasal s.
    "bamboo" s.
    cervical s.
    Charcot's s.
    coccygeal s.
    iliac s.
    lumbar s.
    lumbosacral s.
    "poker" s.
    sacral s.
    "s. sign"
    thoracic s.
    thoracolumbar s.
    tibial s.
spin echo image
Spinnaker sail sign
"spinning top"
    "s. t. test"
    "s. t. urethra"
spinocerebellar
spinocervicothalamic
spinoglenoid

spinogram
spino-olivary
spinothalamic
spinous
    s. plane
    s. process
spinthariscope
spintherometer
spintometer
spiral
spirochetal
spirochete
splanchnic
splayed
splayfoot
splaying
spleen
    accessory s.
    cyanotic s.
    floating s.
    lardaceous s.
    porphyry s.
    sago s.
    speckled s.
    wandering s.
    waxy s.
splenectomy
splenic
    s. angle
    s. arteriography
    s. cyst
    s. dysfunction
    s. flexure
    s. hypofunction
    s. infarction
    s. rupture
    s. sac
    s. vein

splenium
    s. corporis callosi
splenography
splenomegaly
splenoportal
splenoportogram
splenoportography
splenosis
splenunculi
splintered
"split film" radiography
split hand
spondylarthritis
spondylitis
    ankylosing s.
    paratyphoid s.
    psoriatic s.
    tuberculous s.
spondyloarthropathy
spondyloenchondrodysplasia
spondyloepiphyseal
    s. dysplasia
    s. dysplasia congenita
    s. dysplasia tarda
spondylohumerofemoral
    s. hypoplasia
spondylolisthesis
spondylolysis
spondylometaphyseal
    s. dysplasia
spondylosis
    s. deformans
sponge kidney
spongioblastoma
spongy bone
spontaneous radiation

sporadic
sporotrichosis
Sporotrichum
    S. schenckii
spot film study
SPR – scanned projection radiography
Sprengel's deformity
sprue
    nontropical s.
    postgastrectomy s.
spur
spurious
spurring
sputum
squama (squamae)
squamosomastoid
squamosoparietal
squamososphenoid
squamous
    s. cell carcinoma
    s. cell papilloma
    s. portion
    s. suture
squamozygomatic
SQUID – superconducting quantum interference device
SSD –
    source-skin distance
    source-surface distance
SSFP – steady-state-free-precession
stabilizer
stacked coin sign
"staghorn calculi"
staging

standard free air ionization
chamber
Stanford and Wheatstone stereoscope
stannosis
stapedial
stapediovestibular
stapes
staphylococcal
Staphylococcus
S. aureus
star test pattern
stasis
static
s. electricity
s. image display
s. magnetic field
s. marks
statokinetic
stator
stature
status
s. asthmaticus
s. epilepticus
s. marmoratus
s. vertiginosus
Staunig's
method
position
steady-state-free-preces-
sion
steatorrhea
Stecher's
method
position
steerhorn
stellate
stenopthalmia

stenosis
aortic s.
biliary s.
cerebral aqueduct s.
foraminal s.
infundibular subaortic s.
laryngeal s.
medullary s.
mitral s.
pulmonic s.
pyloric s.
renal artery s.
spinal s.
subaortic s.
subglottic s.
tracheal s.
tricuspid s.
tubular s.
Stensen's duct
Stenver's
method
position
view
stephanion
step-wedge (or ladder)
stereocinefluorography
stereofluoroscopy
stereogram
stereograph
stereography
stereometry
stereomicroradiography
stereoradiogram
stereoradiograph
stereoradiography
stereoroentgenography
stereoroentgenometry
stereosalpingography

stereoscope
- direct measuring s.
- monocular s.
- Stanford and Wheatstone s.
- Wheatstone's s.

stereoscopic
- s. binoculars
- s. radiography
- s. view
- s. zonography

stereoscopy
stereoskiagraphy
stereotactic
stereotaxis
stereotrophic
Steripaque-BR
Steripaque-V
sternal
- s. angle
- s. notch
- s. plane

sternoclavicular
sternocleidal
sternocleidomastoid
sternocostal
sternohyoid
sternoid
sternomastoid
sternopericardial
sternoscapular
sternothyroid
sternotomy
sternotracheal
sternovertebral
sternoxiphoid
sternum
steroid

Stewart-Hamilton equation
sthenic
Stieda's fracture
stiffening
"stiff lung"
stippled
stippling
stoma
stomach
- cascade s.
- eutonic s.
- hypotonic s.
- infantile s.
- steerhorn s.

stomatognathic
stone
- Meckel's s.
- milk of calcium s.

stop bath
stopcock
Stout's fibromatosis
straggling
straight back syndrome
strandlike margins
strangulated
strangulation
stratigraphy
streptococcal
Streptococcus
- *S. pneumoniae*
- *S. pyogenes*

streptomycin
stress
- s. film
- s. fracture
- s. incontinence
- s. ulcer
- s. view

stria (striae)
striation
Strickler's method
stricture
stridor
string sign
string test
stripe
     paratracheal s.
stripped atom
stroboscopic
stroma (stromata)
stromal
Strongyloides
strontium (with yttrium 90)
     s. nitrate Sr 85
     s. Sr 87m
strut
     sphenoid s.
struvite
STS – subtrapezial space
study
     air contrast s.
     barium meal s.
     blood flow s.
     cine s.
     double-contrast s.
     dual-contrast s.
     equilibrium s.
     erythrokinetic s.
     flow s.
     horizontal beam s.
     iodized oil s.
     isotope s.
     lumbar, flexion and ex-
       tension s.
     motility s.
     perfusion s.

study *(continued)*
     perirenal air s.
     phonation s.
     quantitative regional
       lung function s.
     quantitative tracer s.
     rapid drip s.
     regional ventilation/per-
       fusion s.
     renal radionuclide s's
     retrococcygeal air s.
     retroperitoneal air s.
     single-contrast s.
     spot film s.
     tracer s.
     ventilation-perfusion
       imaging s.
     ventilation-perfusion nu-
       clear medicine s.
     video tape s.
     washout s.
     xenon-133 ventila-
       tion s.
styloglossus
stylohyoideus
styloid
stylomastoid
stylopharyngeus
subacromial
subacute
subaortic
subarachnoid
     s. hemorrhage
     s. space
subatomic
subcapital
subcapsular
subcarinal

subchondral
>   s. cyst
>   s. osteoporosis
>   s. sclerosis

subclavian
subclavicular
subcortical
subcostal
subcutaneous
subdeltoid
subdiaphragmatic
subdural
subendocardial
>   s. sclerosis

subependymal
subependymoma
subepicranial
subepidermal
subglottic
subglottis
subhepatic
subject
>   s.-film distance
>   s. motion
>   s. unsharpness

sublingual
subluxated
subluxation
subluxed
submandibular
submaxillary
submental
submentovertex
submentovertical
submucosal
subparietal
subperiosteal
subphrenic

subpial
subpleural
subpubic
subpulmonary
subscapular
subscapularis
subsegmental
subshell
substantia (substantiae)
>   s. nigra

substernal
subtalar
subtentorial
subtraction
>   s. angiography
>   film s.
>   first-order s.
>   photographic s.
>   second-order s.
>   s. venography

subtrapezial
subtrochanteric
subungual
>   s. epidermoid carci-
>   noma
>   s. exostosis
>   s. keratoacanthoma

subxiphoid
succinic semialdehyde
sudden infant death syndrome
Sudeck's atrophy
sugar-icing liver
sulcus (sulci)
>   calcarine s.
>   callosal s.
>   central s.
>   s. chiasmatis
>   cingulate s.

sulcus (sulci) *(continued)*
 collateral s.
 frontal lobe s.
 interhemispheric s.
 s. intermedius
 occipital s.
 occipitotemporal s.
 olfactory s.
 s. for optic chiasma
 parieto-occipital s.
 postcalcarine s.
 rhinal s.
 sagittal s.
 sigmoid s.
 subparietal s.
 superior s.
 suprasplenial s.
 transverse s.
sulfate
 barium s.
 barium lead s.
 barium strontium s.
sulfide
sulfite
sulfur
 s. colloid
"sump" ulcer
"sunburst" appearance
"sun-ray" appearance
"sunrise" projection
supercam scintillation scanner
superciliary
superconducting
 s. magnet
 s. quantum interference
  device
superconductive
superconductivity

superimposed
superimposition
superior straight
supernatant
supernumerary
superoinferior
superscan
supervoltage
supinate
supination
supinator
supine
suppuration
suppurative
supraciliary
supraclavicular
supracondylar
 s. ridge
supracondyloid
supradiaphragmatic
supraglottic
supraglottis
supramesocolic
supraoccipital
supraoptic
supraopticohypophyseal
supraorbital
suprapatellar
suprapubic
suprarenal
suprascapular
suprasellar
supraspinous
suprasplenial
suprasternal
supratentorial
supratragal
supratrochlear

supravalvular
surface
    articular s.
    s. coil method
surgical neck
sustentaculum (sustentacula)
    s. lienis
    s. tali
sutural
suture
    arcuate s.
    bregmatomastoid s.
    coronal s.
    cranial s.
    cutaneous s.
    dentate s.
    ethmoidomaxillary s.
    frontoethmoidal s.
    frontolacrimal s.
    frontomalar s.
    frontomaxillary s.
    frontonasal s.
    frontoparietal s.
    frontosphenoid s.
    frontozygomatic s.
    infraorbital s.
    interendognathic s.
    intermaxillary s.
    internasal s.
    interparietal s.
    jugal s.
    lacrimoconchal s.
    lacrimoethmoidal s.
    lacrimomaxillary s.
    lacrimoturbinal s.
    lambdoidal s.
    longitudinal s.
    malomaxillary s.

suture *(continued)*
    mastoid s.
    mendosal s.
    metopic s.
    nasal s.
    nasofrontal s.
    nasomaxillary s.
    occipital s.
    occipitomastoid s.
    occipitoparietal s.
    occipitosphenoidal s.
    palatine s.
    palatoethmoidal s.
    parietal s.
    parietomastoid s.
    parieto-occipital s.
    petrobasilar s.
    petrosphenobasilar s.
    petrospheno-occipital s.
    petrosquamous s.
    premaxillary s.
    rhabdoid s.
    sagittal s.
    sphenoethmoidal s.
    sphenofrontal s.
    sphenomalar s.
    sphenomaxillary s.
    spheno-occipital s.
    spheno-orbital s.
    sphenoparietal s.
    sphenopetrosal s.
    sphenosquamous s.
    sphenotemporal s.
    sphenozygomatic s.
    squamosomastoid s.
    squamosoparietal s.
    squamososphenoid s.
    squamous s.

suture *(continued)*
    temporomalar s.
    temporozygomatic s.
    zygomaticofrontal s.
    zygomaticomaxillary s.
    zygomaticotemporal s.
SV – interventricular septum
SVC – superior vena cava
Swan-Ganz catheter
swan-neck deformity
Swanson's prosthesis
sweat test
Sweet's method
"swimmer's"
    position
    lateral projection
    view
"Swiss Alps" appearance
sylvian
Sylvius'
    aqueduct
    cistern
    fissure
symmetrical
symmetry
sympathetic nervous system
symphalangism
symphysis
    mandibular s.
    s. menti
    s. pubis
synarthrodial
synarthrosis
synchondrodial
synchondrosis (synchondroses)
    sphenoethmoidal s.
synchronization
synchronous

synchrotron
syncope
syncytial
syncytium
    venous epidural s.
syndactylism
syndactyly
syndesmodial
syndesmophyte
syndesmosis
syndrome (for eponyms *see*
    Part III, Eponymic Dis-
    eases and Syndromes)
synechia (synechiae)
synergism
synostosis (synostoses)
    radioulnar s.
synovial
    s. chondromatosis
    s. cyst
    s. fluid
    s. joint
    s. margin
    s. membrane
    s. osteochondromatosis
    s. sarcoma
    s. sheath
    s. thickening
synovioblast
synovioma
synoviosarcoma
synovitis
    villonodular s.
synovium
synpolydactyly
synthesis
syphilis
syphilitic

syringoadenoma
syringobulbia
syringocarcinoma
syringocele
syringocoele
syringocystadenoma
syringocystoma
syringoencephalomyelia
syringoid
syringomelia
syringomeningocele
syringomyelia
syringomyelitis
syringomyelocele
syringomyelus
syringopontia
syrinx
system
    acquisition s.
    automatic processing s.
    British engineering s.
    capacitor discharge s.
    catenary s.
    centimeter-gram-
      second s.
    constant potential s.
    conventional single-
      phase s.
    data acquisition s.
    daylight s.
    dryer s.
    electron transmitter s.
    field emission x-ray s.
    gradient s.
    image intensifier s.
    Jewett-Marshall s.
    linear compartmental s.
    mamillary s.

system *(continued)*
    meter-kilogram-
      second s.
    metric s.
    mobile x-ray s.
    Orbitome tomographic
      s.
    recirculation s.
    rectifying s.
    replenishment s.
    semiautomatic s.
    single-film automatic s.
    single phase s.
    single photon
      counting s.
    three-compartment s.
    three-phase s.
    three-wire s.
    Tomolex tomographic s.
    transport s.
    two-compartment s.
    vacuum cassette s.
    water s.
    whole body proton
      magnetic resonance
      imaging s.
    XY s.
system (anatomical)
    absorbent s.
    adipose s.
    alimentary s.
    autonomic nervous s.
    biliary s.
    biologic amplification s.
    bulbospiral s.
    cardiovascular s.
    central nervous s.
    centrencephalic s.

system *(continued)*
- cerebrospinal s.
- chemoreceptor s.
- chromaffin s.
- circulatory s.
- collecting s.
- conduction s.
- dermal s.
- digestive s.
- endocrine s.
- exteroceptive nervous s.
- extrapyramidal s.
- gastrointestinal s.
- genitourinary s.
- glandular s.
- haversian s.
- hematopoietic s.
- heterogeneous s.
- homogeneous s.
- hormonopoietic s.
- hypophyseoportal s.
- integumentary s.
- interceptive nervous s.
- interrenal s.
- involuntary nervous s.
- keratinizing s.
- labyrinthine s.
- lacrimal s.
- limbic s.
- lymphatic s.
- lymphoid s.
- lymphoreticular s.
- macrophage s.
- malpighian s.
- mamillary s.
- mononuclear phagocyte s.

system *(continued)*
- muscular s.
- musculoskeletal s.
- nervous s.
- parasympathetic nervous s.
- pelvicalyceal s.
- pelviureteric s.
- peripheral nervous s.
- periventricular s.
- pigmentary s.
- pituitary portal s.
- plenum s.
- portal s.
- proprioceptive nervous s.
- replenishment s.
- reproductive s.
- respiratory s.
- reticular activating s.
- reticuloendothelial s.
- sinospiral s.
- skeletal s.
- somatic nervous s.
- stomatognathic s.
- sympathetic nervous s.
- urinary s.
- urogenital s.
- uropoietic s.
- vascular s.
- vasomotor s.
- vertebrobasilar s.
- vestibular s.
- visceral nervous s.

systemic
- s. lupus erythematosus

systole

systolic

T t

T – tesla
T_1 – longitudinal or spin-lattice relaxation time constant
T_2 – transverse or spin-spin relaxation time constant
T_3 – l-3,5,3′-triiodothyronine
T_4 – l-3,5,3′, 5′-tetraiodothyronine
t – transformer
table

Bucky's t.
tachycardia
tachypnea
Taenia

T. echinococcus
T. solium
taenia (taeniae)
t. chorioidea
t. cinerea
t. coli
t. fimbriae
t. hippocampi
t. libera
t. mesocolica
t. omentalis
t. pontis
t. terminalis
t. thalami
t. ventriculi tertii
tagged atom
tagging
tailored excitation
Takayasu's arteritis
talcosis

talipes
t. calcaneovalgus
t. calcaneovarus
t. calcaneus
t. cavus
t. equinovalgus
t. equinovarus
t. equinus
t. valgus
t. varus
talipomanus
talocalcaneal
talocalcaneonavicular
talocrural
talofibular
talonavicular
talotibial
talus
tampon
tamponade
tangent
tangential
Tanner-Whitehouse-Healy method
tannic acid
tantalum
target
t. angle
t.-film distance
"t." reconstruction
resolution t.
rotating anode t.
t.-skin distance
t.-to-nontarget ratio

Tarrant's
    method
    position
tarsal
tarsalia
tarsoepiphyseal
    t. aclasis
tarsometatarsal
tarsophalangeal
tarsophyma
tarsotarsal
tarsotibial
tarsus
tautography
Taylor's
    method
    position
TBG – thyroxine-binding globulin
TBW – total body water
TC – technetium
TCA – tentorium cerebelli attachment
TCAT – transmission computer-assisted tomography
Tc 99m (*see* technetium)
TDV – thoracodorsal vessels
TEA – top of ear attachment
teardrop
    "t." distance
    t. fracture
teat sign
technetium
    t. 99m acetanilidoiminodiacetic acid
    t. 99m aggregated albumin kit
    t. 99m albumin

technetium *(continued)*
    t. 99m albumin microspheres kit
    t. 99m antimony
    t. 99m blood pool study
    t. 99m colloid
    t. 99m diethylenetriamine penta-acetic acid
    t. 99m 2,3 dimercaptosuccinic acid
    t. 99m etidronate sodium kit
    t. 99m ferric hydroxide
    t. 99m generator
    t. 99m glucoheptonate
    t. 99m HAM perfusion scan
    t. 99m imidodiphosphonate
    t. 99m iminodiacetic acid
    t. 99m macroaggregates
    t. 99m medronate sodium kit
    t. 99m methylene diphosphonate
    t. 99m microspheres
    t. 99m pentetate sodium kit
    t. 99m phosphate uptake
    t. 99m phytate
    t. 99m pyridoxylideneglutamate
    t. 99m pyrophosphate

technetium *(continued)*
- t. 99m radiopharma-
  ceutical
- t. 99m serum albumin
  kit
- t. 99m stannous pyro-
  phosphate/polyphos-
  phate kit
- t. 99m sulfur colloid
- t. 99m technetium per-
  technetate

99mtechnetium-labelled pyridoxylideneglutamate (PYG)
99mtechnetium lidofenin
99mtechnetium-labelled 2,6-di-
methylacetanilide iminodiacetic acid (HIDA)
"technical" empyema
Technicare Delta 2020 scanner
technique
- air gap t.
- autoradiographic t.
- chromatographic-fluoro-
  metric t.
- compression t.
- Corbin's t.
- 51Cr-labelled red cell t.
- drip infusion t.
- Klein's t.
- Seldinger's percuta-
  neous t.
- selective excitation irradiation t.
- supervoltage t.
- three-dimensional t.
- time-dependent gra-
  dient t.
- Welin's t.

tectocerebellar
tectum
- t. of mesencephalon
TED – threshold erythema
dose
tegmen (tegmina)
- t. antri
- t. mastoideum
- t. tympani
- t. ventriculi quarti
tegmental
tegmentospinal
tegmentum (tegmenta)
- t. auris
- t. rhombencephali
- subthalmic t.
TEK – total exchangeable potassium
telangiectasia
- capillary t.
telangiectatic
Telebrix
telecobolt
telecardiogram
telecardiography
telefluoroscopy
telemetry
Telepaque
teleradiography
teleroentgenogram
teleroentgenography
teleroentgentherapy
teletherapy
television camera
"tell-tale triangle"
tellurium
Templeton and Zim carpal tunnel projection

temporal
temporalis
temporoauricular
temporofacial
temporofrontal
temporohyoid
temporomalar
temporomandibular
temporomaxillary
temporo-occipital
temporoparietal
temporopontile
temporosphenoid
temporosquamous
temporozygomatic
TENa – total exchangeable sodium
tendinitis
tendinous
    t. ring
tendon
    Achilles' t.
    bowed t.
    calcaneal t.
    common t.
    conjoined t.
    cordiform t.
    coronary t's
    cricoesophageal t.
    extensor t.
    flexor digitorum profundus t.
    Gerlach's t.
    hamstring t.
    Hector's t.
    membranaceous t.
    patellar t.
    t. sheath

tendon *(continued)*
    supraspinatus t.
    trefoil t.
    Zinn's t.
tendonitis
tennis elbow
tenogram
tenography
Tenon's
    capsule
    fascia
tenosynovial
tenosynovitis
tension
tensor
tentorial
    t. incisura
    t. notch
    t. ridge
tentorium
    t. cerebelli attachment
teratoblastoma
teratocarcinoma
teratogen
teratogenetic
teratogenic
teratogenous
teratoma (teratomas or teratomata)
    calvarial t.
    sacrococcygeal t.
teratomatous
terbium
teres
    t. major
    t. minor
Teridax
terminal

terrestrial radiation
tertiary
tesla
test
    bile salt breath t.
    ^{14}C-glycocholic acid t.
    ^{14}C lactose breath t.
    chlormerodrin accumu-
      lation t.
    Dicopac t.
    fat absorption breath t.
    gastrointestinal blood
      loss t.
    gastrointestinal protein
      loss t.
    H_2 breath t.
    hepatic t. of Glass
    ^{125}I-fibrinogen uptake t.
    Lasix t.
    limulus lysate t.
    perchlorate discharge t.
    positive washout t.
    radioimmunoprecipi-
      tation t.
    radioiodine uptake t.
    regional lung function t.
    Schilling t.
    Seidlitz powder t.
    single photon emis-
      sion t.
    "spinning top t."
    string t.
    sweat t.
    thyrotropin-releasing
      hormone t.
    "tilt t."
    triiodothyronine red cell
      uptake t.

test *(continued)*
    triiodothyronine resin t.
    washout t.
    water siphonage t.
testes
testicle
testicular
testis (testes)
testosterone
tetany
"tethered cord" syndrome
tethering
tetrabromophenolphthalein
tetrachloride
tetracycline
tetraiodophenolphthalein
tetraiodothyronine
tetralogy
    Fallot's t.
Teufel's method
TFD – target-film distance
Tg – thyroglobulin
TGC – time gain compensation
TH – thyroid hormone
thalamocortical
thalamoperforate
thalamus
thalassemia
thalidomide
thallium
    t. 201 imaging
    t. myocardial scan
    t. perfusion scintigraphy
    t. 201 stress testing
thallous chloride Tl 201
thanatophoric
theca (thecae)
    t. lutein

thecal
thecoma
thecomatosis
thecostegnosis
thenar
    t. eminence
    t. space
theorem
    Bayes' t.
    dose reciprocity t.
theory
    atomic t.
    Bohr's t.
    Culiner's t.
    electron t.
    Maxwell's t. of radiation
    Planck's quantum t.
    quantum t.
therapeutic
therapy
    beam t.
    deep roentgen ray t.
    megavolt t.
    t. quality
    radiation t.
    t. tube
    x-ray t.
thermal
    t. conductivity
    t. energy
    t. equilibrium
    t. neutron
    t. radiation
thermionic
    t. emission
    t. vacuum tube
thermistor

thermodynamics
thermoelectron
thermogram
thermograph
thermography
thermoluminescent
thermonuclear
thermovision
thesaurosis
thiazide
thiosemicarbazide
thiosemicarbazone
thiosulfate
"third mogul"
Thixokon
Thoms' method
Thomson's scattering
thoracentesis
thoracic
    t. aneurysm
    t. aorta
    t. aortic dissection
    t. aortography
    t. calcification
    t. curve
    t. dehiscence
    t. duct
    t. inlet
    t. kidney
    t. myelography
    t. outlet syndrome
    t.-pelvic-phalangeal dystrophy
    t. plane
    t. spine
    t. vertebra
thoracoabdominal sign
thoracodorsal

thoracolumbar
thoracoplasty
thoracostomy
thoracotomy
Thoraeus' filter
Thoramat
thorax
thoriated tungsten filament
thorium
    t. dioxide
    t. nitrate
    radioactive t.
    t. tartrate
    t. X
Thorotrast
Thorpe's plastic lens
three
    t.-compartment system
    t.-phase bone scanning
    t.-phase circuit
    t.-phase current
    t.-phase generator
    t.-phase system
    t.-vessel angiography
    t.-wire system
three-dimensional
    t.-d. echo planar imaging
    t.-d. Fourier imaging
    t.-d. imaging
    t.-d. KWE direct Fourier imaging
    t.-d. measurement
    t.-d. physiologic flow pattern
    t.-d. projection reconstruction imaging
    t.-d. technique

threshold
    alpha t.
    t. dose
thrombi (*see* thrombus)
thromboangiitis obliterans
thrombocytopenia
    t.-absent radius syndrome
    hypoplastic t.
thromboemboli
thromboembolic
thromboembolism
thromboembolus
thrombophlebitis
thrombosis
    catheter-induced t.
    umbilical t.
    venous t.
thrombotic
thrombus (thrombi)
    cardiac t.
    intracardiac t.
    mural t.
thulium
thumb
    gamekeeper's t.
    "hitchhiker's" t.
    hypoplastic t.
    murderer's t.
    Potter's t.
    t. rule
    stub t.
    triphalangeal t.
"thumbprinting"
Thurston-Holland fracture
thymic
    t. alymphoplasia
    t. wave sign

thymidine
thymolipoma
thymoma
thymosin
thymus
thyratron
thyrocalcitonin
thyrocervical
thyroglobulin
thyroglossal
thyrohyal
thyrohyoid
thyroid
    t. acropachy
    t. adenoma
    t. carcinoma
    t. cyst
    ectopic t.
    t. gland uptake
    t. neoplasia
    t. nodule
    t. scan
    t. storm
    t. uptake
thyroidectomy
thyroiditis
    de Quervain's t.
    focal t.
    Hashimoto's t.
    lymphocytic t.
thyrotoxicosis
thyrotropin releasing hormone
    test
thyroxine
    t.-binding globulin
Thyrx timer
Ti – titanium
TIA – transient ischemic attack

TIBC – total iron-binding capacity
tibia
tibial
    t. condylar fracture
    t. malleolus
    t. plafond fracture
    t. plateau
    proximal t.
    t. pseudarthrosis
    t. shaft fracture
    t. spine
    t. tubercle
    t. tuberosity
tibiocalcanean
tibiofemoral
tibiofibular
tibionavicular
tibiotalar
tibiotarsal
Tillaux's fracture
"tilt test"
time
    t. compensated gain
    t. density curve
    t.-dependent gradient
      technique
    doubling t.
    t. gain compensation
    proton relaxation t.
    recovery t.
    renal transit t.
    spin-lattice relaxation t.
    spin-spin relaxation t.
    transverse relaxation t.
timer
    fluoroscopic t.
    impulse t.

timer *(continued)*
> photoelectric t.
> Thyrx t.

tin (with indium 113m)

tinnitus

tissue
> adipose t.
> t. characterization
> connective t.
> t. discrimination
> t. equivalent detector
> fibrous t.
> glandular t.
> pathologic t.
> t. technique
> t. tolerance dose

titanium

Titterington's
> method
> position

Tl – thallium

TLD –
> thermoluminescent dosimeter
> tumor lethal dose

TM – time motion

TMI – transient myocardial ischemia

TMJ – temporomandibular joint

TMR – topical magnetic resonance

toddler's fracture

Todd's paresis

toe-touch maneuver

tolazoline hydrochloride

toluidine blue

tomogram *(see* tomography)

tomograph

tomographic
> t. multiplane scanner

tomography
> axial transverse t.
> circular t.
> computed t.
> computer assisted t.
> computerized axial t.
> emission computed t.
> focal plane t.
> hypercycloidal t.
> linear t.
> longitudinal section t.
> metrizamide-assisted computed t.
> panoramic t.
> plesiosectional t.
> pluridirectional t.
> polycycloidal t.
> positron emission t.
> positron emission transverse t.
> quantitative computed t.
> radionuclide emission t.
> rotational t.
> simultaneous multifilm t.
> single photon emission computed t.
> skip t.
> transmission computer-assisted t.
> transversal t.
> wide angle t.

tomolaryngography

Tomolex tomographic system

tomoscopy

tonic
tonicity
tonsil
      cerebellar t.
      palatine t.
      pharyngeal t.
tonsillar
tonsillitis
tonsillolith
tonsillomoniliasis
tophus (tophi)
topical
torcular
      t. Herophili
torque
torsion
      femoral t.
      t. fracture
      lobar t.
      testicular t.
torticollis
tortuous
torulosis
torus fracture
tourniquet
Towne's
      position
      view
Townsend's avalanche
toxic
toxicity
Toxoplasma
toxoplasmosis
trabecula (trabeculae)
trabecular
trabeculated
trabeculation
tracer study

trachea
      saber-sheath t.
tracheal
      t. amyloidosis
      t. band
      t. "button"
      t. deviation
      t. dilatation
      t. diverticulum
      t. duplication
      t. intubation
      t. lymph node
      t. perforation
      "t. spill"
      t. stenosis
      t. tube
tracheitis
tracheobronchial
      t. rupture
tracheobronchomalacia
tracheobronchomegaly
tracheobronchopathia
      t. osteochondroplastica
tracheobronchoscopy
tracheoesophageal
tracheoesophagus
tracheoinnominate
tracheolaryngeal
tracheomalacia
tracheopathia
      t. osteoplastica
tracheopharyngeal
tracheostenosis
tracheostomy
trachiectasis
tract
      alimentary t.
      biliary t.

tract *(continued)*
- bulbar t.
- bulbospinal t.
- cerebellar t.
- cerebellorubrospinal t.
- cerebellospinal t.
- cerebellotegmental t.
- cerebellothalamic t.
- cerebrospinal t.
- cornucommissural t.
- corticobulbar t.
- corticocerebellar t.
- corticopontile t.
- corticorubral t.
- corticospinal t.
- corticothalamic t.
- digestive t.
- extracorticospi-
  nal t.
- extrapyramidal t.
- fistulous t.
- foraminous spiral t.
- frontopontine t.
- gastrointestinal t.
- genitourinary t.
- hypothalamicohypo-
  physeal t.
- iliopubic t.
- iliotibial t.
- intestinal t.
- mamillotegmental t.
- olfactory t.
- olivocerebellar t.
- olivospinal t.
- optic t.
- pyramidal t.
- respiratory t.
- rubroreticular t.

tract *(continued)*
- sensory t.
- septomarginal t.
- spinocerebellar t.
- spinocervicothalamic t.
- spino-olivary t.
- spinothalamic t.
- supraopticohypophys-
  eal t.
- tectocerebellar t.
- tegmental t.
- tegmentospinal t.
- temporopontile t.
- thalamocortical t.
- urinary t.
- uveal t.
- ventricular outflow t.
- vestibulocerebellar t.
- vestibulospinal t.

traction
tragal
tragus (tragi)
transabdominal
transaxillary
transcervical
transcondylar
transcranial
transducer
- aspiration t.

transduodenal
transfacial
transfalcine
transferrin
transformation
transformer
- air core t.
- t. coil
- closed core t.

transformer *(continued)*
    Coolidge's t.
    distribution t.
    "doughnut" t.
    t. equation
    filament t.
    high-voltage t.
    t. law
    t. loss
    ratio t.
    step-down t.
    step-up t.
transglottic
transglottis
transhepatic
transient
    t. ischemic attack
    t. response resonance
transillumination
transition
    beta t.
    isomeric t.
transitional cell carcinoma
    t. c. c. stage A
    t. c. c. stage B1
    t. c. c. stage B2
    t. c. c. stage C
    t. c. c. stage D1
    t. c. c. stage D2
translateral
translocation
translucent
translumbar
transmitter
transmural
transmutation
transoral
transorbital

transparent
transplant
transplantation
transport
    t. case
    t. feeder
    t. system
transposition
transpyloric
transradiant
transscaphoid
transtabular
transtentorial
transthoracic
transtracheal
transtubercular
transvenous
transversal tomography
transversalis
transverse
    t. arch
    t. colon
    t. deficiency
    t. foramen
    t. fracture
    t. line
    t. mesocolon
    t. plane
    t. process
    t. relaxation time
    t. relaxation time constant
    t. scanning
    t. section imaging
    t. sinus
    t. sulcus
    t. time constant

trapezioscaphoid
trapezium
trapezoid
trauma
traumatic
tray
    Bucky's t.
TRDN – transient respiratory distress of the newborn
treadmill
"trefoil" appearance
Treitz
    ligament of T.
tremolite talc
tremor
Trendelenburg's
    gait
    position
TRH – thyrotropin releasing hormone
triangle
    aortic t.
    Codman's t.
    femoral t.
    sylvian t.
    "tell-tale t."
triangular
triangulation
trichinosis
trichloroacetic acid
trichomonas
tricho-rhino-phalangeal syndrome
tricuspid
    t. atresia
    t. murmur
    t. regurgitation

tricuspid *(continued)*
    t. stenosis
    t. valve
    t. vertebra
trident hand
trifurcation
trigeminal
trigger finger
triglyceride
trigone
trigonocephaly
trigonum
    t. parietale
triiodinated benzoic acid
triiodobenzoic acid
triiodothyronine
    t. red cell uptake test
    t. resin test
trimalleolar
triode tube
triolein (glyceral trioleate)
    I 131
Triosil
tripartite
triphalangeal
triphalangism
Triphasix generator
triphenyl tetrazolium chloride
triphosphate
"triple line" shadows
triple-voiding cystography
triploidy
"tripod"
    t. fracture
    t. position
triquetrum
trisection
trismus

trisomy
t. G
t. 8 mosaicism syn-
drome
t. 9p
t. 13
t. 18
t. 21
t. 22
trispiral
tritium
triton
trocar
trochanter
greater t.
lesser t.
t. minor
rudimentary t.
t. tertius
trochanteric
trochlea
trochlear
t. nerve
t. notch
t. surface
trochocephaly
trochoid
trophoblast
"tropical ulcer" osteoma
TRP – trichorhinophalangeal
TruCut needle
Truemmerfeld's zone
truncus arteriosus
TSC – technetium sulfur colloid
TSD – target-skin distance
TSH – thyroid stimulating hormone

TTC – triphenyl tetrazolium
chloride
TTD – tissue tolerance dose
TTL – transitor-transitor
logic
T-tube
T-t. cholangiography
tubal
tube
auditory t.
Bilbao-Dotter t.
camera t.
Cantor's t.
cathode ray r.
Coolidge's t.
Crookes' t.
Dotter t.
double focus t.
electron beam t.
electron multiplier t.
endotracheal t.
eustachian t.
fallopian t.
Hittorf's t.
hot cathode x-ray t.
image intensifier t.
image Orthicon t.
Kenotron t.
Lenard's ray t.
Miller-Abbott t.
overcouch t.
photomultiplier t.
pleural drainage t.
plumbicon t.
t. rating charts
rectifying t.
rotating anode t.
t. saturation

tube *(continued)*
 Sengstaken-
  Blakemore t.
 t. shift
 tracheal t.
 tracheostomy t.
 t. travel
 triode t.
 valve t.
 vidicon t.
 t. voltage waveform
 x-ray t.
tuber (tubers or tubera)
 t. cinereum
 t. ischii
 t. vermis
tubercle
 articular t.
 conoid t.
 mental t.
 spinous t.
 tibial t.
 transverse t.
tuberculoid
tuberculoma
tuberculosis
 diaphyseal t.
 fibrocavitary t.
 miliary t.
 multinodular t.
 pulmonary t.
tuberculous
 t. adenitis
 t. arthritis
 t. dactylitis
 t. gumma
 t. lymphadenopathy
 t. meningitis

tuberculous *(continued)*
 t. osteomyelitis
 t. spondylitis
 t. synovitis
tuberculum (tubercula)
 t. selle
tuberosity
 greater t.
 ischial t.
 lesser t.
 tibial t.
tuberous
 t. sclerosis
tubo-ovarian
tubular
tubulation
tubule
 collecting t.
 distal convoluted t.
 lactiferous t.
 proximal convoluted t.
 seminiferous t.
 uriniferous t.
tufts
 phalangeal t.
 sclerotic t.
tularemia
tumefacient
tumefaction
tumefactive
tumentia
 vasomotor t.
tumescence
tumid
tumor
 adenomatous t.
 adrenal t.
 benign t.

tumor *(continued)*
>   biliary t.
>   "brown" t.
>   carcinoid t.
>   carcinomatous t.
>   cystic t.
>   desmoid t.
>   t. dose
>   t. embolus
>   epithelial t.
>   Ewing's t.
>   fibro-osseous t.
>   giant cell t.
>   glial t.
>   glomus jugulare t.
>   glomus tympanicum t.
>   granular cell t.
>   Grawitz's t.
>   "iceberg" t.
>   islet cell t.
>   Klatzkin's t.
>   Krukenberg's t.
>   malignant mixed t.
>   mesodermal t.
>   metastatic t.
>   mucinous t.
>   müllerian t.
>   neurogenic t.
>   nonseminomatous t.
>   Pancoast's t.
>   Perlmann's t.
>   pharyngeal t.
>   polycystic t.
>   postirradiation t.
>   Rathke's pouch t.
>   serous t.
>   third ventricle t.
>   ulcerogenic t.

tumor *(continued)*
>   "vanishing" t.
>   t. volume
>   Warthin's t.
>   Wilms' t.

tumoral

tungstate

tungsten

tunica (tunicae)
>   t. vaginalis

tunnel
>   aortico–left ventricular t.
>   carpal t.
>   cassette t.
>   cervical t's
>   cubital t.
>   flexor t.
>   t. projection
>   tarsal t.

tunneling

turbinate

Turkel needle

Turner's
>   needle
>   phenotype
>   sign

"turret" exostosis

turricephaly

twelve-pulse three-phase generator

Twining's
>   method
>   position

two-dimensional
>   t.-d. echocardiography
>   t.-d. Fourier imaging
>   t.-d. Fourier transformation imaging

two-dimensional *(continued)*
  t.-d. KWE direct Fourier imaging
  t.-d. line integral projection reconstruction
  t.-d. modified KWE direct Fourier imaging
  t.-d. projection reconstruction
tympanic
  t. cavity
  t. sinus

tympanography
tympanosclerosis
tympanum
typhlitis
typhoid fever
typus
  t. degenerativus amstelodamensis
tyropanoate
  t. sodium
tyropanoic acid
tyrosinosis

u

UGI – upper gastrointestinal
UIBC – unsaturated iron-binding capacity
UIQ – upper inner quadrant
ulcer
  anastomotic u.
  atheromatous u.
  u. crater
  decubitus u.
  diabetic u.
  duodenal u.
  esophageal u.
  fistulous u.
  follicular u.
  gastric u.
  gastroduodenal u.
  gouty u.
  jejunal u.

ulcer *(continued)*
  "kissing" u's
  marginal u.
  peptic u.
  perforating u.
  prepyloric u.
  pudendal u.
  pyloric u.
  stress u.
  "sump" u.
  varicose u.
ulceration
  "collar button" u.
ulcerative
ulcerogangrenous
ulcerogenic
ulcerogranuloma
ulceromembranous

ulna
ulnar
    u. deviation
    u. drift syndrome
    u. fossa
    u. groove
    u. hypoplasia
    u. malleolus
    u. nerve
    u. ossicle
    u. styloid
ulnaris
ulnocarpal
ulnoradial
Ultracranio T
ultrasonic
    pulse-echo u's
ultrasonogram
ultrasonograph
ultrasonographic
ultrasonography
    A-mode u.
    cardiovascular u.
    Doppler u.
    gray-scale u.
    real-time u.
ultrasonometry
ultrasound
    Doppler u.
    u. imaging
    u. phantoms
    u. propagation parameters
    real-time u.
    u. resolution
    u. scattering
    u. vibrations
ultraviolet

umbilical
umbilicus
umbra
Umbradil
umbrella filter
unciform
uncinate
unco-ossified
uncovertebral
uncus
undercirculation
underdevelopmental
underhorn
undertoe
undervascularity
undescended
undifferentiated
undifferentiation
undirectional
undulating
uniaxial
unifocal
uniformity
unilateral
unilobar
unilocular
unit
    Angstrom u.
    atomic mass u.
    Bart's abdomino-peripheral angiography u.
    electromagnetic u.
    electrostatic u.
    Hounsfield u.
    Odelca camera u.
    Optiplanimat automated u.
    Orbix x-ray u.

unit *(continued)*
      Video Display u.
univentricle
unlabelled
unmodified scatter
unopacified
unresectable
unsaturated
      u. compounds
      u. iron-binding capa-
        city
unsharpness
unstable
unsymmetrical
UOQ – upper outer quadrant
UPJ – ureteropelvic junction
upper GI series
upper limb–cardiovascular syn-
      drome
uptake
urachal
urachus
uranium
urate
uremia
uremic
uresis
ureter
      circumcaval u.
      ectopic u.
      postcaval u.
      retrocaval u.
      retroiliac u.
ureteral
      u. calculus
      u. obstruction
      u. orifice
ureterectasis

ureteric
      u. reflux
ureteritis
      u. cystica
      u. glandularis
ureterocele
ureterocystography
ureteroduodenal
ureterogram
ureterography
ureteropelvic
ureteropyelography
ureteropyelonephritis
ureterouterine
ureterovaginal
ureterovesical
      u. reflux
urethra
      ''spinning top u.''
urethral
urethritis
urethrocystogram
urethrocystography
urethrogram (*see* urethrography)
urethrography
      excretory u.
      injection u.
      retrograde u.
urethrovaginal
urethrovesical
uric acid
urinalysis
urinary
      u. bladder
      u. extravasation
      u. obstruction
      u. system
      u. tract infection

urine
uriniferous
urinoma
urogenital
Urografin
urogram (*see* urography
urographic
urography
      ascending u.
      descending u.
      drip-infusion u.
      excretory u.
      hypertensive u.
      intravenous u.
      percutaneous ante-
         grade u.
      retrograde u.
urokymography
Uromiro
Uropac
uropathy
      obstructive u.
uropoietic
uroradiology
Uroselectan

urothelial
Urovision
urticaria
      u. pigmentosa
uterine
uterocervical
uterography
uterosalpingogram
uterosalpingography
uterotubography
uterovaginal
uteroventral
uterovesical
uterus
utricle
utriculitis
utriculus (utriculi)
uvea
uveal
uveitis
uveomeningitis
uviform
uvula
uvulitis

V

v – volt
va – volt-ampere
V.A.C. – volts, alternating
   current
vacuum
      v. arthrography

vacuum (*continued*)
      v. cassette system
      "v. phenomenon"
vagina
vaginal
      v. reflux

vaginitis
    atrophic v.
    desquamative inflamma-
      tory v.
    emphysematous v.
    granular v.
    trichomonas v.
vaginocutaneous
vaginogram
vaginography
vaginomycosis
vagus
Valdini's method
valence
    v. bond
    v. electron
    ionic polar v.
    v. shell
valgus
    cubitus v.
    v. deformity
    forefoot v.
    hallux v.
    hindfoot v.
    pes v.
    v. stress film
vallecula (valleculae)
vallecular sign
Valsalva's maneuver
Valvassori's method
valve
    aortic v.
    bicuspid v.
    Bochdalek's v.
    colic v.
    flail v.
    Heister's v.
    ileocecal v.

valve *(continued)*
    mitral v.
    prosthetic v.
    pulmonary v.
    pulmonic v.
    pyloric v.
    spiral v.
    tricuspid v.
    v. tube rectifier
    ureteral v.
valvula (valvulae)
    v. conniventes
valvular
    v. calcification
    v. heart disease
    v. regurgitation
    v. vegetation
vanadium
van Buchem's endosteal hyper-
    ostosis
Van de Graaff's generator
"vanishing tumor"
variable
variac
Varian CT scanner
variceal
varicella
varices
varicocele
varicose
varicosity
varix (varices)
varus
    cubitus v.
    v. deformity
    hallux v.
    humerus v.
    pes v.

varus *(continued)*
    v. stress film
vas (vasa)
    v. aberrans
    v. deferens
    v. nervorum
    v. vasorum
vascular
    v. calcification
    v. collapse
    v. compression
    v. ectasia
    v. foramen
    v. funnel
    v. groove
    v. hypertension
    v. murmur
    v. occlusion
    v. resistance
    v. ring
    v. sclerosis
    v. sling
    v. system
vascularity
vascularization
vasculature
vasculitis
    hypocomplementemic v.
vasculopathy
Vasiodone
vasoactive
vasoconstriction
vasoconstrictive
vasoconstrictor
vasodilation
vasodilator
vasography
vasomotor

vaso-occlusive
Vasopressin
vasospasm
vasospastic disease
vasovagal
VATER association – *v*ertebral anomalies; *a*norectal malformations, particularly anal atresia; *t*racheoesophageal fistula; *e*sophageal atresia; *r*adial and *r*enal anomalies
Vater's
    ampulla
    papilla
VCUG – voiding cystourethrogram
VDU – video display unit
VE – voluntary effort
vector concept
vegetal
vegetation
    adenoid v.
    bacterial v's
    dendritic v.
    valvular v.
    verrucous v's
vein (*see* Part II, Table of Veins)
velocity
    closing v.
    v. distribution function
Velpeau's axillary view
velum (vela)
    medullary v.
vena (venae)
    v. cava inferior
    v. cava occlusion

vena (venae) *(continued)*
    v. cava superior
venacavogram
venereal
venogram (*see* venography)
venography
    epidural v.
    limb v.
    magnified carotid v.
    mediastinal v.
    peripheral v.
    portal v.
    radionuclide v.
    renal v.
    selective v.
    splenoportal v.
    subtraction v.
venolobar syndrome
venous
    v. sclerosis
    v. shunt
ventilation
    collateral v.
    v.-perfusion imaging
      study
    v.-perfusion nuclear
      medicine study
    pulmonary v.
    v. scan
ventilator
    v.-induced gas
    v.-induced pneumoperi-
      cardium
    v.-induced pneumoperi-
      toneum
    v.-induced pneumo-
      thorax
    v. lung

ventilator *(continued)*
    mechanical v.
    volume-regulated v.
ventrad
ventral
ventricle
    auxiliary v.
    cardiac v.
    cerebral v.
    double-outlet right v.
    laryngeal v.
    lateral v.
    terminal v.
    Verga's v.
ventricular
    v. aneurysm
    v. arrhythmia
    v. canal
    v. fibrillation
    v. flutter
    v. hypertrophy
    v. performance studies
    v. pseudoaneurysm
    v. septal defect
    v. tachycardia
ventriculogram
ventriculography
    radionuclide v.
ventriculoperitoneal
    v. shunt
ventriculoradial
    v. dysplasia
ventrolateral
    v. sclerosis
venule
Verga's ventricle
Veripaque
vermiform

vermis
    cerebellar v.
vermography
verrucous
vertebra (vertebrae)
    abdominal v.
    basilar v.
    biconcave v.
    block v.
    "butterfly" v.
    Calvé's v. plana
    cervical v.
    cleft v.
    coccygeal v.
    "codfish" v.
    cranial v.
    "fish" v.
    "H" v.
    "ivory" v.
    lumbar v.
    occipital v.
    odontoid v.
    v. plana
    v. prominens
    sacral v.
    "sandwich" v.
    thoracic v.
    tricuspid v.
    wedge v.
vertebral
vertebrarium
vertebrobasilar
    v. angiography
    v. arteriogra-
      phy
    v. magnification
    v. system
vertebrochondral

vertebrocostal
vertebrofemoral
vertebromammary
vertebrosacral
vertebrosternal
vertex
vertical
verticomental
verticosubmental
Vesalius
    foramen of V.
vesica (vesicae)
    v. prostatica
    v. urinaria
vesical
vesicle
    auditory v.
    cervical v.
    graafian v.
    multilocular v.
    prostatic v.
    seminal v.
vesicoureteral
    v. reflux
    v. regurgitation
vesiculogram
vesiculography
vessel
    epiphyseal v.
    metaphyseal v.
    thoracodorsal v's
vestibular
vestibule
vestibulocerebellar
vestibulocochlear
vestibulospinal
vestibulum (vestibula)
viability

*Judet (ortho)
view*

vibration

Vibrio

    V. fetus

Victoreen dosimeter

video

    v. disk

    v. disk recorder

    v. display camera

    v. display unit

    v. tape head

    v. tape recorder

    v. tape study

    v. taping

videodensitometric

videodensitometry

videometry

videx

vidicon tube

view

    "ball catcher's" v.

    Chaussé's v.

    comparison v.

    coned-down v.

    decubitus v.

    dorsal v.

    frog-leg v.

    Hampton's v.

    kyphotic v.

    lateral v.

    lateral decubitus v.

    Law's v.

    lordotic v.

    Mayer's v.

    normal anteroposterior v.

    oblique v.

    overcouch v.

    panoramic v.

view *(continued)*

    pantomographic v.

    plantar v.

    posterior v.

    profile ray v.

    recumbent v.

    Runström's v.

    "scottie dog" v.

    scout v.

    skyline v.

    Stenver's v.

    stereoscopic v.

    stress v.

    submentovertical v.

    superoinferior v.

    "swimmer's v."

    tangential v.

    Towne's v.

    Velpeau's axillary v.

    Waters' v.

viewbox

vignetting

villard

villi

villonodular

villous

villus (villi)

Vim-Silverman needle

viral

Virchow's plane

virulent

virus

    respiratory syncytial v.

viscera

visceral

viscerography

visceromegaly

visceroptosis

viscid
viscosity
viscus (viscera)
visual
    v. acuity
    v. center
    v. cortex
    v. pathway
visualization
    double-contrast v.
vitelline
vitiate
vitreous
vocal cord
Vogt's bone free projection
voiding
volar
Volkmann's
    canal
    contracture
volt
Volta's effect
voltage
    v. compensator
    v. drop
    effective v.
    filament v.
    forward biased v.
    full-wave rectified v.
    half-wave rectified v.
    inverse v.

voltage *(continued)*
    v. regulator
    root mean square v.
    saturation v.
    v. waveform
voltammeter
voltmeter
volume
    atomic v.
    "v. averaging"
    molar v.
    tumor v.
volumetry
voluntary
volvulus
    midgut v.
    sigmoid v.
vomer
vomerobasilar
vomeronasal
vomerovaginal
vomit
vomitus
Von Sonnenberg's catheter
voxel – volume element
VSD – ventricular septal
    defect
vulvar
vulvouterine
vulvovaginal

W

W – tungsten
w – watt
wagonwheel fracture
Wagstaffe's fracture
Waldenström's macroglobuli-
    nemia
Walker's
        magnet
        sarcoma
wallstand
        Bucky's w.
Walther's fracture
wandering
        w. kidney
        w. spleen
Warburg's effect
warfarin
        sodium w.
Warthin's tumor
"washboard" effect
washout
        w. pyelography
        w. study
        w. test
"wasp waist" indentation
water
        activated w.
        body w.
        w. path scanning
        w. proton
        w. range
        regional extravascular
            lung w.
        w. retention

water *(continued)*
        w. siphonage test
        w.-soluble agent
        w. system
        total body w.
Waters'
        method
        position
        projection
        view
watt
wattmeter
watt-second
wave
        amplitude w.
        diffraction w's
        electromagnetic w's
        w. forms
        frequency w's
        interference w's
        particle w's
        w.-particle duality
        sine w.
        sound w's
waveform
wavelength
        Compton's w.
        de Broglie's w.
        energy w.
waxy
        w. liver
        w. spleen
web
        esophageal w.

267

web *(continued)*
    laryngeal w.
    tracheal w.
webbed fingers
webbing
"weblike" appearance
wedge
    w. arteriography
    w.-shaped lesion
Wedge's filter
Wegener's
    granuloma
    granulomatosis
Wehlin's method
weight
    atomic w.
    w.-bearing
Welin's technique
well counter
well-defined
Westcott needle
Westmark's sign
wet lung disease
wet-pressure sensitization
"wet" reading
wetting agent
Wharton's duct
Wheatstone's stereoscope
wheeze
    w. and crackle
wheezing
    cardiogenic w.
whiplash
whipworm colitis
whistling face syndrome
white
    w. hot
    w. radiation

whole body
    w. b. counter
    w. b. counting
    w. b. proton magnetic
       resonance imaging
       system
    w. b. scan
    w. b. scanner
    w. b. scanning
wide angle tomography
Wigby-Taylor
    method
    position
Williams'
    elfin facies syndrome
    method
Willis'
    antrum
    circle
Wilms' tumor
Wilson's chamber
Wimberger's sign
Winchester's disc
window
    aorticopulmonary w.
    cochlear w.
    oval w.
    radiation w.
    round w.
    vestibular w.
"windswept hand"
"wineglass" appearance
winged scapula
Winslow
    foramen of W.
wire
    Kirschner's w.
Wirsung's duct

Wisconsin
  W. kV.p test cassette
  W. timing and mA.s
    test tool
WL symphalangism-
  brachydactyly syndrome
wolfram
Wolf's method
"wooden shoe" configuration

Wood's lamp
work function
wormian bones
"wormy" appearance
Wratten's 6B filter
wry neck
WT syndrome
Wuchereria
  W. bancrofti

X

X – reactance
xanthochromic
xanthofibroma
xanthogranuloma
xanthogranulomatous
xanthoma
xanthomatosis
xanthomatous
xanthosarcoma
X axis
Xe – xenon
xenon 127
xenon 133 ventilation
  study
xerg
xerogram
xerography
xeromammography
xeroradiogram
xeroradiograph
xeroradiographic
xeroradiography

xerosialography
xerosis
xerostomia
xerotomography
xiphisternal
xiphisternum
xiphocostal
xiphoid
XL – inductive reactance
XO syndrome
x-ray
  x-r. beam
  x-r. bremsstrahlung
  x-r. characteristic
  x-r. circuit
  x-r. detector
  discrete x-r.
  x-r. emission spectrum
  x-r. energy
  x-r. equipment
  x-r. exposure fog
  x-r. film

x-ray *(continued)*
    x-r. generator
    grid controlled x-r.
    hard x-r.
    x-r. image
    x-r. K-characteristic
    monoenergetic x-r.
    x-r. orthovoltage
    x-r. photon
    x-r. pinhole camera
    polyenergetic x-r.
    x-r. remnant
    soft x-r.
    x-r. spectrometer
    x-r. spectrum

x-ray *(continued)*
    x-r. synchronization
    x-r. therapy
    x-r. tube
    x-r. tube housing
    x-r. tube rating chart
XU – excretory urography
Xu – X-unit
XXX syndrome
XXXX syndrome
XXXXY syndrome
xylene
xylose
    D-x.
xy system
XYY syndrome

y

Y – yttrium
yaws
    y. dactylitis
Y axis
Yb – ytterbium
Yersinia
    Y. enterocolitica

yersiniosis
ytterbium
    y. Yb pentetate sodium
yttrium oxysulfide
"Y" winding

Z

Z –
   atomic number
   impedance
Zanelli's
   method
   position
Zeeman's hamiltonian function
Zenker's diverticulum
zero-field splitting
zero potential
zeugmatography
   Fourier transformation z.
Zimmer's method
zinc
   z. cadmium sulfide
   z. sulfide
Zinn's tendon
zipper (on bone scan)
zirconium (with niobium 95)
Zizmor's method
zonal
zone
   epigastric z.
   focal z.
   hypogastric z.
   Looser's transformation z's
   subcostal z.

zone *(continued)*
   Truemmerfeld's z.
   umbilical z.
zone plate
   Fresnel's z. p.
zonogram
zonography
   stereoscopic z.
"zoom"
   z. lens
   z. reconstruction
zoster
Zuckerkandl's fascia
zwitterion
zygapophyseal
zygapophysis (zygapophyses)
zygion (zygia)
zygodactyly
zygoma
zygomatic
   z. arch
   z. process
zygomaticofacial
zygomaticofrontal
zygomaticomaxillary
zygomatico-orbital
zygomaticosphenoid
zygomaticotemporal
zygomaxillare
zygomaxillary

PART II

ANATOMY

Plates and Tables

Ever since Morgagni formulated and defined the idea of pathologic anatomy, perception of alterations in normal structure and function of the body has become the key to effective diagnosis. Hence this section is devoted to a brief synopsis of fundamental anatomy, for knowledge of vocabulary is essential to the understanding of any of the specialties of bioscience. The plates to follow are used by gracious permission of the authors and publisher of Leeson and Leeson: *Human Structure* (W. B. Saunders, 1972), and the tables are adapted from the Twenty-Third Edition of *Dorland's Pocket Medical Dictionary* (W. B. Saunders, 1982).

PLATE 1 – SKIN AND FASCIA   275

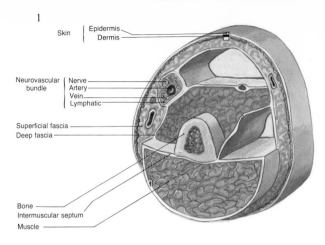

1

Skin { Epidermis
       Dermis

Neurovascular { Nerve
bundle   Artery
                Vein
                Lymphatic

Superficial fascia
Deep fascia

Bone
Intermuscular septum
Muscle

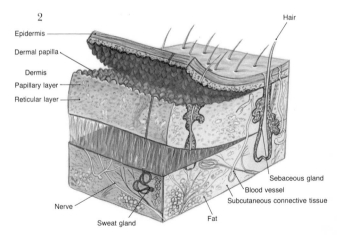

2

Hair

Epidermis

Dermal papilla

Dermis
Papillary layer
Reticular layer

Sebaceous gland
Blood vessel
Subcutaneous connective tissue

Nerve

Sweat gland

Fat

PLATE 1. 1. Diagram of a segment of the upper arm in cross section to show the relationship among skin, superficial fascia and deep fascia. Two muscles have been removed to show the fibro-osseous compartments in which they lie. 2. Diagram of skin and superficial fascia. The tissue has been split to show the slips of fibrous tissue between the dermis and the subcutaneous connective tissue (below) and the dermal papillae at the junction between the epidermis and the dermis (above).

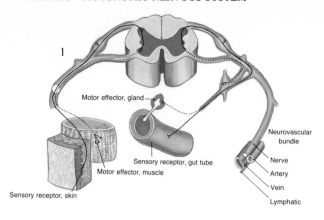

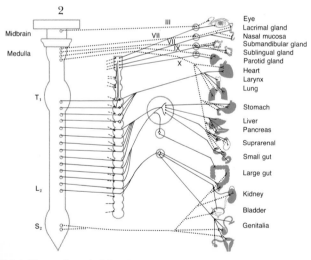

PLATE 2. 1. Diagram of somatic (left) and autonomic (right) reflex arcs. In each, the sensory neuron is illustrated by a solid line with its cell body in the dorsal root ganglion. The connector or internuncial neuron is shown by a dotted line, with its cell body in the posterior horn of grey matter of the spinal cord (somatic) or lateral horn (autonomic), and the motor neuron is shown by a broken line, with its cell body in the anterior horn (somatic) or in a ganglion of the sympathetic trunk (autonomic). 2. Diagram of the general distribution of the autonomic nervous system. Sympathetic fibers are illustrated by solid lines; parasympathetic fibers, by dotted lines.

PLATE 3 – SYMPATHETIC/PARASYMPATHETIC SYSTEMS   277

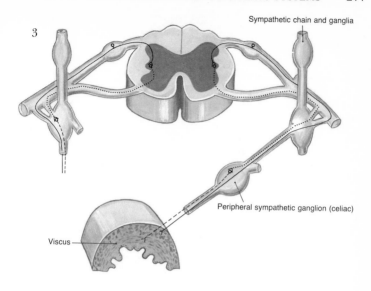

Sympathetic chain and ganglia

3

Peripheral sympathetic ganglion (celiac)

Viscus

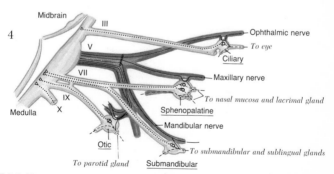

Midbrain

4

III

Ophthalmic nerve

To eye

V

Ciliary

VII

Maxillary nerve

To nasal mucosa and lacrimal gland

IX

Sphenopalatine

Medulla

X

Mandibular nerve

To submandibular and sublingual glands

Otic

To parotid gland   Submandibular

PLATE 3. 3. Diagram of the sympathetic nervous system. Sensory fibers are shown by solid lines; connector neuron fibers, by dotted lines; and motor (postganglionic) fibers, by broken lines. 4. Diagram of the cranial parasympathetic system to show the connections of the four cranial ganglia. Note that only parasympathetic (motor) roots relay in the ganglia.

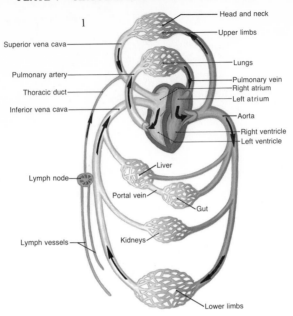

1

Head and neck
Upper limbs
Superior vena cava
Lungs
Pulmonary artery
Pulmonary vein
Thoracic duct
Right atrium
Left atrium
Inferior vena cava
Aorta
Right ventricle
Left ventricle
Liver
Lymph node
Portal vein
Gut
Lymph vessels
Kidneys
Lower limbs

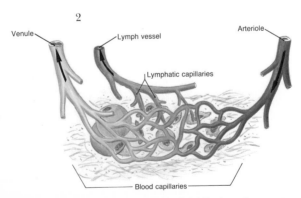

2

Venule
Lymph vessel
Arteriole
Lymphatic capillaries
Blood capillaries

PLATE 4. 1. Diagram of the circulatory system. Darkly shaded blood vessels transport oxygenated blood. 2. Diagrammatic representation of the arrangement of blood and lymphatic capillaries. Note the blind endings of the latter.

PLATE 5 – VERTEBRAL COLUMN   279

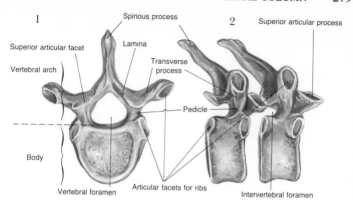

1

Spinous process

Superior articular facet

Vertebral arch

Lamina

Transverse process

Superior articular process

2

Pedicle

Body

Vertebral foramen

Articular facets for ribs

Intervertebral foramen

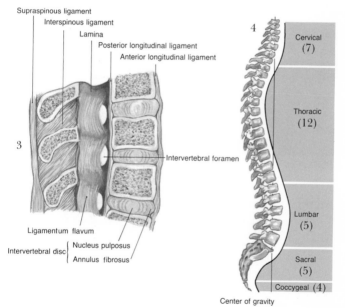

Supraspinous ligament

Interspinous ligament

Lamina

Posterior longitudinal ligament

Anterior longitudinal ligament

3

Intervertebral foramen

Ligamentum flavum

Intervertebral disc { Nucleus pulposus
Annulus fibrosus

4

Cervical (7)

Thoracic (12)

Lumbar (5)

Sacral (5)

Coccygeal (4)

Center of gravity

PLATE 5. Typical vertebra. 1. Superior view. 2. Lateral view. 3. Sagittal section of a part of the vertebral column, showing ligaments and intervertebral discs. 4. Lateral view of vertebral column illustrating curvatures and relative proportions.

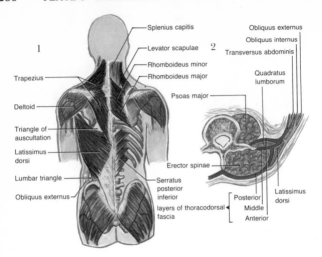

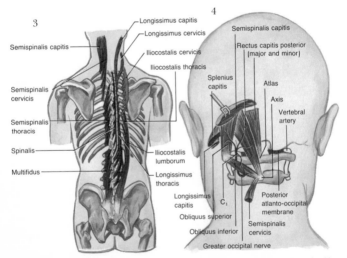

PLATE 6. 1. Diagram of a dissection to display muscles of the back. On the left side, only skin and superficial and deep fasciae have been removed. On the right side, the trapezius and latissimus dorsi have been removed to reveal deeper muscles. 2. A transverse section through the lumbar region to show the components of the thoracodorsal fascia. 3. The deep muscles of the back. On the left, the transversospinalis group; on the right, the erector spinae group. 4. The left suboccipital triangle.

PLATE 7 – THE SKULL   281

1

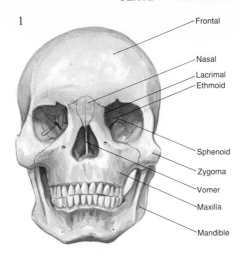

Frontal

Nasal

Lacrimal

Ethmoid

Sphenoid

Zygoma

Vomer

Maxilla

Mandible

2

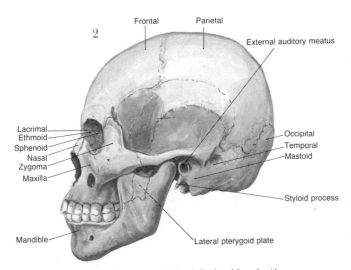

Frontal

Parietal

External auditory meatus

Lacrimal

Ethmoid

Sphenoid

Nasal

Zygoma

Maxilla

Occipital

Temporal

Mastoid

Styloid process

Mandible

Lateral pterygoid plate

PLATE 7. 1. The skull, viewed from the front. 2. The skull, viewed from the side.

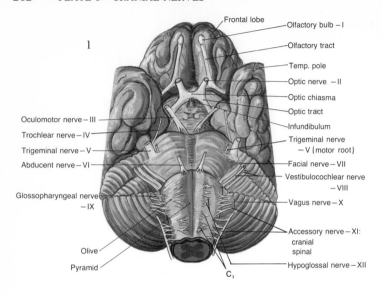

1

Frontal lobe

Olfactory bulb – I

Olfactory tract

Temp. pole

Optic nerve – II

Optic chiasma

Optic tract

Infundibulum

Oculomotor nerve – III

Trochlear nerve – IV

Trigeminal nerve – V

Abducent nerve – VI

Trigeminal nerve
– V (motor root)

Facial nerve – VII

Vestibulocochlear nerve
– VIII

Glossopharyngeal nerve
– IX

Vagus nerve – X

Olive

Pyramid

Accessory nerve – XI:
cranial
spinal

Hypoglossal nerve – XII

C₁

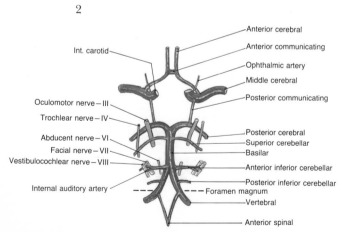

2

Int. carotid

Anterior cerebral

Anterior communicating

Ophthalmic artery

Middle cerebral

Posterior communicating

Oculomotor nerve – III

Trochlear nerve – IV

Abducent nerve – VI

Facial nerve – VII

Vestibulocochlear nerve – VIII

Internal auditory artery

Posterior cerebral

Superior cerebellar

Basilar

Anterior inferior cerebellar

Posterior inferior cerebellar

Foramen magnum

Vertebral

Anterior spinal

PLATE 8. 1. The base of the brain, showing the attachments of the cranial nerves. 2. The arterial supply of the base of the brain. The relationship to some cranial nerves is indicated.

PLATE 9 – THE SCALP AND FACE   283

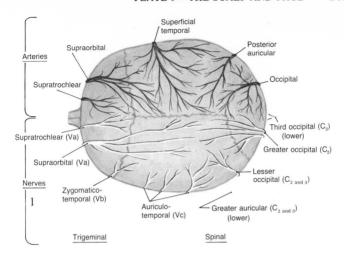

Arteries

- Superficial temporal
- Supraorbital
- Posterior auricular
- Supratrochlear
- Occipital
- Third occipital (C₃) (lower)
- Greater occipital (C₂)

Nerves

- Supratrochlear (Va)
- Supraorbital (Va)
- Zygomatico-temporal (Vb)
- Auriculo-temporal (Vc)
- Lesser occipital (C₂ and 3)
- Greater auricular (C₂ and 3) (lower)

Trigeminal   Spinal

1

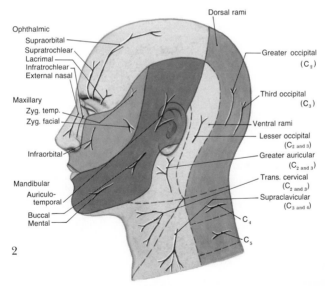

- Dorsal rami
- Ophthalmic
  - Supraorbital
  - Supratrochlear
  - Lacrimal
  - Infratrochlear
  - External nasal
- Maxillary
  - Zyg. temp.
  - Zyg. facial
  - Infraorbital
- Mandibular
  - Auriculo-temporal
  - Buccal
  - Mental
- Greater occipital (C₂)
- Third occipital (C₃)
- Ventral rami
- Lesser occipital (C₂ and 3)
- Greater auricular (C₂ and 3)
- Trans. cervical (C₂ and 3)
- Supraclavicular (C₃ and 4)
- C₄
- C₅

2

PLATE 9. 1. Diagram to illustrate the nervous and arterial supply to the scalp. The origin of the nerves is indicated. Va is the ophthalmic branch of the trigeminal nerve; Vb, the maxillary branch; and Vc, the mandibular branch. 2. Diagram of the sensory nerve supply to the face and neck.

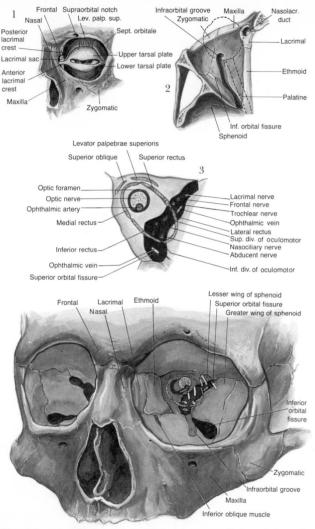

1. Frontal   Supraorbital notch
Nasal
Lev. palp. sup.
Posterior lacrimal crest
Sept. orbitale
Lacrimal sac
Upper tarsal plate
Anterior lacrimal crest
Lower tarsal plate
Maxilla
Zygomatic

2. Infraorbital groove   Maxilla   Nasolacr. duct
Zygomatic
Lacrimal
Ethmoid
Palatine
Inf. orbital fissure
Sphenoid

3. Levator palpebrae superioris
Superior oblique   Superior rectus
Optic foramen
Optic nerve
Ophthalmic artery
Medial rectus
Inferior rectus
Ophthalmic vein
Superior orbital fissure
Lacrimal nerve
Frontal nerve
Trochlear nerve
Ophthalmic vein
Lateral rectus
Sup. div. of oculomotor
Nasociliary nerve
Abducent nerve
Inf. div. of oculomotor

Frontal   Lacrimal   Ethmoid
Nasal
Lesser wing of sphenoid
Superior orbital fissure
Greater wing of sphenoid
Inferior orbital fissure
Zygomatic
Infraorbital groove
Maxilla
Inferior oblique muscle

PLATE 10. 1. Left orbit from front, showing the orbital margin, septum orbitale, tarsal plates and part of the tendon of levator palpebrae superioris. 2. Left bony orbit from above. The eyeball and optic nerve are outlined. 3. Diagram of the left orbit, showing nerves and muscle origins. 4. Diagram to show nerves, vessels and muscle origins at the apex of the left orbit.

PLATE 11 – MUSCLES OF MASTICATION   285

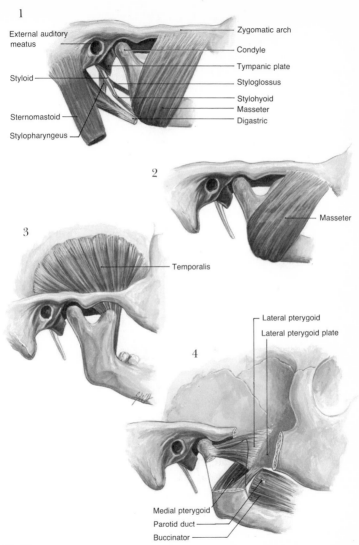

PLATE 11. 1. Diagram to illustrate the parotid bed. 2. Diagram of the masseter muscle. 3. Diagram of temporalis. 4. Diagram of the pterygoid muscles and buccinator.

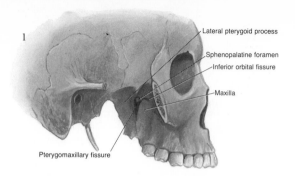

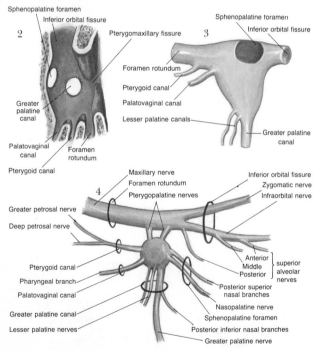

PLATE 12. 1. Lateral view of skull with zygomatic arch removed, showing the pterygopalatine fossa as seen through the pterygomaxillary fissure. 2. Diagrammatic representation of a transverse section through the right pterygopalatine fossa, looking inferiorly. 3. Diagrammatic representation of the right pterygopalatine fossa, as viewed from the lateral side. 4. The right pterygopalatine ganglion and its branches.

PLATE 13 – THE NECK AND ITS TRIANGLES   287

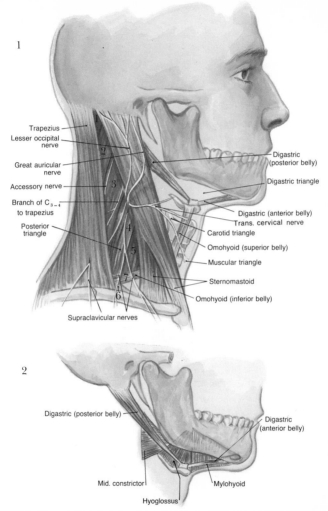

1

- Trapezius
- Lesser occipital nerve
- Great auricular nerve
- Accessory nerve
- Branch of C_{3-4} to trapezius
- Posterior triangle
- Supraclavicular nerves

- Digastric (posterior belly)
- Digastric triangle
- Digastric (anterior belly)
- Trans. cervical nerve
- Carotid triangle
- Omohyoid (superior belly)
- Muscular triangle
- Sternomastoid
- Omohyoid (inferior belly)

2

- Digastric (posterior belly)
- Mid. constrictor
- Hyoglossus
- Digastric (anterior belly)
- Mylohyoid

PLATE 13. 1. Diagram to illustrate the boundaries of the triangles of the neck and details of the posterior triangle. The numbered muscles in the floor of the posterior triangle are: 1, semispinalis capitis; 2, splenius; 3, levator scapulae; 4, scalenus posterior and medius; 5, scalenus anterior; 6, serratus anterior; and 7, inferior belly of omohyoid. 2. Diagram to show the boundaries and floor of the digastric or submandibular triangle.

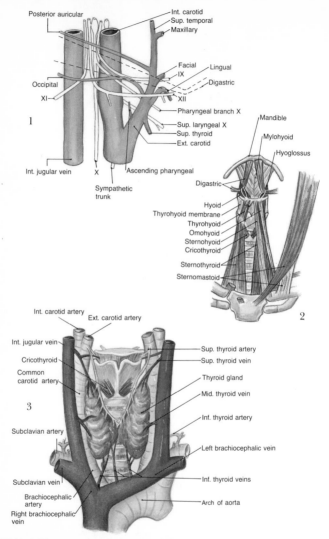

PLATE 14. 1. Diagram to show the branches of the external carotid artery and the relation of nerves. 2. Diagram of the muscular triangle (the anterior region of the neck). 3. Diagram to illustrate the blood supply of the thyroid gland and anterior relationships of the trachea.

PLATE 15 - THE NECK: PREVERTEBRAL REGION   289

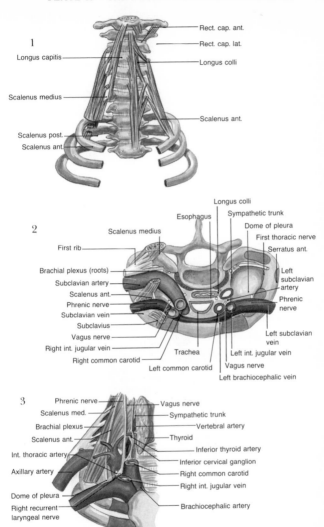

1

Longus capitis

Scalenus medius

Scalenus post.
Scalenus ant.

Rect. cap. ant.
Rect. cap. lat.
Longus colli

Scalenus ant.

2

Longus colli
Esophagus
Sympathetic trunk
Scalenus medius
Dome of pleura
First thoracic nerve
First rib
Serratus ant.
Brachial plexus (roots)
Subclavian artery
Left subclavian artery
Scalenus ant.
Phrenic nerve
Phrenic nerve
Subclavian vein
Subclavius
Vagus nerve
Left subclavian vein
Right int. jugular vein
Trachea
Left int. jugular vein
Right common carotid
Left common carotid
Vagus nerve
Left brachiocephalic vein

3

Phrenic nerve
Vagus nerve
Scalenus med.
Sympathetic trunk
Brachial plexus
Vertebral artery
Scalenus ant.
Thyroid
Int. thoracic artery
Inferior thyroid artery
Axillary artery
Inferior cervical ganglion
Right common carotid
Dome of pleura
Right int. jugular vein
Right recurrent laryngeal nerve
Brachiocephalic artery

PLATE 15. 1. Diagram of the prevertebral and scalene muscles. On the right, scalenus anterior has been removed; on the left, longus capitis. 2. Diagram of a horizontal section at the level of the thoracic inlet. 3. Thoracic inlet and root of neck.

1

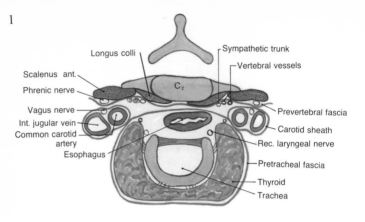

Longus colli

Sympathetic trunk

Vertebral vessels

Scalenus ant.

Phrenic nerve

C₇

Vagus nerve

Prevertebral fascia

Int. jugular vein

Carotid sheath

Common carotid artery

Rec. laryngeal nerve

Esophagus

Pretracheal fascia

Thyroid

Trachea

2

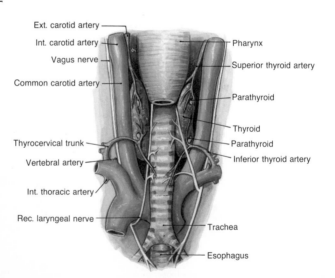

Ext. carotid artery

Int. carotid artery

Pharynx

Vagus nerve

Superior thyroid artery

Common carotid artery

Parathyroid

Thyroid

Thyrocervical trunk

Parathyroid

Vertebral artery

Inferior thyroid artery

Int. thoracic artery

Rec. laryngeal nerve

Trachea

Esophagus

PLATE 16. 1. Diagram of a cross section at the level of C₇ to illustrate relationships of trachea and esophagus. 2. Diagram of the trachea from the posterior aspect.

PLATE 17 – TONGUE AND MOUTH   291

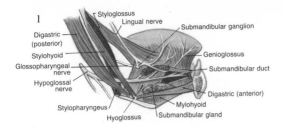

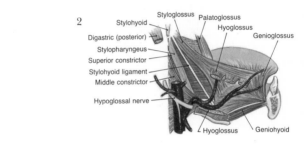

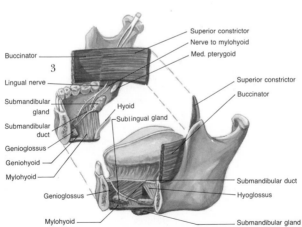

PLATE 17. 1. Diagram of the extrinsic muscles of the tongue with nerves and the submandibular duct shown. 2. Diagram of the extrinsic muscles of the tongue and the lingual artery. The mylohyoid, digastric and stylohyoid muscles and the central part of the hyoglossus have been removed. 3. Diagrams to illustrate the floor of the mouth. Top: The right portion, tongue removed. Bottom: The left portion, tongue intact.

1

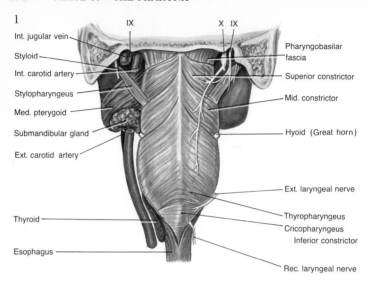

Int. jugular vein
Styloid
Int. carotid artery
Stylopharyngeus
Med. pterygoid
Submandibular gland
Ext. carotid artery

Thyroid

Esophagus

IX   X IX

Pharyngobasilar fascia
Superior constrictor
Mid. constrictor
Hyoid (Great horn)

Ext. laryngeal nerve
Thyropharyngeus
Cricopharyngeus
    Inferior constrictor
Rec. laryngeal nerve

2

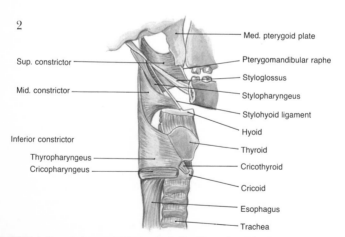

Sup. constrictor
Mid. constrictor

Inferior constrictor
Thyropharyngeus
Cricopharyngeus

Med. pterygoid plate
Pterygomandibular raphe
Styloglossus
Stylopharyngeus
Stylohyoid ligament
Hyoid
Thyroid
Cricothyroid
Cricoid
Esophagus
Trachea

PLATE 18. 1. The posterior aspect of the pharynx. 2. The pharyngeal constrictor muscles from the lateral aspect.

PLATE 19 – THE LARYNX   293

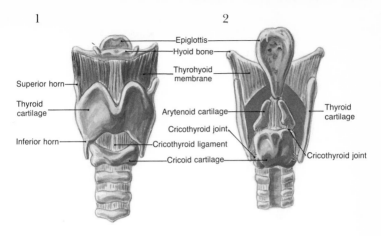

1

- Epiglottis
- Hyoid bone
- Thyrohyoid membrane

Superior horn

Thyroid cartilage

Inferior horn

Arytenoid cartilage

Cricothyroid joint

Cricothyroid ligament

Cricoid cartilage

2

Thyroid cartilage

Cricothyroid joint

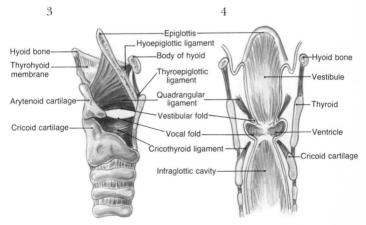

3

Hyoid bone

Thyrohyoid membrane

Arytenoid cartilage

Cricoid cartilage

- Epiglottis
- Hyoepiglottic ligament
- Body of hyoid
- Thyroepiglottic ligament
- Quadrangular ligament
- Vestibular fold
- Vocal fold
- Cricothyroid ligament

Infraglottic cavity

4

Hyoid bone

Vestibule

Thyroid

Ventricle

Cricoid cartilage

PLATE 19. The laryngeal skeleton. 1. Anterior view. 2. Posterior view. 3. Diagrammatic representation of a sagittal section of the larynx to demonstrate the two components of the fibroelastic membrane of the larynx. 4. A coronal section through the larynx and the superior portion of the trachea, illustrating the three divisions of the laryngeal cavity.

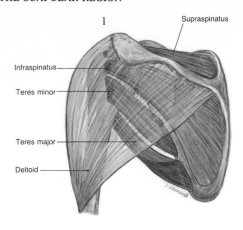

1

Supraspinatus

Infraspinatus

Teres minor

Teres major

Deltoid

2

Suprascapular artery   Deep branch of transverse cervical artery

Supraspinatus tendon

Infraspinatus

Teres minor

Posterior humeral
circumflex artery

Deltoid

Supraspinatus

Infraspinatus

Teres minor

Teres major

Quadrangular space

Circumflex scapular artery

Triangular space

Triceps (long head)

PLATE 20. 1. Intrinsic muscles of the left shoulder, from behind. 2. The anastomoses and intermuscular spaces in relation to the scapula. Dorsal aspect of left shoulder.

PLATE 21 – THE AXILLA; THE BRACHIAL PLEXUS   295

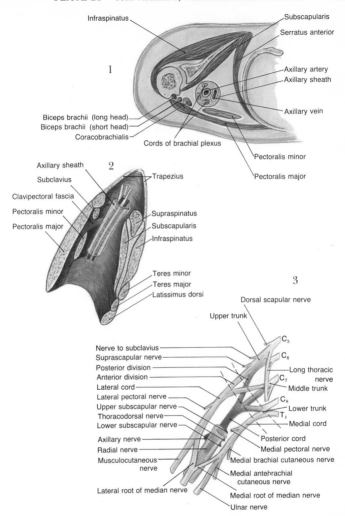

Infraspinatus

Subscapularis

Serratus anterior

1

Axillary artery

Axillary sheath

Axillary vein

Biceps brachii (long head)

Biceps brachii (short head)

Coracobrachialis

Cords of brachial plexus

Pectoralis minor

Pectoralis major

Axillary sheath   2

Trapezius

Subclavius

Clavipectoral fascia

Pectoralis minor

Pectoralis major

Supraspinatus

Subscapularis

Infraspinatus

Teres minor

Teres major

Latissimus dorsi

3

Dorsal scapular nerve

Upper trunk

C_5

C_6

Nerve to subclavius

Suprascapular nerve

Posterior division

Anterior division

Lateral cord

Lateral pectoral nerve

Upper subscapular nerve

Thoracodorsal nerve

Lower subscapular nerve

Axillary nerve

Radial nerve

Musculocutaneous nerve

Lateral root of median nerve

Long thoracic nerve

C_7

Middle trunk

C_8

Lower trunk

T_1

Medial cord

Posterior cord

Medial pectoral nerve

Medial brachial cutaneous nerve

Medial antebrachial cutaneous nerve

Medial root of median nerve

Ulnar nerve

PLATE 21. 1. Cross section through the axilla, to show the boundaries and the contents. The view is toward the base of the right axilla. 2. Schematic vertical section through the axilla to show the anterior and posterior walls and contents. The diagram represents the right axilla as viewed from the medial side. 3. The brachial plexus. Posterior divisions of the plexus and the posterior cord are shown in heavy shading. The approximate level of the clavicle is shown by the interrupted lines and the position of the axillary artery is indicated.

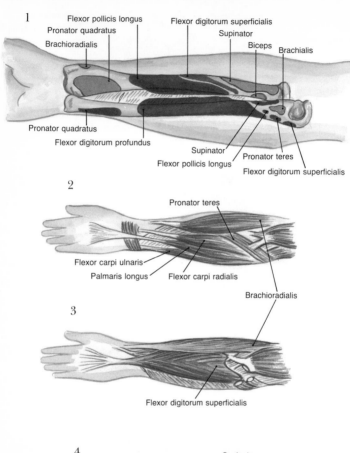

1

Flexor pollicis longus
Pronator quadratus
Brachioradialis

Flexor digitorum superficialis
Supinator
Biceps
Brachialis

Pronator quadratus
Flexor digitorum profundus

Supinator
Flexor pollicis longus
Pronator teres
Flexor digitorum superficialis

2

Pronator teres

Flexor carpi ulnaris
Palmaris longus
Flexor carpi radialis

Brachioradialis

3

Flexor digitorum superficialis

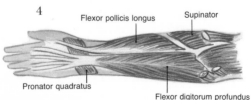

4

Flexor pollicis longus
Supinator

Pronator quadratus
Flexor digitorum profundus

PLATE 22. 1. Anterior view of bones of forearm, showing muscular attachments. Muscles of the anterior compartment. 2. Superficial. 3. Intermediate. 4. Deep.

PLATE 23 – THE FOREARM; POSTERIOR VIEW 297

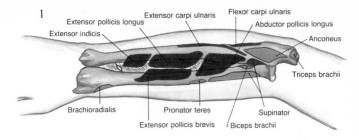

1

Extensor carpi ulnaris
Flexor carpi ulnaris
Extensor pollicis longus
Abductor pollicis longus
Extensor indicis
Anconeus
Triceps brachii
Brachioradialis
Pronator teres
Supinator
Extensor pollicis brevis
Biceps brachii

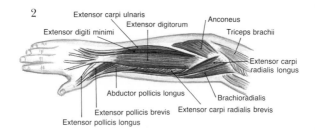

2

Extensor carpi ulnaris
Extensor digitorum
Anconeus
Extensor digiti minimi
Triceps brachii
Extensor carpi radialis longus
Abductor pollicis longus
Brachioradialis
Extensor pollicis brevis
Extensor carpi radialis brevis
Extensor pollicis longus

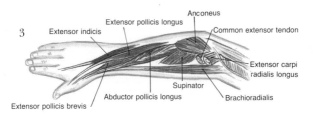

3

Anconeus
Extensor pollicis longus
Common extensor tendon
Extensor indicis
Extensor carpi radialis longus
Supinator
Abductor pollicis longus
Brachioradialis
Extensor pollicis brevis

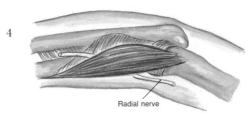

4

Radial nerve

PLATE 23. 1. Posterior view of bones of forearm, showing muscular attachments. 2. Superficial muscles of posterior compartment. 3. Deep muscles of posterior compartment. 4. Supinator muscle.

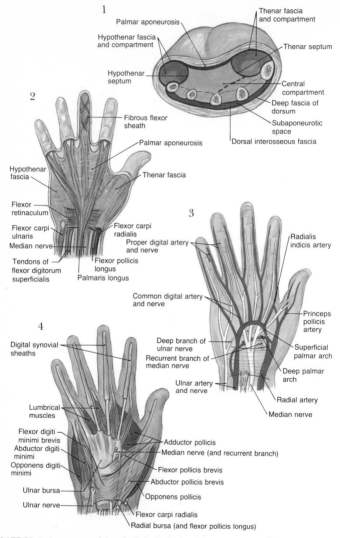

PLATE 24. 1. Arrangement of deep fascia in the hand and the compartments of the palm, as seen in a transverse section. 2. The deep fascia of the palm. 3. The principal nerves and arteries of the palm. 4. The palm of the hand: Thenar and hypothenar muscles, synovial sheaths, and lumbrical muscles.

PLATE 25 – SHOULDER JOINTS   299

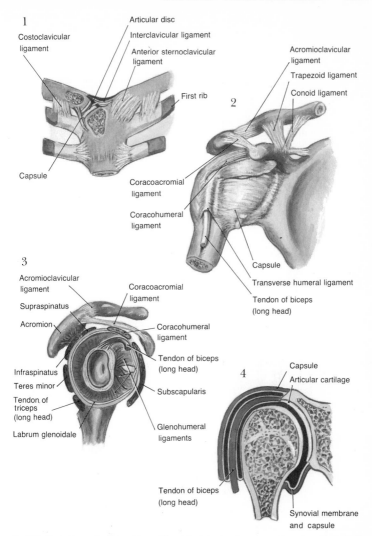

1

Costoclavicular ligament

Articular disc

Interclavicular ligament

Anterior sternoclavicular ligament

First rib

Capsule

Acromioclavicular ligament

Trapezoid ligament

Conoid ligament

2

Coracoacromial ligament

Coracohumeral ligament

Capsule

Transverse humeral ligament

Tendon of biceps (long head)

3

Acromioclavicular ligament

Supraspinatus

Acromion

Infraspinatus

Teres minor

Tendon of triceps (long head)

Labrum glenoidale

Coracoacromial ligament

Coracohumeral ligament

Tendon of biceps (long head)

Subscapularis

Glenohumeral ligaments

Capsule

Articular cartilage

4

Tendon of biceps (long head)

Synovial membrane and capsule

PLATE 25. 1. Sternoclavicular joints. The right joint has been opened to show the articular disc. 2. Acromioclavicular and shoulder joints. The conoid and trapezoid ligaments together form the coracoclavicular ligament. 3. Interior of shoulder joint. 4. Coronal section through shoulder joint. Note the reflections of synovial membrane.

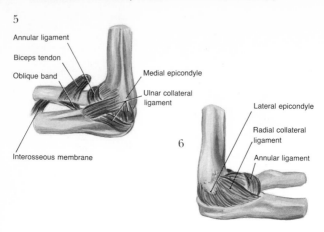

5

Annular ligament

Biceps tendon

Oblique band

Medial epicondyle

Ulnar collateral ligament

Interosseous membrane

6

Lateral epicondyle

Radial collateral ligament

Annular ligament

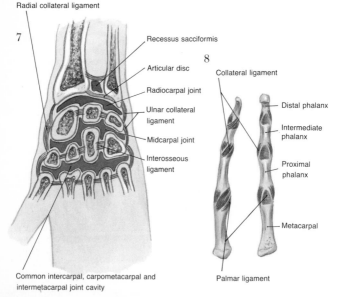

7

Radial collateral ligament

Recessus sacciformis

8

Articular disc

Collateral ligament

Radiocarpal joint

Distal phalanx

Ulnar collateral ligament

Intermediate phalanx

Midcarpal joint

Proximal phalanx

Interosseous ligament

Metacarpal

Common intercarpal, carpometacarpal and intermetacarpal joint cavity

Palmar ligament

PLATE 26. 5. Right elbow joint, viewed from the medial side. 6. Right elbow joint, viewed from the lateral side. 7. Vertical (coronal) section through the right wrist. 8. Metacarpophalangeal and interphalangeal joints.

PLATE 27 – THE THORACIC CAGE   301

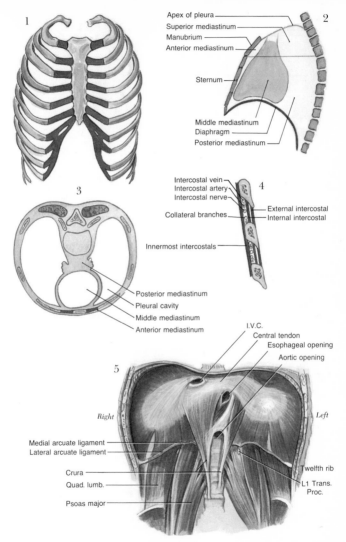

1

2
Apex of pleura
Superior mediastinum
Manubrium
Anterior mediastinum

Sternum

Middle mediastinum
Diaphragm
Posterior mediastinum

3

4
Intercostal vein
Intercostal artery
Intercostal nerve
Collateral branches
External intercostal
Internal intercostal

Innermost intercostals

Posterior mediastinum
Pleural cavity
Middle mediastinum
Anterior mediastinum

I.V.C.
Central tendon
Esophageal opening
Aortic opening

5

Right   *Left*

Medial arcuate ligament
Lateral arcuate ligament

Crura
Quad. lumb.
Psoas major

Twelfth rib
L1 Trans. Proc.

PLATE 27. 1. The thoracic cage. 2. Diagram of a sagittal section of the thorax to show its boundaries and subdivisions. 3. Diagram of a horizontal section of the thorax. 4. Diagram of two intercostal spaces. 5. Diagram of the posterior portion of the diaphragm.

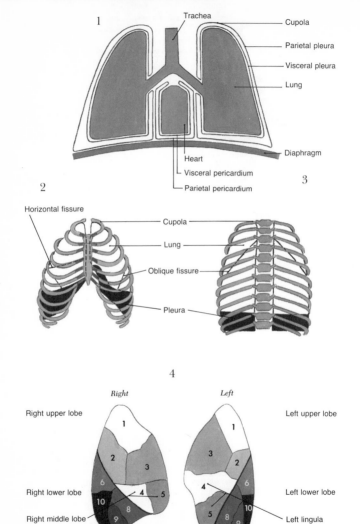

PLATE 28. 1. Diagram to illustrate pleurae and pericardium. 2. Anterior view to show extent of pleurae and lungs. 3. Posterior view to show extent of pleurae and lungs. 4. Anterior view of lungs to show bronchopulmonary segments.

PLATE 29 – LUNGS; BRONCHIAL TREE 303

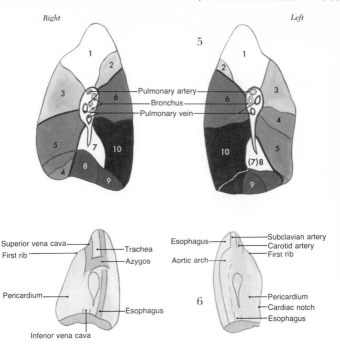

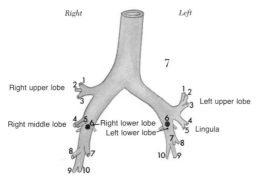

PLATE 29. 5. Medial aspect of lungs. 6. Diagrams to illustrate medial relations of the lungs. 7. Diagram of the bronchial tree.

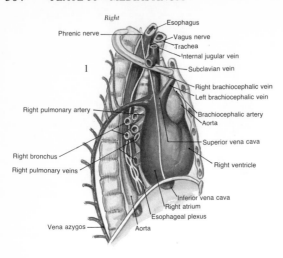

Right

Phrenic nerve
Esophagus
Vagus nerve
Trachea
Internal jugular vein
Subclavian vein

1

Right brachiocephalic vein
Left brachiocephalic vein

Right pulmonary artery

Brachiocephalic artery
Aorta

Superior vena cava

Right bronchus
Right pulmonary veins

Right ventricle

Inferior vena cava
Right atrium
Esophageal plexus

Vena azygos
Aorta

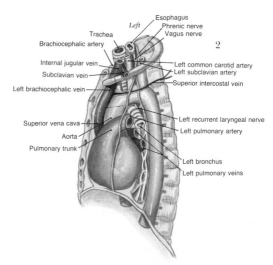

Left
Esophagus
Phrenic nerve
Vagus nerve

Trachea

Brachiocephalic artery

2

Internal jugular vein
Left common carotid artery
Left subclavian artery

Subclavian vein
Superior intercostal vein

Left brachiocephalic vein

Superior vena cava
Left recurrent laryngeal nerve
Left pulmonary artery

Aorta
Pulmonary trunk
Left bronchus
Left pulmonary veins

PLATE 30. 1. Diagram of the right surface of the mediastinum (mediastinal pleura removed). 2. Diagram of the left surface of the mediastinum (mediastinal pleura removed).

PLATE 31 – THE HEART   305

3

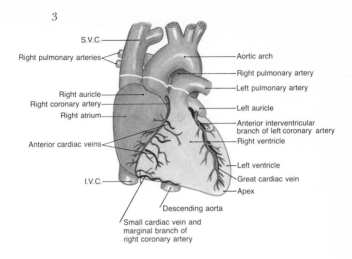

S.V.C.

Right pulmonary arteries

Right auricle
Right coronary artery
Right atrium

Anterior cardiac veins

I.V.C.

Aortic arch
Right pulmonary artery
Left pulmonary artery
Left auricle
Anterior interventricular
branch of left coronary artery
Right ventricle

Left ventricle
Great cardiac vein
Apex

Descending aorta

Small cardiac vein and
marginal branch of
right coronary artery

4

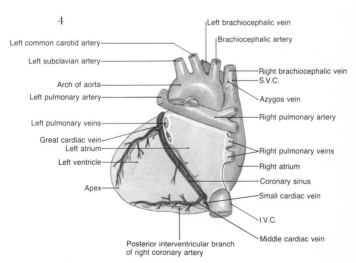

Left common carotid artery

Left subclavian artery

Arch of aorta
Left pulmonary artery

Left pulmonary veins

Great cardiac vein
Left atrium
Left ventricle

Apex

Left brachiocephalic vein
Brachiocephalic artery

Right brachiocephalic vein
S.V.C.

Azygos vein

Right pulmonary artery

Right pulmonary veins

Right atrium
Coronary sinus
Small cardiac vein

I.V.C.

Middle cardiac vein

Posterior interventricular branch
of right coronary artery

PLATE 31. 3. Diagram of the anterior surface of the heart. 4. Diagram of the posterior aspect of the heart.

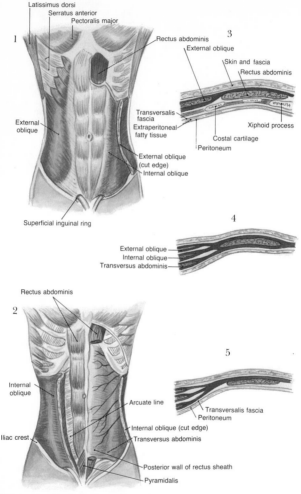

Latissimus dorsi
Serratus anterior
Pectoralis major
Rectus abdominis
External oblique
Skin and fascia
Rectus abdominis
External oblique
Transversalis fascia
Extraperitoneal fatty tissue
Xiphoid process
Costal cartilage
Peritoneum
External oblique (cut edge)
Internal oblique
Superficial inguinal ring

External oblique
Internal oblique
Transversus abdominis

Rectus abdominis
Internal oblique
Arcuate line
Iliac crest
Transversalis fascia
Peritoneum
Internal oblique (cut edge)
Transversus abdominis
Posterior wall of rectus sheath
Pyramidalis

1
2
3
4
5

PLATE 32. Anterior abdominal wall. 1. Skin and fasciae removed on the right side to show the external oblique muscle. The external oblique removed on the left to show the internal oblique. 2. The external oblique removed on the right side and the internal oblique reflected laterally to expose the rectus abdominis muscle. On the left the internal oblique and rectus abdominis have been removed to show the transversus abdominis and the posterior rectus sheath. Transverse sections show the constituents of the rectus sheath at different levels. 3. Above the costal margin. 4. Upper three-quarters of the abdominal wall. 5. Lower one-quarter of the wall.

PLATE 33 – ABDOMINOPELVIC CAVITY   307

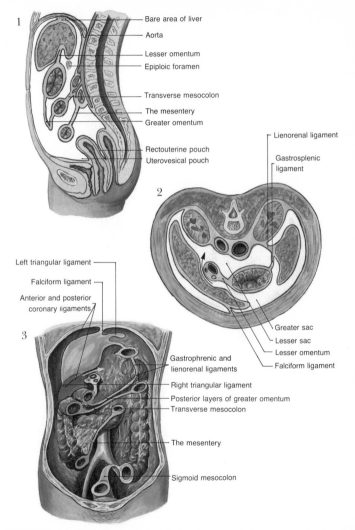

1

Bare area of liver
Aorta
Lesser omentum
Epiploic foramen
Transverse mesocolon
The mesentery
Greater omentum
Rectouterine pouch
Uterovesical pouch

Lienorenal ligament
Gastrosplenic ligament

2

Left triangular ligament
Falciform ligament
Anterior and posterior coronary ligaments

3

Greater sac
Lesser sac
Lesser omentum
Falciform ligament

Gastrophrenic and lienorenal ligaments
Right triangular ligament
Posterior layers of greater omentum
Transverse mesocolon

The mesentery

Sigmoid mesocolon

PLATE 33. 1. A sagittal section through the abdominopelvic cavity. 2. A transverse section through the abdominal cavity at the level of the epiploic foramen. The arrow lies within the epiploic foramen. 3. The posterior abdominal wall, showing the lines of peritoneal reflection. The arrow lies within the epiploic foramen.

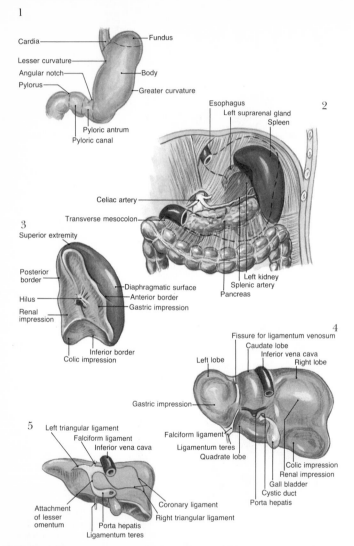

1

Cardia
Fundus
Lesser curvature
Angular notch
Body
Pylorus
Greater curvature
Pyloric antrum
Pyloric canal

2

Esophagus
Left suprarenal gland
Spleen
Celiac artery
Transverse mesocolon
Left kidney
Splenic artery
Pancreas

3

Superior extremity
Posterior border
Diaphragmatic surface
Hilus
Anterior border
Renal impression
Gastric impression
Inferior border
Colic impression

4

Fissure for ligamentum venosum
Caudate lobe
Inferior vena cava
Right lobe
Left lobe
Gastric impression
Falciform ligament
Ligamentum teres
Quadrate lobe
Colic impression
Renal impression
Gall bladder
Cystic duct
Porta hepatis

5

Left triangular ligament
Falciform ligament
Inferior vena cava
Falciform ligament
Attachment of lesser omentum
Coronary ligament
Right triangular ligament
Porta hepatis
Ligamentum teres

PLATE 34. 1. Parts of the stomach. 2. The "stomach bed." 3. The borders and visceral relations of the spleen. 4. Visceral surface of the liver. 5. Posterior view of liver to show peritoneal reflections.

PLATE 35 – DUODENUM AND PANCREAS; BLOOD VESSELS   309

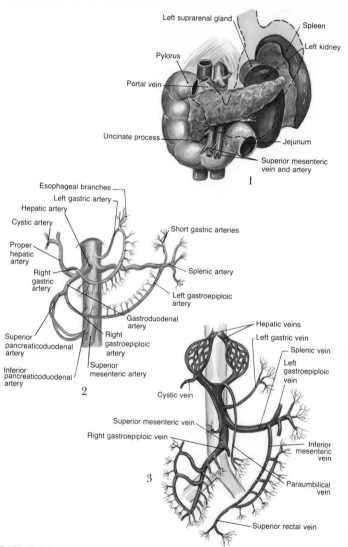

PLATE 35. 1. Duodenum and pancreas. The position of the stomach is indicated in outline. 2. Celiac artery and its branches. 3. Portal vein and its tributaries.

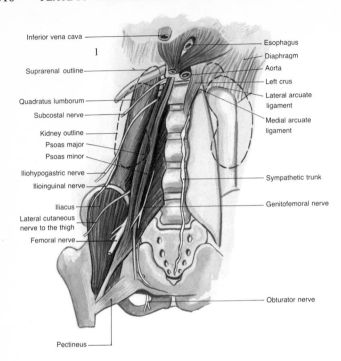

Inferior vena cava

Suprarenal outline

Quadratus lumborum

Subcostal nerve

Kidney outline

Psoas major

Psoas minor

Iliohypogastric nerve

Ilioinguinal nerve

Iliacus

Lateral cutaneous nerve to the thigh

Femoral nerve

Pectineus

Esophagus

Diaphragm

Aorta

Left crus

Lateral arcuate ligament

Medial arcuate ligament

Sympathetic trunk

Genitofemoral nerve

Obturator nerve

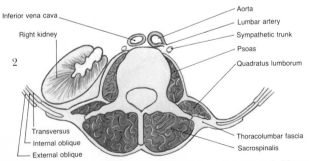

Inferior vena cava

Right kidney

Transversus

Internal oblique

External oblique

Aorta

Lumbar artery

Sympathetic trunk

Psoas

Quadratus lumborum

Thoracolumbar fascia

Sacrospinalis

PLATE 36. 1. Diagram of the muscles and nerves of the posterior abdominal wall. 2. Diagram of a horizontal section through the upper lumbar region to show thoracolumbar (lumbar) fascia.

PLATE 37 – ABDOMINAL WALL: VESSELS/NERVES   311

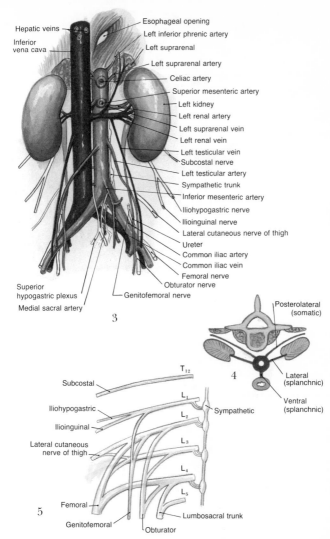

Hepatic veins

Inferior
vena cava

Esophageal opening
Left inferior phrenic artery
Left suprarenal
Left suprarenal artery
Celiac artery
Superior mesenteric artery
Left kidney
Left renal artery
Left suprarenal vein
Left renal vein
Left testicular vein
Subcostal nerve
Left testicular artery
Sympathetic trunk
Inferior mesenteric artery
Iliohypogastric nerve
Ilioinguinal nerve
Lateral cutaneous nerve of thigh
Ureter
Common iliac artery
Common iliac vein
Femoral nerve
Obturator nerve
Genitofemoral nerve

Superior
hypogastric plexus
Medial sacral artery

3

Posterolateral
(somatic)

4

Lateral
(splanchnic)

Ventral
(splanchnic)

Sympathetic

T_{12}

Subcostal

L_1

Iliohypogastric

L_2

Ilioinguinal

L_3

Lateral cutaneous
nerve of thigh

L_4

L_5

5

Femoral

Genitofemoral

Obturator

Lumbosacral trunk

PLATE 37. 3. Diagram of the vessels of the posterior abdominal wall. The positions of the nerves are indicated also. 4. Diagram to illustrate the three main groups of branches of the abdominal aorta. 5. Diagram of the lumbar plexus and the subcostal nerve.

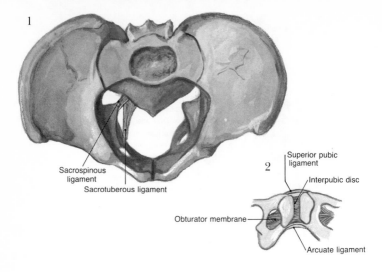

1

Sacrospinous
ligament

Sacrotuberous ligament

2

Superior pubic
ligament

Interpubic disc

Obturator membrane

Arcuate ligament

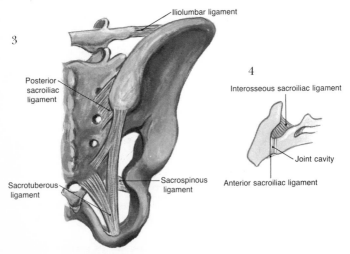

3

Iliolumbar ligament

Posterior
sacroiliac
ligament

Sacrotuberous
ligament

Sacrospinous
ligament

4

Interosseous sacroiliac ligament

Joint cavity

Anterior sacroiliac ligament

PLATE 38. 1. Female pelvis from above. 2. Pubic symphysis. 3. Posterior aspect, sacroiliac joint. 4. Horizontal section through sacroiliac joint.

PLATE 39 – PELVIC VISCERA   313

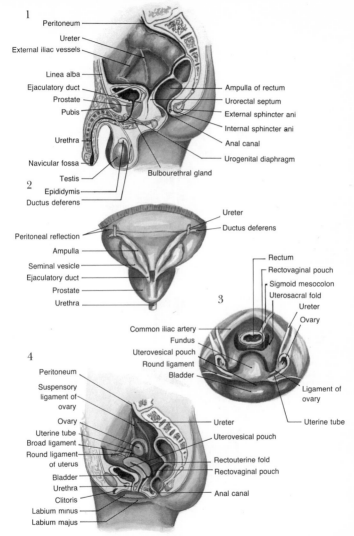

1

Peritoneum
Ureter
External iliac vessels

Linea alba
Ejaculatory duct
Prostate
Pubis

Urethra

Navicular fossa

2
Testis
Epididymis
Ductus deferens

Ampulla of rectum
Urorectal septum
External sphincter ani
Internal sphincter ani
Anal canal
Urogenital diaphragm

Bulbourethral gland

Ureter
Ductus deferens

Peritoneal reflection
Ampulla
Seminal vesicle
Ejaculatory duct
Prostate
Urethra

3

Rectum
Rectovaginal pouch
Sigmoid mesocolon
Uterosacral fold
Ureter
Ovary

Common iliac artery
Fundus
Uterovesical pouch
Round ligament
Bladder

Ligament of ovary

Uterine tube

4
Peritoneum
Suspensory ligament of ovary
Ovary
Uterine tube
Broad ligament
Round ligament of uterus
Bladder
Urethra
Clitoris
Labium minus
Labium majus

Ureter
Uterovesical pouch

Rectouterine fold
Rectovaginal pouch

Anal canal

PLATE 39. 1. Diagram of a midsagittal section of the male pelvis. 2. Diagram of the bladder and associated structures in the male, posterior aspect. 3. Diagram of the female pelvis from above, peritoneum intact. 4. Diagram of a midsagittal section of the female pelvis.

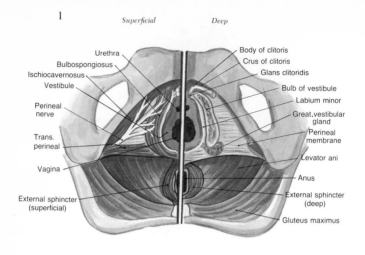

1

Superficial   *Deep*

Urethra
Bulbospongiosus
Ischiocavernosus
Vestibule
Perineal nerve
Trans. perineal
Vagina
External sphincter (superficial)

Body of clitoris
Crus of clitoris
Glans clitoridis
Bulb of vestibule
Labium minor
Great. vestibular gland
Perineal membrane
Levator ani
Anus
External sphincter (deep)
Gluteus maximus

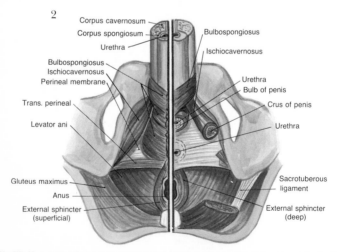

2

Corpus cavernosum
Corpus spongiosum
Urethra
Bulbospongiosus
Ischiocavernosus
Perineal membrane
Trans. perineal
Levator ani
Gluteus maximus
Anus
External sphincter (superficial)

Bulbospongiosus
Ischiocavernosus
Urethra
Bulb of penis
Crus of penis
Urethra
Sacrotuberous ligament
External sphincter (deep)

PLATE 40. 1. Left: Inferior aspect of the female perineum after removal of the skin and fascia. Right: Inferior aspect of the female perineum after removal of some contents of the superficial perineal pouch. 2. Left: Inferior aspect of the male perineum, scrotum removed. Right: Inferior aspect of the male perineum, a deeper dissection.

PLATE 41 – INTERNAL ILIAC ARTERY; SACRAL PLEXUS   315

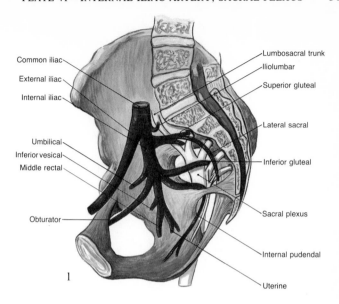

Common iliac
External iliac
Internal iliac

Umbilical
Inferior vesical
Middle rectal

Obturator

Lumbosacral trunk
Iliolumbar
Superior gluteal

Lateral sacral

Inferior gluteal

Sacral plexus

Internal pudendal

Uterine

1

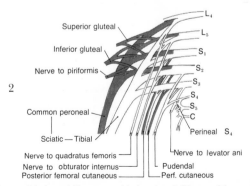

Superior gluteal

Inferior gluteal

Nerve to piriformis

2

Common peroneal

Sciatic — Tibial

Nerve to quadratus femoris
Nerve to obturator internus
Posterior femoral cutaneous

L₄
L₅
S₁
S₂
S₃
S₄
S₅
C
Perineal S₄

Nerve to levator ani

Pudendal
Perf. cutaneous

PLATE 41. 1. Diagram of the internal iliac artery and its branches. 2. Diagram of the sacral plexus.

316   PLATE 42 – GLUTEAL REGION

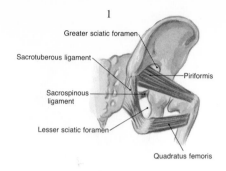

1

Greater sciatic foramen

Sacrotuberous ligament

Sacrospinous
ligament

Lesser sciatic foramen

Piriformis

Quadratus femoris

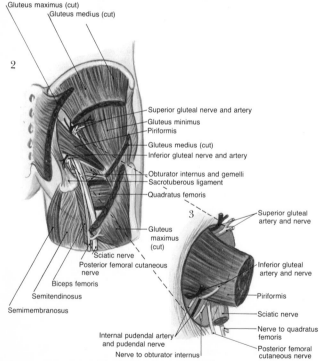

2

Gluteus maximus (cut)
Gluteus medius (cut)

Superior gluteal nerve and artery
Gluteus minimus
Piriformis
Gluteus medius (cut)
Inferior gluteal nerve and artery
Obturator internus and gemelli
Sacrotuberous ligament
Quadratus femoris

3

Superior gluteal
artery and nerve

Inferior gluteal
artery and nerve

Piriformis

Sciatic nerve

Nerve to quadratus
femoris

Posterior femoral
cutaneous nerve

Gluteus
maximus
(cut)

Sciatic nerve
Posterior femoral cutaneous
nerve

Biceps femoris

Semitendinosus

Semimembranosus

Internal pudendal artery
and pudendal nerve
Nerve to obturator internus

PLATE 42. 1. The greater and lesser sciatic foramina and the position of piriformis. 2. The gluteal region. Intermediate portions of gluteus maximus and gluteus medius have been removed. 3. The relationships of structures emerging from the greater sciatic foramen.

PLATE 43 – THE THIGH   317

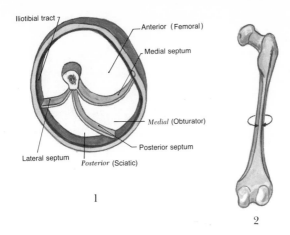

Iliotibial tract

Anterior (Femoral)

Medial septum

Medial (Obturator)

Posterior septum

Lateral septum

Posterior (Sciatic)

1

2

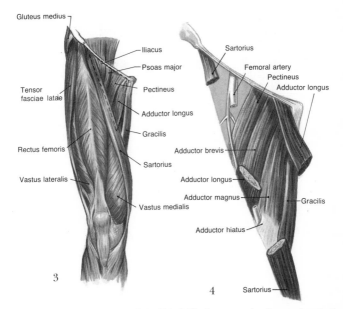

Gluteus medius

Iliacus

Psoas major

Pectineus

Adductor longus

Gracilis

Sartorius

Tensor fasciae latae

Rectus femoris

Vastus lateralis

Vastus medialis

3

Sartorius

Femoral artery

Pectineus

Adductor longus

Adductor brevis

Adductor longus

Adductor magnus

Gracilis

Adductor hiatus

Sartorius

4

PLATE 43. 1. The three compartments of the thigh. 2. The femur, posterior view, to show the linea aspera and its continuations superiorly and inferiorly. 3. Muscles on the front of the thigh. Note the boundaries (outlined) and floor of the femoral triangle. 4. Medial (adductor) compartment of the thigh.

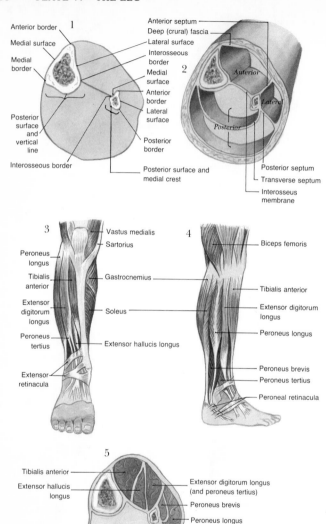

1

Anterior border
Medial surface
Medial border
Posterior surface and vertical line
Interosseous border

2

Anterior septum
Deep (crural) fascia
Lateral surface
Interosseous border
Medial surface
Anterior border
Lateral surface
Posterior border
Posterior surface and medial crest

Anterior
Lateral
Posterior

Posterior septum
Transverse septum
Interosseus membrane

3

Vastus medialis
Sartorius
Peroneus longus
Tibialis anterior
Gastrocnemius
Extensor digitorum longus
Soleus
Peroneus tertius
Extensor hallucis longus
Extensor retinacula

4

Biceps femoris
Tibialis anterior
Extensor digitorum longus
Peroneus longus
Peroneus brevis
Peroneus tertius
Peroneal retinacula

5

Tibialis anterior
Extensor hallucis longus
Extensor digitorum longus (and peroneus tertius)
Peroneus brevis
Peroneus longus

PLATE 44. 1. Transverse section of the leg to illustrate borders and surfaces of the tibia and fibula. 2. Compartments of the leg. 3. Muscles of anterior compartment. 4. Muscles of lateral compartment. 5. Transverse section of leg showing muscles of anterior and lateral compartments.

PLATE 45 – THE FOOT   319

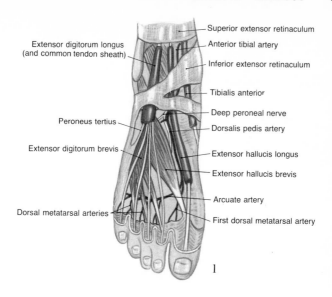

Superior extensor retinaculum
Anterior tibial artery
Extensor digitorum longus (and common tendon sheath)
Inferior extensor retinaculum
Tibialis anterior
Deep peroneal nerve
Peroneus tertius
Dorsalis pedis artery
Extensor digitorum brevis
Extensor hallucis longus
Extensor hallucis brevis
Arcuate artery
Dorsal metatarsal arteries
First dorsal metatarsal artery

1

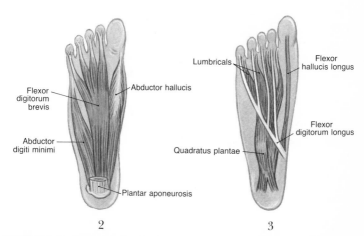

Lumbricals
Flexor hallucis longus
Flexor digitorum brevis
Abductor hallucis
Abductor digiti minimi
Flexor digitorum longus
Quadratus plantae
Plantar aponeurosis

2   3

PLATE 45. 1. The dorsum of the foot. Muscles of the sole of the foot: 2. First layer. 3. Second layer.

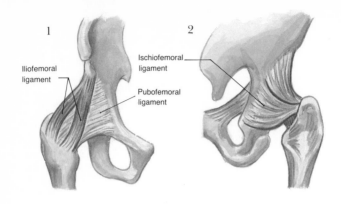

1

Iliofemoral
ligament

2

Ischiofemoral
ligament

Pubofemoral
ligament

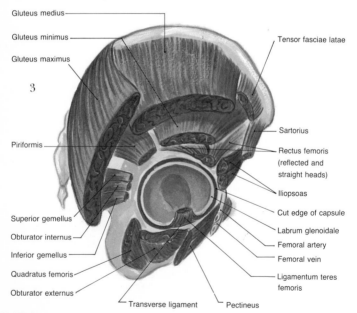

Gluteus medius

Gluteus minimus

Gluteus maximus

3

Piriformis

Superior gemellus

Obturator internus

Inferior gemellus

Quadratus femoris

Obturator externus

Transverse ligament

Pectineus

Tensor fasciae latae

Sartorius

Rectus femoris
(reflected and
straight heads)

Iliopsoas

Cut edge of capsule

Labrum glenoidale

Femoral artery

Femoral vein

Ligamentum teres
femoris

PLATE 46. 1. Hip joint, anterior view. 2. Hip joint, posterior view. 3. Diagrammatic representation of the right hip joint, viewed from the lateral side after disarticulation and removal of the femur. Note the muscular relationships.

PLATE 47 – KNEE JOINT 321

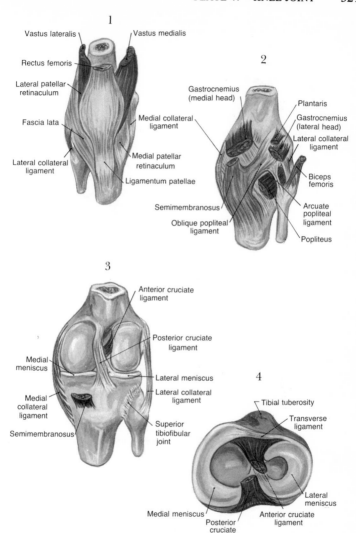

1

Vastus lateralis

Vastus medialis

Rectus femoris

Lateral patellar retinaculum

Fascia lata

Lateral collateral ligament

Medial collateral ligament

Medial patellar retinaculum

Ligamentum patellae

2

Gastrocnemius (medial head)

Plantaris

Gastrocnemius (lateral head)

Lateral collateral ligament

Biceps femoris

Arcuate popliteal ligament

Popliteus

Semimembranosus

Oblique popliteal ligament

3

Anterior cruciate ligament

Posterior cruciate ligament

Medial meniscus

Lateral meniscus

Medial collateral ligament

Lateral collateral ligament

Semimembranosus

Superior tibiofibular joint

4

Tibial tuberosity

Transverse ligament

Lateral meniscus

Medial meniscus

Posterior cruciate ligament

Anterior cruciate ligament

PLATE 47. The knee joint. 1. Anterior view. 2. Posterior view. 3. Posterior view after removal of capsule, to show menisci and cruciate ligaments. 4. Upper end of tibia, showing menisci and inferior attachments of cruciate ligaments.

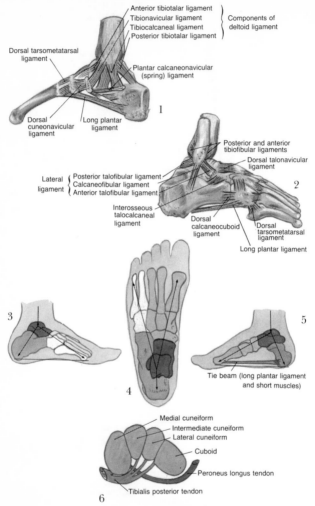

PLATE 48. Ligaments of the ankle and foot: 1. Medial view. 2. Lateral view. Arches of the foot: 3. Lateral view of longitudinal arch. 4. Dorsal view of longitudinal arch. The talus (dark shading) is the keystone. The posterior pillar is the calcaneus (medium shading). The anterior pillar is in two columns: the medial column (light shading) is formed by the navicular, the three cuneiforms and the medial three metatarsals; the lateral column (unshaded) is formed by the cuboid and the lateral two metatarsals. 5. Medial view of longitudinal arch. 6. Transverse arch at the level of the distal row of tarsal bones.

T A B L E   O F   A R T E R I E S

Common Name	Origin	Branches
alveolar a's, anterior, superior (aa. alveolares superiores anteriores)	infraorbital a.	dental branches
alveolar a., inferior (a. alveolaris inferior)	maxillary a.	dental, mylohyoid branches, mental a.
alveolar a., posterior, superior (a. alveolaris superior posterior)	maxillary a.	dental branches
angular a. (a. angularis)	facial a.	
aorta (aorta) abdominal aorta (aorta abdominalis)	left ventricle lower portion of descending aorta, from aortic hiatus of diaphragm	inferior phrenic, lumbar, median sacral, superior and inferior mesenteric, middle suprarenal, renal, and testicular or ovarian a's, celiac trunk
arch of aorta (arcus aortae)	continuation of ascending aorta	brachiocephalic trunk, left common carotid and left subclavian a's; continues as descending thoracic aorta
ascending aorta (aorta ascendens)	proximal portion of aorta, arising from left ventricle	right and left coronary a's
thoracic aorta (aorta thoracica)	continuation from arch of aorta to aortic hiatus of diaphragm	bronchial, esophageal, pericardiac, and mediastinal branches, superior phrenic a's, posterior intercostal a's, subcostal a's, continues as abdominal aorta

NOTES: After the common or anglicized names are given in parentheses the official NA equivalents. In the table the following abbreviations are used: a. = artery; a's = arteries; a. [L] = arteria; aa. [L] = arteriae.

Table continued on following page

T A B L E   O F   A R T E R I E S   --   continued

Common Name	Origin	Branches
appendicular a. (a. appendicularis)	ileocolic a.	dorsal metatarsal a's
arcuate a. of foot (a. arcuata pedis)	dorsal artery of foot	
arcuate a's of kidney (aa. arcuatae renis)	interlobar a.	interlobar a's, arterioles of kidney
auricular a., deep (a. auricularis profunda)	maxillary a.	temporomandibular branch
auricular a., posterior (a. auricularis posterior)	external carotid a.	auricular and occipital branches, stylomastoid a.
axillary a. (a. axillaris)	continuation of subclavian a.	subscapular branches, highest thoracic, thoracoacromial, lateral thoracic, subscapular, and anterior and posterior circumflex humeral a's
basilar a. (a. basilaris)	from junction of right and left vertebral a's	pontine branches, anterior inferior cerebellar, labyrinthine, superior cerebellar, posterior cerebral a's
brachial a. (a. brachialis)	continuation of axillary a. at distal margin of tendon	deep brachial, nutrient of humerus, superior and inferior ulnar collateral, radial, ulnar a's
brachial a., deep (a. profunda brachii)	brachial a.	nutrient of humerus, deltoid branch, middle and radial collateral a's
brachial a., superficial (a. brachialis superficialis)	variant brachial a.	see brachial a.
brachiocephalic trunk (truncus brachiocephalicus)	arch of aorta	right common carotid, right subclavian a's

TABLE OF ARTERIES - continued

Common Name	Origin	Branches
buccal a. (a. buccalis)	maxillary a.	
a. of bulb of penis (a. bulbi penis)	internal pudendal a.	
a. of bulb of vaginal vestibule (a. bulbi vestibuli vaginae)	internal pudendal a.	
carotid a., common (a. carotis communis)	brachiocephalic trunk (right), arch of aorta (left)	external and internal carotid a's
carotid a., external (a. carotis externa)	common carotid a.	superior thyroid, ascending pharyngeal, lingual, facial, occipital, posterior auricular, superficial temporal, maxillary a's
carotid a., internal (a. carotis interna)	common carotid a.	caroticotympanic branches, ophthalmic, posterior communicating, anterior choroid, anterior cerebral, middle cerebral a's
celiac trunk (truncus celiacus)	abdominal aorta	left gastric, common hepatic, splenic a's
central a. of retina (a. centralis retinae)	ophthalmic a.	
cerebellar a., inferior, anterior (a. cerebelli inferior anterior)	basilar a.	a. of labyrinth
cerebellar a., inferior, posterior (a. cerebelli inferior posterior)	vertebral a.	
cerebellar a., superior (a. cerebelli superior)	basilar a.	
cerebral a., anterior (a. cerebri anterior)	internal carotid a.	cortical, anterior choroidal, and central branches and anterior communicating a.

Table continued on following page

T A B L E   O F   A R T E R I E S -- continued

Common Name	Origin	Branches
cerebral a., middle (a. cerebri media)	internal carotid a.	cortical and central branches
cerebral a., posterior (a. cerebri posterior)	terminal bifurcation of basilar a.	cortical, central, and choroid branches
cervical a., ascending (a. cervicalis ascendens)	inferior thyroid a.	spinal branches
cervical a., deep (a. cervicalis profunda)	costocervical trunk	
cervical a., transverse (a. transversa colli)	subclavian a.	deep and superficial branches
choroid a., anterior (a. choroidea anterior)	internal carotid or middle cerebral a.	
ciliary a's, anterior (aa. ciliares anteriores)	ophthalmic and lacrimal a's	episcleral and anterior conjunctival a's
ciliary a's, posterior, long (aa. ciliares posteriores longae)	ophthalmic a.	
ciliary a's, posterior, short (aa. ciliares posteriores breves)	ophthalmic a.	
circumflex femoral a., lateral (a. circumflexa femoris lateralis)	deep femoral a.	ascending, descending, and transverse branches
circumflex femoral a., medial (a. circumflexa femoris medialis)	deep femoral a.	deep, ascending, transverse, and acetabular branches
circumflex humeral a., anterior (a. circumflexa humeri anterior)	axillary a.	

TABLE OF ARTERIES -- continued

Common Name	Origin	Branches
circumflex humeral a., posterior (a. circumflexa humeri posterior)	axillary a.	ascending branches
circumflex iliac a., deep (a. circumflexa ilium profunda)	external iliac a.	
circumflex iliac a., superficial (a. circumflexa ilium superficialis)	femoral a.	
circumflex a. of scapula (a. circumflexa scapulae)	subscapular a.	
colic a., left (a. colica sinistra)	inferior mesenteric a.	
colic a., middle (a. colica media)	superior mesenteric a.	
colic a., right (a. colica dextra)	superior mesenteric a.	
collateral a., middle (a. collateralis media)	deep brachial a.	
collateral a., radial (a. collateralis radialis)	deep brachial a.	
collateral a., ulnar, inferior (a. collateralis ulnaris inferior)	brachial a.	
collateral a., ulnar, superior (a. collateralis ulnaris superior)	brachial a.	
communicating a., of cerebrum, anterior (a. communicans anterior cerebri)	interconnects anterior cerebral a's	
communicating a., of cerebrum, posterior (a. communicans posterior cerebri)	interconnects internal carotid and posterior cerebral a's	

Table continued on following page

TABLE OF ARTERIES -- continued

Common Name	Origin	Branches
conjunctival a's, anterior (aa. conjunctivales anteriores)	anterior ciliary a's	
conjunctival a's, posterior (aa. conjunctivales posteriores)	medial palpebral a.	
coronary a., left (a. coronaria sinistra)	left aortic sinus	anterior interventricular and circumflex branches
coronary a., right (a. coronaria dextra)	right aortic sinus	posterior interventricular branch
costocervical trunk (truncus costo-cervicalis)	subclavian a.	deep cervical and highest intercostal a's
cremasteric a. (a. cremasterica)	inferior epigastric a.	
cystic a. (a. cystica)	right branch of hepatic a.	
deep a. of clitoris (a. profunda clitoridis)	internal pudendal a.	
deep a. of penis (a. profunda penis)	internal pudendal a.	
digital a's of foot, dorsal (aa. digitales dorsales pedis)	dorsal metatarsal a's	
digital a's of hand, dorsal (aa. digitales dorsales manus)	dorsal metacarpal a's	
digital a's, palmar, common (aa. digitales palmares communes)	superficial palmar arch	proper palmar digital a's
digital a's, palmar, proper (aa. digitales palmares propriae)	common palmar digital a's	
digital a's, plantar, common (aa. digitales plantares communes)	plantar metatarsal a's	proper plantar digital a's

TABLE OF ARTERIES -- continued

Common Name	Origin	Branches
digital a's, plantar, proper (aa. digitales plantares propriae)	common plantar digital a's	
dorsal a. of clitoris (a. dorsalis clitoridis)	internal pudendal a.	
dorsal a. of nose (a. dorsalis nasi)	ophthalmic a.	lacrimal branch
dorsal a. of penis (a. dorsalis penis)	internal pudendal a.	
dorsalis pedis a. (a. dorsalis pedis)	continuation of anterior tibial a.	lateral and medial tarsal, and arcuate a's
a. of ductus deferens (a. ductus deferentis)	umbilical a.	ureteral a.
epigastric a., inferior (a. epigastrica inferior)	external iliac a.	pubic branch, cremasteric a., a. of round ligament of uterus
epigastric a., superficial (a. epigastrica superficialis)	femoral a.	
epigastric a., superior (a. epigastrica superior)	internal thoracic a.	
episcleral a's (aa. episclerales)	anterior ciliary a.	
ethmoidal a., anterior (a. ethmoidalis anterior)	ophthalmic a.	anterior meningeal a.
ethmoidal a., posterior (a. ethmoidalis posterior)	ophthalmic a.	
facial a. (a. facialis)	external carotid a.	ascending palatine, submental, inferior and superior labial and angular a's; tonsillar and glandular branches

Table continued on following page

T A B L E   O F   A R T E R I E S -- continued

Common Name	Origin	Branches
facial a., transverse (a. transversa faciei)	superficial temporal a.	
femoral a. (a. femoralis)	continuation of external iliac a.	superficial epigastric, superficial circumflex iliac, external pudendal, deep femoral, and descending genicular a's
femoral a., deep (a. profunda femoris)	femoral a.	medial and lateral circumflex femoral a's, perforating a's
gastric a., left (a. gastrica sinistra)	celiac trunk	esophageal branches
gastric a., right (a. gastrica dextra)	common hepatic a.	
gastric a's, short (aa. gastricae breves)	splenic a.	
gastroduodenal a. (a. gastro-duodenalis)	common hepatic a.	superior pancreaticoduodenal and right gastroepiploic a's
gastroepiploic a., left (a. gastro-epiploica sinistra)	splenic a.	epiploic branches
gastroepiploic a., right (a. gastro-epiploica dextra)	gastroduodenal a.	epiploic branches
genicular a., descending (a. genus descendens)	femoral a.	saphenous and articular branches
genicular a., inferior, lateral (a. genus inferior lateralis)	popliteal a.	
genicular a., inferior, medial (a. genus inferior medialis)	popliteal a.	

TABLE OF ARTERIES -- continued

Common Name	Origin	Branches
genicular a., middle (a. genus media)	popliteal a.	
genicular a., superior, lateral (a. genus superior lateralis)	popliteal a.	
genicular a., superior, medial (a. genus superior medialis)	popliteal a.	
gluteal a., inferior (a. glutea inferior)	internal iliac a.	sciatic a.
gluteal a., superior (a. glutea superior)	internal iliac a.	superficial and deep branches
helicine a's of penis (a. helicinae penis)	deep and dorsal a's of penis	
hepatic a., common (a. hepatica communis)	celiac trunk	right gastric, gastroduodenal, proper hepatic a's
hepatic a., proper (a. hepatica propria)	common hepatic a.	right and left hepatic branches
hyaloid a. (a. hyaloidea)	fetal ophthalmic a.	
ileal a's (aa. ilei)	superior mesenteric a.	
ileocolic a. (a. ileocolica)	superior mesenteric a.	ascending, anterior, and posterior cecal branches, appendicular a.
iliac a., common (a. iliaca communis)	abdominal aorta	internal and external iliac a's
iliac a., external (a. iliaca externa)	common iliac a.	inferior epigastric, circumflex iliac a's
iliac a., internal (a. iliaca interna)	continuation of common iliac a.	iliolumbar, obturator, superior and inferior gluteal, umbilical, inferior vesical, uterine, middle rectal, and internal pudendal a's

Table continued on following page

T A B L E   O F   A R T E R I E S   --   continued

Common Name	Origin	Branches
iliolumbar a. (a. iliolumbalis)	internal iliac a.	iliac and lumbar branches, lateral sacral a's
infraorbital a. (a. infraorbitalis)	maxillary a.	anterior superior alveolar a's
intercostal a., highest (a. intercostalis suprema)	costocervical trunk	posterior intercostal a's
intercostal a's, posterior (aa. intercostalis posteriores)	thoracic artery	collateral, intercostal, muscular, cutaneous, and mammary branches
interlobar a's of kidney (aa. interlobares renis)	renal a.	arcuate a's of kidney
interlobular a's of kidney (aa. interlobulares renis)	arcuate a's of kidney	
interlobular a's of liver (aa. interlobulares hepatis)	right or left branch of proper hepatic a.	
interosseous a., anterior (a. interossea anterior)	posterior or common interosseous a.	median a.
interosseous a., common (a. interossea communis)	ulnar a.	anterior and posterior interosseous a's
interosseous a., posterior (a. interossea posterior)	common interosseous a.	recurrent interosseous a.
interosseous a., recurrent (a. interossea recurrens)	posterior or common interosseous a.	
intestinal a's (aa. intestinales)	mesenteric, pancreaticoduodenal, jejunal, ileal, ileocolic, and colic a's	

TABLE OF ARTERIES -- continued

Common Name	Origin	Branches
jejunal a's (aa. jejunales)	superior mesenteric a.	
labial a., inferior (a. labialis inferior)	facial a.	
labial a., superior (a. labialis superior)	facial a.	septal and alar branches
a. of labyrinth (a. labyrinthi)	basilar or anterior inferior cerebellar a.	vestibular and cochlear branches
lacrimal a. (a. lacrimalis)	ophthalmic a.	lateral palpebral a.
laryngeal a., inferior (a. laryngea inferior)	inferior thyroid a.	
laryngeal a., superior (a. laryngea superior)	superior thyroid a.	
lingual a. (a. lingualis)	external carotid a.	suprahyoid, dorsal lingual, and deep lingual branches
lumbar a's (aa. lumbales)	abdominal aorta	dorsal and spinal branches
lumbar a., lowest (a. lumbalis ima)	median sacral a.	
malleolar a., anterior, lateral (a. malleolaris anterior lateralis)	anterior tibial a.	
malleolar a., anterior, medial (a. malleolaris anterior medialis)	anterior tibial a.	
masseteric a. (a. masseterica)	maxillary a.	
maxillary a. (a. maxillaris)	external carotid a.	deep auricular, anterior tympanic, inferior alveolar, middle meningeal, masseteric, deep temporal, buccal, and sphenopalatine a's

Table continued on following page

TABLE OF ARTERIES -- continued

Common Name	Origin	Branches
median a. (a. mediana)	anterior interosseous a.	
meningeal a., anterior (a. meninges anterior)	anterior ethmoidal a.	
meningeal a., middle (a. meningea media)	maxillary a.	accessory meningeal and petrous branches, and superior tympanic a.
meningeal a., posterior (a. meningea posterior)	ascending pharyngeal a.	
mental a. (a. mentalis)	inferior alveolar a.	
mesenteric a., inferior (a. mesenterica inferior)	abdominal aorta	left colic, sigmoid, and superior rectal a's
mesenteric a., superior (a. mesenterica superior)	abdominal aorta	inferior pancreaticoduodenal, jejunal, ileal, ileocolic, right and middle colic a's
metacarpal a's, dorsal (aa. metacarpeae dorsales)	radial a.	dorsal digital a's
metacarpal a's, palmar (aa. metacarpeae palmares)	deep palmar arch	
metatarsal a's, dorsal (aa. metatarseae dorsales)	arcuate a. of foot	dorsal digital a's
metatarsal a's, plantar (aa. metatarseae plantares)	plantar arch	perforating branches, common and proper plantar digital a's
musculophrenic a. (a. musculophrenica)	internal thoracic a.	anterior, intercostal, phrenic and muscular branches

TABLE OF ARTERIES -- continued

Common Name	Origin	Branches
nasal a's, posterior, lateral and septal (aa. nasales posteriores laterales et septi)	sphenopalatine a.	
nutrient a's of humerus (aa. nutriciae humeri)	brachial and deep brachial a's	
obturator a. (a. obturatoria)	internal iliac a.	pubic, acetabular, anterior and posterior branches
occipital a. (a. occipitalis)	external carotid a.	auricular, meningeal, mastoid, descending, occipital, and sternocleidomastoid branches
ophthalmic a. (a. ophthalmica)	internal carotid a.	lacrimal and supraorbital a's, central a. of retina, ciliary, ethmoidal, palpebral, supratrochlear, and dorsal nasal a's
ovarian a. (a. ovarica)	abdominal aorta	
palatine a., ascending (a. palatina ascendens)	facial a.	ureteral branches
palatine a., descending (a. palatina descendens)	maxillary a.	greater and lesser palatine a's
palatine a., greater (a. palatina major)	descending palatine a.	
palatine a's, lesser (aa. palatinae minores)	descending palatine a.	
palpebral a's, lateral (aa. palpebrales laterales)	lacrimal a.	

Table continued on following page

TABLE OF ARTERIES -- continued

Common Name	Origin	Branches
palpebral a's, medial (aa. palpebrales mediales)	ophthalmic a.	posterior conjunctival a's
pancreaticoduodenal a's, inferior (aa. pancreaticoduodenales inferiores)	superior mesenteric a.	
pancreaticoduodenal a., superior (a. pancreaticoduodenalis superior)	gastroduodenal a.	
perforating a's (aa. perforantes)	deep femoral a.	
pericardiacophrenic a. (a. pericardiacophrenica)	internal thoracic a.	
perineal a. (a. perinealis)	internal pudendal a.	
peroneal a. (a. peronea)	posterior tibial a.	perforating, communicating, calcaneal, and malleolar branches
pharyngeal a., ascending (a. pharyngea ascendens)	external carotid a.	posterior meningeal, pharyngeal, inferior tympanic branches
phrenic a's, inferior (aa. phrenicae inferiores)	abdominal aorta	superior suprarenal a's
phrenic a's, superior (aa. phrenicae superiores)	thoracic aorta	
plantar a., lateral (a. plantaris lateralis)	posterior tibial a.	plantar arch, plantar metatarsal a's
plantar a., medial (a. plantaris medialis)	posterior tibial a.	deep and superficial branches
popliteal a. (a. poplitea)	continuation of femoral a.	lateral and medial superior genicular, middle genicular, sural, lateral and medial inferior genicular, anterior and posterior tibial a's

T A B L E   O F   A R T E R I E S   --   continued

Common Name	Origin	Branches
princeps pollicis a. (a. princeps pollicis)	radial a.	radial index a.
profunda linguae a. (a. profunda linguae)	lingual a.	
a. of pterygoid canal (a. canalis pterygoidei)	maxillary a.	
pudendal a's, external (aa. pudendae externae)	femoral a.	anterior scrotal or anterior labial branches
pudendal a., internal (a. pudenda interna)	internal iliac a.	posterior scrotal or posterior labial branches, inferior rectal, perineal, urethral a's, a. of bulb of penis or vestibule, deep a. and dorsal a. of penis or clitoris
pulmonary trunk (truncus pulmonalis)	right ventricle	right and left pulmonary a's
pulmonary a., left (a. pulmonalis sinistra)	pulmonary trunk	numerous branches named according to segments of lung to which they distribute unaerated blood
pulmonary a., right (a. pulmonalis dextra)	pulmonary trunk	numerous branches named according to segments of lung to which they distribute unaerated blood
radial a. (a. radialis)	brachial a.	palmar carpal, superficial palmar and dorsal carpal branches; recurrent radial a., princeps pollicis a.
radialis indicis a. (a. radialis indicis)	princeps pollicis a.	
rectal a., inferior (a. rectalis inferior)	internal pudendal a.	

Table continued on following page

T A B L E   O F   A R T E R I E S -- continued

Common Name	Origin	Branches
rectal a., middle (a. rectalis media)	internal iliac a.	
rectal a., superior (a. rectalis superior)	inferior mesenteric a.	
recurrent a., radial (a. recurrens radialis)	radial a.	
recurrent a., tibial, anterior (a. recurrens tibialis anterior)	anterior tibial a.	
recurrent a., tibial, posterior (a. recurrens tibialis posterior)	anterior tibial a.	
recurrent a., ulnar (a. recurrens ulnaris)	ulnar a.	anterior and posterior branches
renal a. (a. renalis)	abdominal aorta	ureteral branches, inferior suprarenal a.
a. of round ligament of uterus (a. ligamenti teretis uteri)	inferior epigastric a.	
sacral a's, lateral (aa. sacrales laterales)	iliolumbar a.	spinal branches
sacral a., median (a. sacralis mediana)	central continuation of abdominal aorta	lowest lumbar a.
sciatic a. (a. comitans nervi ischiadici)	inferior gluteal a.	
sigmoid a's (aa. sigmoideae)	inferior mesenteric a.	
sphenopalatine a. (a. sphenopalatina)	maxillary a.	lateral and septal posterior nasal a's
spinal a., anterior (a. spinalis anterior)	vertebral a.	

TABLE OF ARTERIES -- continued

Common Name	Origin	Branches
spinal a., posterior (a. spinalis posterior)	vertebral a.	
splenic a. (a. lienalis)	celiac trunk	pancreatic and splenic branches, left gastroepiploic, short gastric a's
stylomastoid a. (a. stylomastoidea)	posterior auricular a.	mastoid and stapedial branches, posterior tympanic a.
subclavian a. (a. subclavia)	brachiocephalic trunk	vertebral, internal thoracic a's, thyro-cervical and costocervical trunks
subcostal a. (a. subcostalis)	thoracic aorta	dorsal and spinal branches
sublingual a. (a. sublingualis)	lingual a.	
submental a. (a. submentalis)	facial a.	
subscapular a. (a. subscapularis)	axillary a.	thoracodorsal and circumflex scapular a's
supraorbital a. (a. supraorbitalis)	ophthalmic a.	
suprarenal a., inferior (a. suprarenalis inferior)	renal a.	
suprarenal a., middle (a. suprarenalis media)	abdominal aorta	
suprarenal a's, superior (aa. supra-renales superiores)	inferior phrenic a.	
suprascapular a. (a. suprascapularis)	thyrocervical trunk	acromial branch
supratrochlear a. (a. supratrochlearis)	ophthalmic a.	
sural a's (aa. surales)	popliteal a.	

Table continued on following page

TABLE OF ARTERIES -- continued

Common Name	Origin	Branches
tarsal a., lateral (a. tarsea lateralis)	dorsal artery of foot	
tarsal a's, medial (aa. tarseae mediales)	dorsal artery of foot	
temporal a's, deep (aa. temporales profundae)	maxillary a.	
temporal a., middle (a. temporalis media)	superficial temporal a.	
temporal a., superficial (a. temporalis superficialis)	external carotid a.	parotid, anterior auricular, frontal and parietal branches; transverse facial, zygomaticoorbital, middle temporal a's
testicular a. (a. testicularis)	abdominal aorta	ureteral branches
thoracic a., highest (a. thoracica suprema)	axillary a.	
thoracic a., internal (a. thoracica interna)	subclavian a.	mediastinal, thymic, bronchial, sternal, perforating, lateral costal and anterior intercostal branches; pericardiacophrenic, musculophrenic, superior epigastric a's
thoracic a., lateral (a. thoracica lateralis)	axillary a.	mammary branches
thoracoacromial a. (a. thoracoacromialis)	axillary a.	clavicular, pectoral, deltoid, and acromial branches
thoracodorsal a. (a. thoracodorsalis)	subscapular a.	
thyrocervical trunk (truncus thyrocervicalis)	subclavian a.	inferior thyroid, suprascapular and transverse cervical a's

T A B L E   O F   A R T E R I E S   --   continued

Common Name	Origin	Branches
thyroid a., inferior (a. thyroidea inferior)	thyrocervical trunk	pharyngeal, esophageal, tracheal branches; inferior laryngeal, ascending cervical a's
thyroid a., superior (a. thyroidea superior)	external carotid a.	hyoid, sternocleidomastoid, superior laryngeal, cricothyroid, muscular, and glandular branches
thyroidea ima a. (a. thyroidea ima)	arch of aorta, brachiocephalic trunk	
tibial a., anterior (a. tibialis anterior)	popliteal a.	anterior tibial recurrent a's, lateral and medial anterior malleolar a's
tibial a., posterior (a. tibialis posterior)	popliteal a.	fibular circumflex branch; peroneal, medial plantar, lateral plantar a's
tympanic a., anterior (a. tympanica anterior)	maxillary a.	
tympanic a., inferior (a. tympanica inferior)	ascending pharyngeal a.	
tympanic a., posterior (a. tympanica posterior)	stylomastoid a.	
tympanic a., superior (a. tympanica superior)	middle meningeal a.	
ulnar a. (a. ulnaris)	brachial a.	palmar carpal, dorsal carpal, and deep palmar branches; ulnar recurrent and common interosseous a's; superficial palmar arch

Table continued on following page

TABLE OF ARTERIES -- continued

Common Name	Origin	Branches
umbilical a. (a. umbilicalis)	internal iliac a.	a. of spermatic duct, superior vesical a's
urethral a. (a. urethralis)	internal pudendal a.	
uterine a. (a. uterina)	internal iliac a.	ovarian and tubal branches; vaginal a.
vaginal a. (a. vaginalis)	uterine a.	
vertebral a. (a. vertebralis)	subclavian a.	spinal and meningeal branches; posterior inferior cerebellar, basilar, anterior, and posterior spinal a's
vesical a., inferior (a. vesicalis inferior)	internal iliac a.	
vesical a's, superior (aa. vesicales superiores)	umbilical a.	
zygomaticoorbital a. (a. zygomaticoorbitalis)	superficial temporal a.	

TABLE OF BONES

Name	Region	Description	Articulation With
atlas (atlas)	neck	first cervical vertebra	occipital b. and axis
axis (axis)	neck	second cervical vertebra	atlas above and third cervical vertebra below
calcaneus (calcaneus)	foot	largest of the tarsal bones	talus and cuboid b.
capitate b. (o. capitatum)	wrist	largest of the carpal b's	second, third, and fourth metacarpal b's, and lunate, trapezoid, and scaphoid b's
carpal b's (oss. carpi)	wrist	eight b's arranged in two rows	
clavicle (clavicula)	shoulder	elongated, curved bone lying horizontally at root of neck	sternum, scapula and cartilage of first rib
coccyx (o. coccygis)	lower back	triangular bone formed by fusion of last 4 rudimentary vertebrae	sacrum
concha, inferior nasal (concha nasalis inferior)	skull	thin, rough plate of bone attached by one edge to side of each nasal cavity	ethmoid and palatine b's and maxilla
cuboid b. (o. cuboideum)	foot	pyramidal bone, on lateral side of foot	calcaneus, lateral cuneiform b., fourth and fifth metatarsal b's
cuneiform b., intermediate (o. cuneiforme intermedium)	foot	smallest of 3 cuneiform b's, located between medial and lateral cuneiform b's	navicular, medial and lateral cuneiform b's, and second metatarsal b.
cuneiform b., lateral (o. cuneiforme laterale)	foot	intermediate-sized bone at lateral side of foot	cuboid, navicular, intermediate cuneiform b's and second, third, and fourth metatarsal b's

NOTES: After the common or anglicized name appears its NA equivalent in parentheses. In the table the following abbreviations are used: b. = bone; b's = bones; o. = os [L]; oss. = ossa [L].

Table continued on following page

TABLE OF BONES -- continued

Name	Region	Description	Articulation With
cuneiform b., medial (o. cuneiforme mediale)	foot	largest of 3 cuneiform b's, at medial side of foot	navicular, intermediate cuneiform, and first and second metatarsal b's
ethmoid b. (o. ethmoidale)	skull	unpaired bone forming part of nasal septum and superior and medial conchae of nose	sphenoid and frontal b's, vomer, and both lacrimal, nasal, and palatine b's, maxillae, and inferior nasal conchae
fabella (fabella)	knee	sesamoid b. in lateral head of gastrocnemius muscle	femur
femur (femur)	thigh	longest, strongest, heaviest bone of the body	hip b., distally with patella and tibia
fibula (fibula)	leg	lateral b. of leg	tibia, distally with tibia and talus
frontal b. (o. frontale)	skull	constituting anterior part of skull	ethmoid and sphenoid b's, and both parietal, nasal, lacrimal, and zygomatic b's
hamate b. (o. hamatum)	wrist	most medial of 4 bones of distal row of carpal b's	metacarpal, lunate, capitate, and triquetral b's
hip b. (o. coxae)	pelvis and hip	broadest bone of skeleton forming the greater part of the pelvis	femur, anteriorly with its fellow, posteriorly with sacrum
humerus (humerus)	arm	long bone of upper arm	scapula, radius and ulna b's
hyoid b. (o. hyoideum)	neck	U-shaped bone at root of tongue, between mandible and larynx	none; attached by ligaments and muscles to skull
ilium (o. ilium)	pelvis	broad expanded part of hip bone	sacrum, femur, ischium, pubis
incus (incus)	ear	middle ossicle of chain in the middle ear	malleus and stapes

TABLE OF BONES -- continued

Name	Region	Description	Articulation With
ischium (o. ischii)	pelvis	interior and dorsal part of hip bone	
lacrimal b. (o. lacrimale)	skull	thin, fragile bone near rim of medial wall of each orbit	ethmoid and frontal b's
lunate b. (o. lunatum)	wrist	one of 4 bones of proximal row of carpus	radius, and capitate, hamate, scaphoid, and triquetral b's
malleus (malleus)	ear	most lateral ossicle of chain in middle ear	incus; fibrous attachment to tympanic membrane
mandible (mandibula)	lower jaw	horseshoe-shaped bone carrying lower teeth	temporal b's
maxilla (maxilla)	upper jaw	paired large bone, carrying upper teeth	ethmoid, frontal vomer, fellow maxilla b's and ipsilateral inferior nasal concha and lacrimal, nasal, palatine, and zygomatic b's
metacarpal b's (oss. metacarpalia)	hand	five miniature long bones of hand proper, slightly concave on palmar surface, each consisting of a body and two extremities	first: trapezium and proximal phalanx of thumb; second: third metacarpal b., trapezium, trapezoid, capitate, and proximal phalanx of index finger; third: second and fourth metacarpal b's, capitate and proximal phalanx of middle finger; fourth: third and fifth metacarpal b's, capitate, hamate, and proximal phalanx of ring finger; fifth: fourth metacarpal b., hamate b. and proximal phalanx of little finger

Table continued on following page

TABLE OF BONES -- continued

Name	Region	Description	Articulation With
metatarsal b's (oss. metatarsalia)	foot	five miniature long bones of foot, concave on plantar and slightly convex on dorsal surface, each consisting of a body and two extremities	first: medial cuneiform b., proximal phalanx of great toe, and occasionally with second metatarsal b.; second: intermediate, and lateral cuneiform b's, third and occasionally with first metatarsal b., and proximal phalanx of second toe; third: lateral cuneiform b., second and fourth metatarsal b's and proximal phalanx of third toe; fourth: lateral cuneiform b., cuboid b., third and fifth metatarsal b's, and proximal phalanx of fourth toe; fifth: cuboid b., fourth metatarsal b., and proximal phalanx of fifth toe
nasal b. (o. nasale)	skull	paired bone, the two uniting to form bridge of nose	frontal and ethmoid b's, fellow of opposite side, and ipsilateral maxilla
navicular b. (o. naviculare)	foot	bone at medial side of tarsus, between talus and cuneiform b's	talus and 3 cuneiform b's, occasionally with cuboid b.
occipital b. (o. occipitale)	skull	bone forming posterior part of cranium	sphenoid b. and atlas and both parietal and temporal b's
palatine b. (o. palatinum)	skull	paired bone, the two forming posterior portion of hard palate and lateral wall of nasal cavity	ethmoid and sphenoid b's, vomer, fellow of opposite side, and ipsilateral inferior nasal concha and maxilla
parietal b. (o. parietale)	skull	paired bone between frontal and occipital b's, forming sides and roof of cranium	frontal, occipital, sphenoid, fellow parietal, and ipsilateral temporal b's
patella (patella)	knee	small, irregularly rectangular compressed bone over kneecap	femur

T A B L E   O F   B O N E S   --   continued

Name	Region	Description	Articulation With
phalanges of foot (oss. digitorum pedis)	toes	miniature long bones, two only in great toe, three in each of the other toes	proximal phalanx of each digit with corresponding metacarpal or metatarsal b., and phalanx distal to it
phalanges of hand (oss. digitorum manus)	hand	miniature long bones, two only in thumb, three in each of the other fingers	proximal phalanx of each digit with corresponding metacarpal or metatarsal b., and phalanx distal to it
pisiform b. (o. pisiforme)	wrist	medial and palmar of 4 bones of proximal row of carpal b's	triquetral b.
pubic b. (o. pubis)	pelvis	anterior portion of hip bone	ilium, ischium, femur
radius (radius)	forearm	lateral and shorter of 2 bones of forearm	proximally with humerus and ulna; distally with ulna and lunate and scaphoid b's
ribs (costae)	chest	12 pairs of thin, narrow, curved long bones, forming posterior and lateral walls of chest	all posteriorly with thoracic vertebrae; upper 7 pairs with sternum; lower 5 pairs by costal cartilages, with rib above or unattached anteriorly
sacrum (o. sacrum)	lower back	wedge-shaped bone formed usually by fusion of 5 vertebrae below lumbar vertebrae, constituting posterior wall of pelvis	fifth lumbar vertebra above, coccyx below, and with ilium at each side
scaphoid (o. scaphoideum)	wrist	most lateral of 4 bones of proximal row of carpal b's	radius, trapezium, and trapezoid, capitate and lunate b's
scapula (scapula)	shoulder	wide, thin, triangular bone opposite second to seventh ribs in upper part of back	ipsilateral clavicle and humerus

Table continued on following page

T A B L E   O F   B O N E S   -- continued

Name	Region	Description	Articulation With
sesamoid b's (oss. sesa-moidea)	extremities	small, flat, round bones related to joints between phalanges or between digits and metacarpal or metatarsal b's; including also 2 at knee (fabella and patella)	
sphenoid b. (o. sphenoidale)	base of skull	unpaired, irregularly shaped bone, constituting part of sides and base of skull and part of lateral wall of orbit	frontal, occipital, and ethmoid b's, vomer and both parietal, temporal, palatine, and zygomatic b's
stapes (stapes)	ear	most medial ossicle of chain in middle ear	incus; ligamentous attachment to the window of inner ear
sternum (sternum)	chest	elongated flat bone, forming anterior wall of chest	both clavicles and upper 7 pairs of ribs
talus (talus)	ankle	the "ankle bone," second largest of tarsal b's	tibia, fibula, calcaneus, and navicular b.
tarsal b's (oss. tarsi)	foot	the 7 bones of the instep	
temporal b. (o. temporale)	skull	irregularly shaped bone, one on either side, forming part of side and base of skull, and containing middle and inner ear	occipital, sphenoid, mandible, and ipsilateral parietal and zygomatic b's
tibia (tibia)	leg	medial and larger of 2 bones of lower leg	proximally with femur and fibula, distally with talus and fibula
trapezium (o. trapezium)	wrist	most lateral of 4 bones of distal carpal b's	first and second metacarpal b's and trapezoid and scaphoid b's
trapezoid b. (o. trapezoideum)	wrist	second from thumb side of 4 bones of distal row of carpal b's	second metacarpal b. and capitate, trapezium, and scaphoid b's

TABLE OF BONES -- continued

Name	Region	Description	Articulation With
triquetral b. (o. tri- quetrum)	wrist	third from thumb side of 4 bones of proximal row of carpal b's	hamate, lunate, and pisiform b's and articular disk
ulna (ulna)	forearm	medial and longer of 2 bones of forearm	proximally with humerus and radius, distally with radius and articular disk
vertebrae, cervical (vertebrae cervicales)	back of neck	7 segments of the vertebral column -- smallest of the true vertebrae	first with skull, all others with adjoining vertebrae
vertebrae, lumbar (vertebrae lumbales)	lower back	5 segments of the vertebral column, the largest bones of the movable portion of the column	adjoining vertebrae, fifth with sacrum
vertebrae, thoracic (vertebrae thoracicae)	back	12 segments of the vertebral column	adjoining vertebrae, heads of ribs and tubercles of ribs
vomer (vomer)	skull	thin bone forming posterior and posteroinferior part of nasal septum	ethmoid and sphenoid b's and both maxillae and palatine b's
zygomatic b. (o. zygo- maticum)	skull	bone forming hard part of cheek and lower, lateral aspects of orbit	frontal and sphenoid b's and ipsilateral maxilla and temporal b.

TABLE OF LIGAMENTS

Common Name	NA Designation	Description
accessory l.		any ligament that strengthens or supports another, especially one on the lateral surface of a joint
acromioclavicular l.	l. acromioclaviculare	ligament extending from the acromion process to the scapula of the clavicle
alar l's	ligg. alaria	rounded cords connecting the second vertebra to the skull
alar l's of knee	plicae alares	folds of the synovial membrane of the knee
alveolodental l.		periodontal ligament
annular l's	ligg. anularia	any ligaments encircling a structure
apical odontoid l.	l. apicis dentis axis	ligament extending from the apex of the odontoid process to the anterior margin of the foramen magnum
arcuate l's	ligg. arcuata	the arched ligaments connecting the dia-phragm with the lowest ribs and the first lumbar vertebra

NOTES: The following abbreviations are used: l. = ligament; l's = ligaments; l. [L] = ligamentum; ligg. [L] = ligamenta. The word "process" in the table is used to mean any prominence extending from an anatomic structure, usually for attachment of ligaments or muscles.

TABLE OF LIGAMENTS -- continued

Common Name	NA Designation	Description
arcuate l., median	l. arcuatum mediale	ligament between the crura of the diaphragm
arcuate l. of pubis	l. arcuatum pubis	a thick band of fibers situated along the inferior margin of the symphysis pubis
Barkow's l's		anterior and posterior ligaments of the elbow joint
Bérard's l.		the suspensory ligament of the pericardium
Bertin's l. or Bigelow's l.	l. iliofemorale	fibers forming the upper and anterior portion of the capsular ligament of the hip joint
Botallo's l.	l. arteriosum	fibromuscular cord extending from the pulmonary artery to the aortic arch
Bourgery's l.	l. popliteum obliquum	a band of fibers extending from the medial condyle of the tibia across the back of the knee joint to the epicondyle of the femur
broad l. of uterus	l. latum uteri	a broad fold of peritoneum supporting the uterus
Brodie's l.		transverse humeral ligament
Burns' l.	margo falciformis hiatus saphenus	falciform process
Campbell's l.		suspensory ligament of axilla
Camper's l.	diaphragma urogenitale	urogenital diaphragm
capsular l.	capsula articularis	the fibrous membrane of a joint capsule

Table continued on following page

T A B L E   O F   L I G A M E N T S -- continued

Common Name	NA Designation	Description
cardinal l.		a thickening of the visceral pelvic fascia beside the cervix and vagina
Colles' l.	l. inguinale reflexum	a triangular band of fibers arising from the lacunar ligament and pubic bone and passing to the linea alba
conoid l.	l. conoideum	the posteromedial portion of the coraco-clavicular ligament
Cooper's suspensory l's	ligg. suspensoria mammae	pectineal ligaments
coracoclavicular l.	l. coracoclaviculare	a band joining the coracoid process of the scapula and the acromial extremity of the clavicle
costotransverse l.	l. costotransversarium	one of the ligaments that connect a rib to the transverse process of the vertebrae
cotyloid l.	labrum acetabulare	a ring of fibrocartilage connected with the rim of the acetabulum
cricothyroid l.	l. cricothyroideum	a band of elastic tissue extending from the superior border of the cricoid cartilage to the inferior border of the thyroid cartilage
cruciate l's of knee	ligg. cruciatum genus	X-shaped ligaments that arise from the femur and pass through the intercondylar space to attach to the tibia
cruciform l. of atlas	l. cruciforme atlantis	X-shaped ligament that arches across the ring of the first vertebra and divides the ring into anterior and posterior parts
crural l.	l. inguinale	inguinal ligament

T A B L E   O F   L I G A M E N T S   — continued

Common Name	NA Designation	Description
Cruveilhier's l's	ligg. palmaria	palmar ligaments
cysticoduodenal l.		an anomalous fold of peritoneum extending between the gallbladder and duodenum
deltoid l., medial	l. mediale	the medial reinforcing ligament of the ankle joint
diaphragmatic l.		the urogenital ridge that becomes the suspensory ligament of the ovary
falciform l. of liver	l. falciforme hepatis	a sickle-shaped sagittal fold of peritoneum that helps attach the liver to the diaphragm
fibular collateral l.		a strong fibrous cord on the lateral side of the knee joint, it is attached from the lateral condyle of the femur to the head of the fibula
flaval l.	l. flavum	one of a series of elastic cords that band together the laminae of adjacent vertebrae
Flood's l.		the superior glenohumeral ligament
fundiform l. of penis	l. fundiforme penis	a fibroelastic tissue adherent to the linea alba and the pubic symphysis
Gerdy's l.		suspensory ligament of axilla
Gimbernat's l.	l. lacunare	lacunar ligament
glenohumeral l's	ligg. glenohumeralia	bands on the inner surface of the articular capsule of the humerus
glenoid l's	ligg. plantaria articulationum metatarsophalangearum	dense bands on the plantar surfaces of the metacarpophalangeal joints

Table continued on following page

T A B L E   O F   L I G A M E N T S -- continued

Common Name	NA Designation	Description
Henle's l.	falx inguinalis	a lateral expansion of the edge of the rectus abdominis attached to the pubic bone
Hey's l.	margo falciformis hiatus saphenus	falciform process
hyoepiglottic l.	l. hyoepiglotticum	a triangular elastic band uniting the epiglottis to the upper part of the hyoid bone
iliofemoral l.	l. iliofemorale	a Y-shaped band covering the anterior and superior portions of the hip joint
iliotrochanteric l.		a portion of the articular capsule of the hip joint
inguinal l.	l. inguinale	a fibrous band running from the anterior superior spine of the ilium to the spine of the pubis
interfoveolar l.	l. interfoveolare	the thickened portion of the transverse fascia lying medial to the deep inguinal ring and connecting the transverse muscle of the abdomen to the inguinal ligament
interspinal l.	l. interspinale	short bands of fibrous tissue that interconnect the spinous processes of adjacent vertebrae
lacunar l.	l. lacunare	triangular bands extending from the inguinal ligament to the iliopectineal line of the pubis
Lisfranc's l.		a fibrous band extending from the medial cuneiform to the second metatarsal

T A B L E   O F   L I G A M E N T S — continued

Common Name	NA Designation	Description
Lockwood's l.		a suspensory sheath supporting the eyeball
longitudinal l., anterior	l. longitudinale anterius	a flat band of fibers extending along the anterior surface of the vertebral bodies from the axis to the sacrum
longitudinal l., posterior	l. longitudinale posterius	a flat band of fibers in the vertebral canal extending from the second vertebra to the axis
medial l.	l. mediale	a large fan-shaped ligament on the medial side of the ankle
meniscofemoral l.	l. meniscofemorale	bands of the knee joint attached to the meniscus
nephrocolic l.		fasciculi from the fatty capsule of the kidney passing on the right to the posterior wall of the ascending colon and on the left to the posterior wall of the descending colon
nuchal l.	l. nuchae	a membranous septum in the back of the neck extending to the occipital crest
ovarian l.	l. ovarii proprium	a bundle of fibers joining the uterine end of the ovary to the lateral margin of the uterus
palmar l.'s	ligg. palmaria	the ligaments of the hollow of the hand
palpebral l., medial	l. palpebrale mediale	fibrous bands that connect the medial ends of the tarsi to the frontal process of the maxilla
patellar l.	l. patellae	the continuation of the central portion of the tendon of the quadriceps femoris muscle to the patella

Table continued on following page

TABLE OF LIGAMENTS -- continued

Common Name	NA Designation	Description
pectineal l.	l. pectineale	the lateral continuation of the lacunar ligament along the pectineal line of the pubis
periodontal l.		the connective tissue structure that surrounds the roots of the teeth and holds them in place
Petit's l.		uterosacral l.
phrenicocolic l.	l. phrenicocolicum	a peritoneal fold passing from the left colic flexure to the adjacent diaphragm
Poupart's l.		inguinal ligament
pulmonary l.	l. pulmonale	a vertical fold extending from the hilus to the base of the lung
radial collateral l.	l. collaterale carpi radiale	a bundle of fibers that crosses the lateral side of the elbow joint and is attached to the lateral epicondyle of the humerus
reflected inguinal l.		a small triangular sheet, sometimes absent, extending from the inguinal ring to the linea alba
rhomboid l.	l. costoclaviculare	a ligament connecting cartilage of the first rib to the clavicular undersurface
Robert's l.	l. meniscofemorale posterius	a band extending upward from the posterior part of the lateral meniscus
round l. of liver	l. teres hepatis	a fibrous cord extending from the navel to the anterior border of the liver
round l. of uterus	l. teres uteri	a fibromuscular cord extending from the uterus to the labium majus

T A B L E   O F   L I G A M E N T S — continued

Common Name	NA Designation	Description
sacrospinous l.	l. sacrospinale	a triangular ligament attached to the spine of the ischium and to the sacrum and coccyx
sacrotuberous l.	l. sacrotuberale	a ligament extending from the tuberosity of the ischium to the lateral part of the sacrum and coccyx
Schlemm's l's		two ligamentous bands strengthening the capsule of the shoulder joint
sphenomandibular l.	l. sphenomandibulare	a thin band extending from the spine of the sphenoid bone to the lingula of the lower jaw
spring l.	l. calcaneonaviculare plantare	the ligament joining the calcaneus and navicular bone
stylomandibular l.	l. stylomandibulare	a band of cervical fascia extending from the apex of the styloid process to the border of angle of the lower jaw
subflaval l.	l. flavum	any of the yellow elastic bands between the ventral portions of the laminae of adjacent vertebrae
suspensory l. of axilla		fascia ensheathing the pectoralis minor muscle
suspensory l's of breast	ligg. suspensoria mammae	numerous fibrous bands distributed between the lobes of the mammary glands
suspensory l. of lens	zonula ciliaris	the suspensory apparatus of the crystalline lens
suspensory l. of ovary	l. suspensorium ovarii	a band of peritoneum arising from the ovary, extending upward over the iliac vessels, and containing the ovarian nerves

Table continued on following page

T A B L E   O F   L I G A M E N T S -- continued

Common Name	NA Designation	Description
sutural l.		a band of fibrous tissue between the opposed bones of a suture or immovable joint
synovial l.		a large synovial fold
tendinotrochanteric l.		a portion of the capsule of the hip joint
thyroepiglottic l.	l. thyroepiglotticum	the ligament attaching the pedicle of the epiglottis to the thyroid cartilage
tibial collateral l.		a membranous band of the knee joint
transverse humeral l.		a band of fibers bridging the inter-tubercular groove of the humerus and holding the tendon in place
trapezoid l.	l. trapezoideum	the anterolateral portion of the coraco-clavicular ligament
l. of Treitz	musculus suspensorius duodeni	the suspensory muscle of the duodenum
ulnar carpal collateral l.	l. collaterale carpi ulnare	a fibrous band that passes from the tip of the styloid process to the ulna
ulnar collateral l.	l. collaterale ulnare	a thick band of fibers crossing the medial side of the elbow joint and attached to the medial epicondyle of the humerus
umbilical l., medial, or vesicoumbilical l.	l. umbilicale mediale	a fibrous cord, remnant of the obliterated umbilical artery, that runs beside the bladder to the umbilicus

T A B L E   O F   L I G A M E N T S -- continued

Common Name	NA Designation	Description
uteropelvic l's		expansions of muscular tissue in the broad ligament of the uterus radiating from the fascia to the side of the uterus and the vagina
uterosacral l.		part of the thickening of the visceral pelvic fascia beside the cervix and vagina
ventricular or vestibular l. of larynx	l. vestibulare	the membrane extending from the thyroid cartilage to the anterolateral surface of the arytenoid cartilage
vesicoumbilical l.		umbilical ligament, medial
vesicouterine l.		a ligament extending from the anterior aspect of the uterus to the bladder
vocal l.		the elastic tissue membrane extending from the thyroid cartilage to the vocal process of the arytenoid cartilage
Weitbrecht's l.	chorda obliqua membranae interosseae antebrachii	a small ligamentous band extending from the ulnar tuberosity to the radius
Wrisberg's l.		meniscofemoral ligament

TABLE OF MUSCLES

Common Name	Origin [Description]	Action
abductor m. of great toe (m. abductor hallucis)	medial tubercle of calcaneus, plantar fascia	abducts, flexes great toe
abductor m. of little finger (m. abductor digiti minimi manus)	pisiform bone, tendon of ulnar flexor m. of wrist	abducts little finger
abductor m. of little toe (m. abductor digiti minimi pedis)	medial and lateral tubercle of calcaneus, plantar fascia	abducts little toe
abductor m. of thumb, long (m. abductor pollicis longus)	posterior surfaces of radius and ulna	abducts, extends thumb
abductor m. of thumb, short (m. abductor pollicis brevis)	tubercles of scaphoid and trapezium, flexor retinaculum of hand	abducts thumb
adductor m., great (m. adductor magnus)	*deep part* -- inferior ramus of pubis, ramus of ischium; *superficial part* -- ischial tuberosity	*deep part* -- adducts thigh; *superficial part* -- extends thigh
adductor m. of great toe (m. adductor hallucis)	*oblique head* -- long plantar ligament; *transverse head* -- plantar ligaments	flexes, adducts great toe
adductor m., long (m. adductor longus)	body of pubis	adducts, rotates, flexes thigh
adductor m., short (m. adductor brevis)	body and inferior ramus of pubis	adducts, rotates, flexes thigh

NOTES: After the common or anglicized names, their official NA (*Nomina Anatomica*) equivalents are given in parentheses. Occasionally descriptions rather than origins of muscles will be given under the heading Origin. Such descriptions are set off in brackets. The following abbreviations are used: m. = muscle; m's = muscles; m.[L] = musculus; mm.[L] = musculi.

TABLE OF MUSCLES -- continued

Common Name	Origin [Description]	Action
adductor m. of thumb (m. adductor pollicis)	*oblique head* -- second metacarpal, capitate, and trapezoid; *transverse head* -- front of third metacarpal	adducts, opposes thumb
anconeus m. (m. anconeus)	back of lateral epicondyle of humerus	extends forearm
antitragus m. (m. antitragicus)	outer part of antitragus	
arrector m's of hair (mm. arrectores pilorum)	dermis	elevate hairs of skin
articular m. of elbow (m. articularis cubiti)	[fibers of the deep surface of the triceps m. of arm that insert into the posterior ligament and synovial membrane of the elbow joint]	
articular m. of knee (m. articularis genus)	front of lower part of femur	raises capsule of knee joint
aryepiglottic m. (m. aryepiglotticus)	[inconstant fibers of oblique arytenoid m., from apex of arytenoid cartilage to lateral margin of epiglottis]	closes inlet of larynx
arytenoid m., oblique (m. arytenoideus obliquus)	muscular process of arytenoid cartilage	
arytenoid m., transverse (m. arytenoideus transversus)	medial surface of arytenoid cartilage	approximates arytenoid cartilage
auricular m., anterior (m. auricularis anterior)	superficial temporal fascia	draws auricle forward
auricular m., posterior (m. auricularis posterior)	mastoid process	draws auricle backward
auricular m., superior (m. auricularis superior)	galea aponeurotica	raises auricle

Table continued on following page

TABLE OF MUSCLES -- continued

Common Name	Origin [Description]	Action
biceps m. of arm (m. biceps brachii)	*long head* -- supraglenoid tubercle of scapula; *short head* -- apex of coracoid process	flexes, supinates forearm
biceps m. of thigh (m. biceps femoris)	*long head* -- ischial tuberosity; *short head* -- linea aspera of femur	flexes, rotates leg laterally, extends thigh
brachial m. (m. brachialis)	anterior aspect of humerus	flexes forearm
brachioradial m. (m. brachio-radialis)	lateral supracondylar ridge of humerus	flexes forearm
bronchoesophageal m. (m. bronchoesophageus)	[muscle fibers arising from wall of left bronchus]	
buccinator m. (m. buccinator)	buccinator ridge of mandible, alveolar processes of maxilla, pterygomandibular ligament	compresses cheek and retracts angle of mouth
bulbocavernous m. (m. bulbo-cavernosus, m. bulbospongiosus)	tendinous center of perineum, median raphe of bulb	constricts urethra in male, vagina in female
canine m. *See* levator m. of angle of mouth		
ceratocricoid m. (m. ceratocricoideus)	[muscle fibers from cricoid cartilage to interior horn of thyroid cartilage]	
chin m. (m. mentalis)	incisive fossa of mandible	wrinkles skin of chin
chondroglossus m. (m. chondroglossus)	lesser horn and body of hyoid bone	depresses, retracts tongue
ciliary m. (m. ciliaris)	*longitudinal part* -- scleral spur; *circular part* -- sphincter of ciliary body	makes lens more convex in visual accommodation
coccygeus m. (m. coccygeus)	ischial spine	supports and raises coccyx

T A B L E   O F   M U S C L E S -- continued

Common Name	Origin [Description]	Action
constrictor m. of pharynx, inferior (m. constrictor pharyngis inferior)	undersurfaces of cricoid and thyroid cartilages	constricts pharynx
constrictor m. of pharynx, middle (m. constrictor pharyngis medius)	horns of hyoid bone, stylohyoid ligament	constricts pharynx
constrictor m. of pharynx, superior (m. constrictor pharyngis superior)	pterygoid plate, pterygomandibular raphe, mylohyoid ridge of mandible, mucous membrane of floor of mouth	constricts pharynx
coracobrachial m. (m. coracobrachialis)	coracoid process of scapula	flexes, adducts arm
corrugator m., superciliary (m. corrugator supercilii)	medial end of superciliary arch	draws eyebrow downward and medially
cremaster m. (m. cremaster)	inferior margin of internal oblique m. of abdomen	elevates testis
cricoarytenoid m., lateral (m. cricoarytenoideus)	lateral surface of cricoid cartilage	approximates vocal folds
cricoarytenoid m., posterior (m. cricoarytenoideus posterior)	back of lamina of cricoid cartilage	separates vocal folds
cricothyroid m. (m. cricothyroideus)	front and side of cricoid cartilage	tenses vocal folds
deltoid m. (m. deltoideus)	clavicle, acromion, spine of scapula	abducts, flexes, or extends arm
depressor m. of angle of mouth (m. depressor anguli oris)	lateral border of mandible	pulls down angle of mouth
depressor m. of lower lip (m. depressor labii inferioris)	anterior surface of lower border of mandible	depresses lower lip
depressor m. of septum of nose (m. depressor septi nasi)	incisive fossa of maxilla	constricts nostril and depresses ala

Table continued on following page

TABLE OF MUSCLES -- continued

Common Name	Origin [Description]	Action
depressor m., superciliary (m. depressor supercilii)	[a name applied to a few fibers of orbital part of orbicular m. of eye that are inserted into the eyebrow, which they depress]	
detrusor urinae. See pubo-vesical m.		
diaphragm (diaphragma)	xiphoid process, surfaces of lower 6 costal cartilages and lower 4 ribs, lateral arcuate ligaments, upper lumbar vertebrae	increases volume of thorax in inspiration
digastric m. (m. digastricus)	digastric notch at mastoid process	elevates hyoid bone, lowers jaw
dilator m. of pupil (m. dilator pupillae)	[fibers extending radially from sphincter of pupil to ciliary margin]	dilates iris
epicranial m. (m. epicranius)	[muscular covering of scalp, including occipito-frontal and temporoparietal m's]	
erector m. of spine (m. erector spinae)	[fibers of deep muscles of back, originating from sacrum, spines of lumbar and eleventh and twelfth thoracic vertebrae, and iliac crest]	
extensor m. of fingers (m. extensor digitorum)	lateral epicondyle of humerus	extends wrist joint and phalanges
extensor m. of great toe, long (m. extensor hallucis longus)	front of fibula, interosseous membrane	extends great toe, dorsi-flexes ankle joint
extensor m. of great toe, short (m. extensor hallucis brevis)	[a name applied to portion of short extensor m. of toes that goes to great toe]	
extensor m. of index finger (m. extensor indicis)	posterior surface of ulna, interosseous membrane	extends index finger
extensor m. of little finger (m. extensor digiti minimi)	lateral epicondyle of humerus	extends little finger

T A B L E   O F   M U S C L E S -- continued

Common Name	Origin [Description]	Action
extensor m. of thumb, long (m. extensor pollicis longus)	posterior surface of ulna and interosseous membrane	extends, adducts thumb
extensor m. of thumb, short (m. extensor pollicis brevis)	posterior surface of radius	extends thumb
extensor m. of toes, long (m. extensor digitorum longus)	anterior surface of fibula, lateral condyle of tibia, interosseous membrane	extends toes
extensor m. of toes, short (m. extensor digitorum brevis)	upper surface of calcaneus	extends toes
extensor m. of wrist, radial, long (m. extensor carpi radialis longus)	lateral supracondylar ridge of humerus	extends, abducts wrist joint
extensor m. of wrist, radial, short (m. extensor carpi radialis brevis)	lateral epicondyle of humerus	extends, abducts wrist joint
extensor m. of wrist, ulnar (m. extensor carpi ulnaris)	*humeral head* -- lateral epicondyle of humerus; *ulnar head* -- posterior border of ulna	extends, abducts wrist joint
fibular m. *See* peroneal m.		
flexor m. of fingers, deep (m. flexor digitorum profundus)	shaft of ulna, coronoid process, interosseous membrane	flexes distal phalanges
flexor m. of fingers, superficial (m. flexor digitorum superficialis)	*humeroulnar head* -- medial epicondyle of humerus, coronoid process of ulna; *radial head* -- anterior border of radius	flexes middle phalanges
flexor m. of great toe, long (m. flexor hallucis longus)	posterior surface of fibula	flexes great toe
flexor m. of great toe, short (m. flexor hallucis brevis)	undersurface of cuboid, lateral cuneiform	flexes great toe

Table continued on following page

T A B L E   O F   M U S C L E S -- continued

Common Name	Origin [Description]	Action
flexor m. of little finger, short (m. flexor digiti minimi manus)	hook of hamate bone, transverse carpal ligament	flexes little finger
flexor m. of little toe, short (m. flexor digiti minimi brevis pedis)	sheath of long peroneal	flexes little toe
flexor m. of thumb, long (m. flexor pollicis longus)	anterior surface of radius, medial epicondyle of humerus, coronoid process of ulna	flexes thumb
flexor m. of thumb, short (m. flexor pollicis brevis)	tubercle of trapezium, flexor retinaculum	flexes, adducts thumb
flexor m. of toes, long (m. flexor digitorum longus pedis)	posterior surface of shaft of tibia	flexes toes, extends foot
flexor m. of toes, short (m. flexor digitorum brevis pedis)	medial tuberosity of calcaneus, plantar fascia	flexes toes
flexor m. of wrist, radial (m. flexor carpi radialis)	medial epicondyle of humerus	flexes, abducts wrist joint
flexor m. of wrist, ulnar (m. flexor carpi ulnaris)	*humeral head* -- medial epicondyle of humerus; *ulnar head* -- olecranon and posterior border of ulna	flexes, adducts wrist joint
gastrocnemius m. (m. gastrocnemius)	*medial head* -- popliteal surface of femur, upper part of medial condyle, capsule of knee; *lateral head* -- lateral condyle, capsule of knee	plantar flexes foot, flexes knee joint
gemellus m., inferior (m. gemellus inferior)	tuberosity of ischium	rotates thigh laterally
gemellus m., superior (m. gemellus superior)	spine of ischium	rotates thigh laterally

TABLE OF MUSCLES -- continued

Common Name	Origin [Description]	Action
genioglossus m. (m. genioglossus)	superior genial tubercle	protrudes, depresses tongue
geniohyoid m. (m. geniohyoideus)	inferior genial tubercle	draws hyoid bone forward
glossopalatine m. See palato-glossus m.		
gluteus maximus m., (gluteal m., greatest) (m. gluteus maximus)	dorsal aspect of ilium, dorsal surfaces of sacrum, coccyx, sacrotuberous ligament	extends, abducts, rotates thigh laterally
gluteus medius m., (gluteal m., middle) (m. gluteus medius)	dorsal aspect of ilium between anterior and posterior gluteal lines	abducts, rotates thigh medially
gluteus minimus m., (gluteal m., least) (m. gluteus minimus)	dorsal aspect of ilium between anterior and posterior gluteal lines	abducts, rotates thigh medially
gracilis m. (m. gracilis)	body and inferior ramus of pubis	adducts thigh, flexes knee joint
helix m., greater (m. helicis major)	spine of helix	tenses skin of acoustic meatus
helix m., smaller (m. helicis minor)	anterior rim of helix	
hyoglossus m. (m. hyoglossus)	body and greater horn of hyoid bone	depresses, retracts tongue
iliac m. (m. iliacus)	iliac fossa, ala of sacrum	flexes thigh, trunk on limb
iliococcygeus m. (m. ilio-coccygeus)	[posterior portion of levator ani m., including fibers originating as far forward as obturator canal]	
iliocostal m. (m. iliocostalis)	[lateral division of erector m. of spine]	
iliocostal m. of loins (m. iliocostalis lumborum)	iliac crest	extends lumbar spine

Table continued on following page

T A B L E   O F   M U S C L E S -- continued

Common Name	Origin [Description]	Action
iliocostal m. of neck (m. iliocostalis cervicis)	angles of third, fourth, fifth, and sixth ribs	extends cervical spine
iliocostal m. of thorax (m. iliocostalis thoracis)	upper borders of angles of 6 lower ribs	keeps thoracic spine erect
iliopsoas m. (m. iliopsoas)	[iliac and greater psoas m's]	
incisive m's of inferior lip (mm. incisivi labii inferioris)	incisive fossae of mandible	make vestibule of mouth shallow
incisive m's of superior lip (mm. incisivi labii superioris)	incisive fossae of maxilla	make vestibule of mouth shallow
m. of incisure of helix (m. incisurae helicis)	[inconstant slips of fibers continuing from m. of tragus to bridge notch of cartilaginous part of meatus]	
infraspinous m. (m. infraspinatus)	infraspinous fossa of scapula	rotates arm laterally
intercostal m's (mm. intercostales)	[the layer of muscle fibers separated from the internal intercostal m's by the intercostal nerves and vessels]	
intercostal m's, external (mm. intercostales externi)	inferior border of rib	elevate ribs in inspiration
intercostal m's, internal (mm. intercostales interni)	inferior border of rib and costal cartilage	act on ribs in expiration
interosseous m's of foot, dorsal (mm. interossei dorsales pedis)	sides of adjacent metatarsal bones	flex, abduct toes
interosseous m's of hand, dorsal (mm. interossei dorsales manus)	each by two heads from adjacent sides of meta- carpal bones	abduct, flex proximal, extend middle and distal phalanges
interosseous m's, palmar (mm. interossei palmares)	sides of first, second, fourth, and fifth metacarpal bones	adduct, flex proximal, extend middle and distal phalanges

T A B L E   O F   M U S C L E S -- continued

Common Name	Origin [Description]	Action
interosseous m's, plantar (mm. interossei plantares)	medial side of third, fourth, and fifth metatarsal bones	flex, abduct toes
interspinal m's (mm. inter-spinales)	[short bands of muscle fibers extending on each side between spinous processes of contiguous vertebrae]	extend vertebral column
intertransverse m's (mm. intertransversarii)	[small muscles passing between transverse processes of adjacent vertebrae]	bend vertebral column laterally
ischiocavernous m. (m. ischiocavernosus)	ramus of ischium	maintains erection of penis or clitoris
latissimus dorsi m. (m. latissimus dorsi)	spines of lower thoracic vertebrae and spines of lumbar and sacral vertebrae	adducts, extends, rotates humerus medially
levator m. of angle of mouth (m. levator anguli oris)	canine fossa of maxilla	raises angle of mouth
levator ani m. (m. levator ani)	[important muscular components of pelvic diaphragm, arising mainly from back of body of pubis and running backward toward coccyx]	helps support pelvic viscera and resist increases in intra-abdominal pressure
levator m. of palatine velum (m. levator veli palatini)	apex of pars petrosa of temporal bone and cartilage of auditory tube	raises and draws back soft palate
levator m. of prostate (m. levator prostatae)	[part of anterior portion of pubococcygeus m.]	supports, compresses prostate, helps control micturition
levator m's of ribs (mm. levatores costarum)	transverse processes of seventh cervical and first 11 thoracic vertebrae	aid elevation of ribs in respiration
levator m. of scapula (m. levator scapulae)	transverse processes of 4 upper cervical vertebrae	raises scapula
levator m. of thyroid gland (m. levator glandulae thyroideae)	isthmus or pyramidal lobule of thyroid gland	

Table continued on following page

TABLE OF MUSCLES -- continued

Common Name	Origin [Description]	Action
levator m. of upper eyelid (m. levator palpebrae superioris)	sphenoid bone above optic foramen	raises upper eyelid
levator m. of upper lip (m. levator labii superioris)	lower margin of orbit	raises upper lip
levator m. of upper lip and ala of nose (m. levator labii superioris alaeque nasi)	frontal process of maxilla	raises upper lip, dilates nostril
long m. of head (m. longus capitis)	transverse processes of third to sixth cervical vertebrae	flexes head
long m. of neck (m. longus colli)	*superior oblique portion* -- transverse processes of third to fifth cervical vertebrae; *inferior oblique portion* -- bodies of first to third thoracic vertebrae; *vertical portion* -- bodies of 3 upper thoracic and 3 lower cervical vertebrae	flexes, supports cervical vertebrae
longissimus m. of head (m. longissimus capitis)	transverse processes of 4 or 5 upper thoracic vertebrae, articular processes of 3 or 4 lower cervical vertebrae	draws head backward, rotates head
longissimus m. of neck (m. longissimus cervicis)	transverse processes of 4 or 5 upper thoracic vertebrae	extends cervical vertebrae
longissimus m. of thorax (m. longissimus thoracis)	transverse and articular processes of lumbar vertebrae and thoracolumbar fascia	extends thoracic vertebrae
longitudinal m. of tongue, inferior (m. longitudinalis inferior linguae)	undersurface of tongue at base	changes shape of tongue in mastication and deglutition
longitudinal m. of tongue, superior (m. longitudinalis superior linguae)	submucosa and septum of tongue	changes shape of tongue in mastication and deglutition

TABLE OF MUSCLES -- continued

Common Name	Origin [Description]	Action
lumbrical m's of foot (mm. lumbricales pedis)	tendons of long flexor m. of toes	flex metatarsophalangeal joints, extend distal phalanges
lumbrical m's of hand (mm. lumbricales manus)	tendons of deep flexor m. of fingers	flex metacarpophalangeal joints, extend middle and distal phalanges
masseter m. (m. masseter)	*superficial part* -- zygomatic process of maxilla, lower border of zygomatic arch; *deep part* -- lower border and medial surface of zygomatic arch	raises mandible, closes jaws
multifidus m's (mm. multifidi)	sacrum, sacroiliac ligament, mamillary processes of lumbar, transverse processes of thoracic and lower cervical vertebrae	extend, rotate vertebral column
mylohyoid m. (m. mylohyoideus)	mylohyoid line of mandible	elevates hyoid bone, supports floor of mouth
nasal m. (m. nasalis)	maxilla	*alar part* -- aids in widening nostril; *transverse part* -- depresses cartilage of nose
oblique m. of abdomen, external (m. obliquus externus abdominis)	lower 8 ribs at costal cartilages	flexes, rotates vertebral column, compresses abdominal viscera
oblique m. of abdomen, internal (m. obliquus internus abdominis)	thoracolumbar fascia, iliac crest, iliac fascia, inguinal fascia	flexes, rotates vertebral column, compresses abdominal viscera
oblique m. of auricle (m. obliquus auriculae)	cranial surface of concha	
oblique m. of eyeball, inferior (m. obliquus inferior bulbi)	orbital surface of maxilla	abducts, rotates eyeball upward and outward
oblique m. of eyeball, superior (m. obliquus superior bulbi)	lesser wing of sphenoid above optic foramen	abducts, rotates eyeball downward and outward

Table continued on following page

372 TABLE OF MUSCLES

TABLE OF MUSCLES -- continued

Common Name	Origin [Description]	Action
oblique m. of head, inferior (m. obliquus capitis inferior)	spinous process of axis	rotates atlas and head
oblique m. of head, superior (m. obliquus capitis superior)	transverse process of atlas	extends and moves head laterally
obturator m., external (m. obturatorius externus)	pubis, ischium, external surface of obturator membrane	rotates thigh laterally
obturator m., internal (m. obturatorius internus)	pelvic surface of hip bone and obturator membrane, margin of obturator foramen	rotates thigh laterally
occipitofrontal m. (m. occipitofrontalis)	*frontal* -- galea aponeurotica; *occipital* -- highest nuchal line of occipital bone	*frontal belly* -- raises eyebrow; *occipital belly* -- draws scalp backward
omohyoid m. (m. omohyoideus)	superior border of scapula	depresses hyoid bone
opposing m. of little finger (m. opponens digiti minimi manus)	hook of hamate bone	abducts, flexes, rotates fifth metacarpal
opposing m. of thumb (m. opponens pollicis)	tubercle of trapezium, flexor retinaculum	flexes, opposes thumb
orbicular m. of eye (m. orbicularis oculi)	*orbital part* -- medial margin of orbit; *palpebral part* -- medial palpebral ligament; *lacrimal part* -- posterior lacrimal crest	closes eyelids, wrinkles forehead, compresses lacrimal sac
orbicular m. of mouth (m. orbicularis oris)	[complicated sphincter muscle of mouth, comprising 2 parts: *labial part* -- fibers restricted to lips; *marginal part* -- fibers blending with those of adjacent muscles]	closes, protrudes lips
orbital m. (m. orbitalis)	[bridges inferior orbital fissure]	protrudes eye
palatoglossus m. (m. palatoglossus)	undersurface of soft palate	elevates tongue, constricts fauces

TABLE OF MUSCLES -- continued

Common Name	Origin [Description]	Action
palatopharyngeal m. (m. palatopharyngeus)	posterior border of bony palate, palatine, aponeurosis	constricts pharynx, aids swallowing
palmar m., long (m. palmaris longus)	medial epicondyle of humerus	tenses palmar aponeurosis
palmar m., short (m. palmaris brevis)	palmar aponeurosis	assists in deepening hollow of palm
papillary m's (mm. papillares)	[conical muscular projections from walls of cardiac ventricles, attached to cusps of atrioventricular valves]	steady and strengthen atrio-ventricular valves and prevent eversion of their cusps
pectinate m's (mm. pectinati)	[columns projecting from the inner walls of cardiac auricles]	
pectineal m. (m. pectineus)	pectineal line of pubis	flexes, adducts thigh
pectoral m., greater (m. pectoralis major)	clavicle, sternum, 6 upper costal cartilages, aponeurosis of external oblique m. of abdomen	adducts, flexes, rotates arm medially
pectoral m., smaller (m. pectoralis minor)	second, third, fourth, and fifth ribs	draws shoulder forward and downward, raises third, fourth, and fifth ribs in forced inspiration
peroneal m., long (m. peroneus longus)	lateral condyle of tibia, head of fibula, lateral surface of fibula	plantar flexes, everts, abducts foot
peroneal m., short (m. peroneus brevis)	lateral surface of fibula	everts, abducts, plantar flexes foot
peroneal m., third (m. peroneus tertius)	anterior surface of fibula, interosseous membrane	everts, dorsiflexes foot

Table continued on following page

T A B L E   O F   M U S C L E S -- continued

Common Name	Origin [Description]	Action
piriform m. (m. piriformis)	ilium, second to fourth sacral vertebrae	rotates thigh laterally
plantar m. (m. plantaris)	popliteal surface of femur	plantar flexes foot, flexes leg
platysma (platysma)	[a platelike muscle originating from the fascia of cervical region and inserting on mandible]	wrinkles skin of neck, depresses jaw
pleuroesophageal m. (m. pleuroesophageus)	[a bundle of smooth muscle fibers, usually connecting esophagus with left mediastinal pleura]	
popliteal m. (m. popliteus)	lateral condyle of femur, lateral meniscus	flexes leg, rotates leg medially
procerus m. (m. procerus)	fascia over nasal bones	draws medial angle of eyebrows down
pronator m., quadrate (m. pronator quadratus)	anterior surface and border of distal third or fourth of shaft of ulna	pronates forearm
pronator m., round (m. pronator teres)	*humeral head* -- medial epicondyle of humerus; *ulnar head* -- coronoid process of ulna	pronates and flexes forearm
psoas m., greater (m. psoas major)	lumbar vertebrae	flexes thigh or trunk
psoas m., smaller (m. psoas minor)	last thoracic and first lumbar vertebrae	assists greater psoas m.
pterygoid m., lateral (external) (m. pterygoideus lateralis)	*upper head* -- infratemporal surface of greater wing of sphenoid, infratemporal crest; *lower head* -- lateral surface of lateral pterygoid plate	protrudes mandible, opens jaws, moves mandible from side to side
pterygoid m., medial (internal) (m. pterygoideus medialis)	medial surface of lateral pterygoid plate, tuber of maxilla	closes jaws

T A B L E   O F   M U S C L E S -- continued

Common Name	Origin [Description]	Action
pubococcygeus m. (m. pubococcygeus)	[anterior portion of levator ani m. originating in front of obturator canal and inserting in anococcygeal ligament]	helps support pelvic viscera and resist increases in intra-abdominal pressure
puboprostatic m. (m. pubo-prostaticus)	[smooth muscle fibers contained within medial puboprostatic ligament and passing from prostate anteriorly to pubis]	
puborectal m. (m. puborectalis)	[portion of levator ani m., with a more lateral origin from pubic bone]	helps support pelvic viscera and resist increases in intra-abdominal pressure
pubovaginal m. (m. pubovaginalis)	[part of anterior portion of pubococcygeus m., which is inserted into urethra and vagina]	helps control micturition
pubovesical m. (m. pubovesicalis)	[smooth muscle fibers extending from neck of urinary bladder to pubis]	
pyramidal m. (m. pyramidalis)	body of pubis	tenses abdominal wall
pyramidal m. of auricle (m. pyramidalis auriculae)	[inconstant prolongation of fibers of m. of tragus to spine of helix]	
quadrate m. of loins (m. quadratus lumborum)	iliac crest, thoracolumbar fascia	flexes trunk laterally
quadrate m. of lower lip. See depressor m. of lower lip		
quadrate m. of sole (m. quadratus plantae)	calcaneus, plantar fascia	aids in flexing toes
quadrate m. of thigh (m. quadratus femoris)	tuberosity of ischium	adducts, rotates thigh laterally
quadrate m. of upper lip. See levator m. of upper lip		

Table continued on following page

T A B L E   O F   M U S C L E S -- continued

Common Name	Origin [Description]	Action
quadriceps m. of thigh (m. quadriceps femoris)	[rectus m. of thigh and intermediate, lateral and medial vastus m's]	extends leg upon thigh
rectococcygeus m. (m. recto-coccygeus)	[smooth muscle fibers originating on anterior surface of second and third coccygeal vertebrae]	retracts, elevates rectum
rectourethral m. (m. recto-urethralis)	[band of smooth muscle fibers in male, extending from perineal flexure of rectum to membranous part of urethra]	
rectouterine m. (m. rectouterinus)	[band of fibers in female, running between cervix uteri and rectum, in rectouterine fold]	
rectovesical m. (m. rectovesicalis)	[band of fibers in male, connecting longitudinal musculature of rectum with external muscular coat of bladder]	
rectus m. of abdomen (m. rectus abdominis)	pubic crest and symphysis	flexes lumbar vertebrae, supports abdomen
rectus m. of eyeball, inferior (m. rectus inferior bulbi)	common tendinous ring	adducts, rotates eyeball down-ward and medially
rectus m. of eyeball, lateral (m. rectus lateralis bulbi)	common tendinous ring	abducts eyeball
rectus m. of eyeball, medial (m. rectus medialis bulbi)	common tendinous ring	adducts eyeball
rectus m. of eyeball, superior (m. rectus superior bulbi)	common tendinous ring	adducts, rotates eyeball upward and medially
rectus m. of head, anterior (m. rectus capitis anterior)	lateral mass of atlas	flexes, supports head
rectus m. of head, lateral (m. rectus capitis lateralis)	transverse process of atlas	flexes, supports head

TABLE OF MUSCLES -- continued

Common Name	Origin [Description]	Action
rectus m. of head, posterior, greater (m. rectus capitis posterior major)	spinous process of axis	extends head
rectus m. of head, posterior, smaller (m. rectus capitis posterior minor)	posterior tubercle of atlas	extends head
rectus m. of thigh (m. rectus femoris)	anterior inferior iliac spine, rim of acetabulum	extends leg, flexes thigh
rhomboid m., greater (m. rhomboideus major)	spinous processes of second, third, fourth, and fifth thoracic vertebrae	retracts and fixes scapula
rhomboid m., smaller (m. rhomboideus minor)	spinous processes of seventh cervical and first thoracic vertebrae, lower part of nuchal ligament	retracts and fixes scapula
risorius m. (m. risorius)	fascia over masseter	draws angle of mouth laterally
rotator m's (mm. rotatores)	[a series of small muscles deep in groove between spinous and transverse processes of vertebrae]	extend and rotate vertebral column toward opposite side
sacrococcygeal m., dorsal (posterior) (m. sacrococcygeus dorsalis)	[muscular slip passing from dorsal surface of sacrum to coccyx]	
sacrococcygeal m., ventral (anterior) (m. sacrococcygeus ventralis)	[musculotendinous slip passing from lower sacral vertebra to coccyx]	
sacrospinal m. See erector m. of spine		
salpingopharyngeal m. (m. salpingopharyngeus)	cartilage of auditory tube	raises pharynx
sartorius m. (m. sartorius)	anterior superior iliac spine	flexes thigh and leg

Table continued on following page

T A B L E   O F   M U S C L E S -- continued

Common Name	Origin [Description]	Action
scalene m., anterior (m. scalenus anterior)	transverse processes of third to sixth cervical vertebrae	raises first rib, flexes cervical vertebrae laterally
scalene m., middle (m. scalenus medius)	transverse processes of first to seventh cervical vertebrae	raises first rib, flexes cervical vertebrae laterally
scalene m. of pleura. See scalene m., smallest		
scalene m., posterior (m. scalenus posterior)	transverse processes of fourth to sixth cervical vertebrae	raises first and second ribs, flexes cervical vertebrae laterally
scalene m., smallest (m. scalenus minimus)	[muscular band occasionally found between anterior and middle scalene m's]	
semimembranous m. (m. semimembranosus)	tuberosity of ischium	flexes leg, extends thigh
semispinal m. of head (m. semispinalis capitis)	transverse processes of upper thoracic and lower cervical vertebrae	extends head
semispinal m. of neck (m. semispinalis cervicis)	transverse processes of upper thoracic vertebrae	extends, rotates vertebral column
semispinal m. of thorax (m. semispinalis thoracis)	transverse processes of lower thoracic vertebrae	extends, rotates vertebral column
semitendinous m. (m. semitendinosus)	tuberosity of ischium	flexes and rotates leg medially, extends thigh
serratus m., anterior (m. serratus anterior)	8 upper ribs	draws scapula forward, rotates scapula to raise shoulder in abduction of arm
serratus m., posterior, inferior (m. serratus posterior inferior)	spines of lower thoracic and upper lumbar vertebrae	lowers ribs in expiration

T A B L E   O F   M U S C L E S -- continued

Common Name	Origin [Description]	Action
serratus m., posterior, superior (m. serratus posterior superior)	nuchal ligament, spinous processes of upper thoracic vertebrae	raises ribs in inspiration
soleus m. (m. soleus)	fibula, tendinous arch, tibia	plantar flexes foot
sphincter m. of anus, external (m. sphincter ani externus)	tip of coccyx, anococcygeal ligament	closes anus
sphincter m. of anus, internal (m. sphincter ani internus)	[a thickening or circular layer of muscular tunic at caudal end of rectum]	
sphincter m. of bile duct (m. sphincter ductus choledochi)	[annular sheath of muscle fibers investing bile duct within wall of duodenum]	
sphincter m. of hepatopancreatic ampulla (m. sphincter ampullae hepatopancreaticae)	[annular band of muscle fibers investing hepato-pancreatic ampulla]	
sphincter m. of pupil (m. sphincter pupillae)	[circular fibers of iris]	constricts pupil
sphincter m. of pylorus (m. sphincter pylori)	[a thickening of circular muscle of stomach around its opening into duodenum pylorus]	
sphincter m. of urethra (m. sphincter urethrae)	inferior ramus of pubis	compresses membranous urethra
sphincter m. of urinary bladder (m. sphincter vesicae urinariae)	[circular layer of fibers surrounding internal urethral orifice]	closes internal orifice of urethra
spinal m. of head (m. spinalis capitis)	spinous processes of upper thoracic and lower cervical vertebrae	extends head
spinal m. of neck (m. spinalis cervicis)	spinous process of seventh cervical vertebra, nuchal ligament	extends vertebral column

Table continued on following page

TABLE OF MUSCLES -- continued

Common Name	Origin [Description]	Action
spinal m. of thorax (m. spinalis thoracis)	spinous processes of upper lumbar and lower thoracic vertebrae	extends vertebral column
splenius m. of head (m. splenius capitis)	lower half of nuchal ligament, spinous processes of seventh cervical and upper thoracic vertebrae	extends, rotates head
splenius m. of neck (m. splenius cervicis)	spinous process of upper thoracic vertebrae	extends, rotates head and neck
stapedius m. (m. stapedius)	interior of pyramidal eminence of tympanic cavity	dampens movement of stapes
sternal m. (m. sternalis)	[muscular band occasionally found parallel to sternum on sternocostal head of greater pectoral m.]	
sternocleidomastoid m. (m. sternocleidomastoideus)	*sternal head* -- manubrium; *clavicular head* -- medial third of clavicle	flexes vertebral column, rotates head to opposite side
sternocostal m. See transverse m. of thorax		
sternohyoid m. (m. sternohyoideus)	manubrium sterni and/or clavicle	depresses hyoid bone and larynx
sternothyroid m. (m. sternothyroideus)	manubrium sterni	depresses thyroid cartilage
styloglossus m. (m. styloglossus)	styloid process	raises, retracts tongue
stylohyoid m. (m. stylohyoideus)	styloid process	draws hyoid bone and tongue upward and backward
stylopharyngeus m. (m. stylopharyngeus)	styloid process	raises, dilates pharynx

T A B L E   O F   M U S C L E S -- continued

Common Name	Origin [Description]	Action
subclavius m. (m. subclavius)	first rib and its cartilage	depresses lateral end of clavicle
subcostal m's (mm. subcostales)	lower border of ribs	raise ribs in inspiration
subscapular m. (m. subscapularis)	subscapular fossa of scapula	rotates arm medially
supinator m. (m. supinator)	lateral epicondyle of humerus, ligaments of elbow	supinates forearm
supraspinous m. (m. supra-spinatus)	supraspinous fossa of scapula	abducts arm
suspensory m. (m. suspensorius)	[flat band of smooth muscle fibers originating from left crus of diaphragm and inserting with muscular coat of duodenum]	
tarsal m., inferior (m. tarsalis inferior)	inferior rectus m. of eyeball	widens palpebral fissure
tarsal m., superior (m. tarsalis superior)	levator m. of upper eyelid	widens palpebral fissure
temporal m. (m. temporalis)	temporal fossa and fascia	closes jaws
temporoparietal m. (m. temporo-parietalis)	temporal fascia above ear	tightens scalp
tensor m. of fascia lata (m. tensor fasciae latae)	iliac crest	flexes, rotates thigh medially
tensor m. of palatine velum (m. tensor veli palatini)	scaphoid fossa and spine of sphenoid	tenses soft palate, opens auditory tube
tensor m. of tympanum (m. tensor tympani)	cartilaginous portion of auditory tube	tenses tympanic membrane
teres major m. (m. teres major)	inferior angle of scapula	adducts, extends, and rotates arm medially

Table continued on following page

382   TABLE OF MUSCLES

T A B L E   O F   M U S C L E S -- continued

Common Name	Origin [Description]	Action
teres minor m. (m. teres minor)	lateral margin of scapula	rotates arm laterally
thyroarytenoid m. (m. thyro-arytenoideus)	medial surface of lamina of thyroid cartilage	relaxes, shortens vocal folds
thyroepiglottic m. (m. thyro-epiglotticus)	lamina of thyroid cartilage	closes inlet to larynx
thyrohyoid m. (m. thyrohyoideus)	lamina of thyroid cartilage	raises and changes form of larynx
tibial m., anterior (m. tibialis anterior)	lateral condyle and surface of tibia, interosseous membrane	dorsiflexes, inverts foot
tibial m., posterior (m. tibialis posterior)	tibia, fibula, interosseous membrane	plantar flexes, inverts foot
tracheal m. (m. trachealis)	[transverse smooth muscle fibers filling gap at back of each cartilage of trachea]	lessens caliber of trachea
m. of tragus (m. tragicus)	[short, flattened vertical band on lateral surface of tragus, innervated by auriculotemporal and posterior auricular nerves]	
transverse m. of abdomen (m. transversus abdominis)	lower 6 costal cartilages, thoracolumbar fascia, iliac crest	compresses abdominal viscera
transverse m. of auricle (m. transversus auriculae)	cranial surface of auricle	retracts helix
transverse m. of chin (m. transversus menti)	[superficial fibers of depressor m. of angle of mouth]	
transverse m. of nape (m. transversus nuchae)	[small occasional muscle passing from occipital pro-tuberance to posterior auricular m.]	
transverse m. of perineum, deep (m. transversus perinei pro-fundus)	ramus of ischium	fixes tendinous center of perineum

TABLE OF MUSCLES -- continued

Common Name	Origin [Description]	Action
transverse m. of perineum, superficial (m. transversus perinei superficialis)	ramus of ischium	fixes tendinous center of perineum
transverse m. of thorax (m. transversus thoracis)	posterior surface of body of sternum and of xiphoid process	perhaps narrows chest
transverse m. of tongue (m. transversus linguae)	median septum of tongue	changes shape of tongue in mastication and swallowing
transversospinal m. (m. transversospinalis)	[semispinal, multifidus, and rotator m's]	
trapezius m. (m. trapezius)	occipital bone, nuchal ligament, spinous processes of seventh cervical and all thoracic vertebrae	elevates shoulder, rotates scapula to raise shoulder in abduction of arm, draws scapula backward
triangular m. *See* depressor m. of angle of mouth		
triceps m. of arm (m. triceps brachii)	*Long head* -- infraglenoid tubercle of scapula; *Lateral head* -- posterior surface of humerus; *medial head* -- posterior surface of humerus	extends forearm; *long head* adducts, extends arm
triceps m. of calf (m. triceps surae)	[gastrocnemius and soleus m's]	
m. of uvula (m. uvulae)	posterior nasal spine of palatine bone and aponeurosis of soft palate	raises uvula
vastus m., intermediate (m. vastus intermedius)	anterior and lateral surfaces of femur	extends leg
vastus m., lateral (m. vastus lateralis)	lateral aspect of femur	extends leg

Table continued on following page

TABLE OF MUSCLES -- continued

Common Name	Origin [Description]	Action
vastus m., medial (m. vastus medialis)	medial aspect of femur	extends leg
vertical m. of tongue (m. verticalis linguae)	dorsal fascia of tongue	changes shape of tongue in mastication and deglutition
vocal m. (m. vocalis)	angle between laminae of thyroid cartilage	causes local variations in tension of vocal fold
zygomatic m., greater (m. zygomaticus major)	zygomatic bone	draws angle of mouth upward and backward
zygomatic m., smaller (m. zygomaticus minor)	zygomatic bone	draws upper lip upward and laterally

T A B L E O F N E R V E S

Common Name [Modality]	NA Designation	Branches
abducent n. (6th cranial) [motor]	n. abducens	filaments
accessory n. (11th cranial) [parasympathetic, motor]	n. accessorius	external branch
acoustic n. *See* vestibulocochlear n.		
alveolar n., inferior [motor, general sensory]	n. alveolaris inferior	inferior dental, mental, and inferior gingival nerves; mylohyoid n.
alveolar n's, superior	nn. alveolares superiores	filaments
ampullary n., anterior	n. ampullaris anterior	filaments
ampullary n., inferior. *See* ampullary n., posterior		
ampullary n., lateral	n. ampullaris lateralis	filaments
ampullary n., posterior	n. ampullaris posterior	filaments
ampullary n., superior. *See* ampullary n., anterior		
anococcygeal n's [general sensory]	nn. anococcygei	filaments
auditory n. *See* vestibulococh- lear n.		

NOTES: The following abbreviations are used: n. = nerve; n's = nerves; n.[L] = nervus; nn.[L] = nervi.

Table continued on following page

T A B L E   O F   N E R V E S — continued

Common Name [Modality]	NA Designation	Branches
auricular n's, anterior [general sensory]	nn. auriculares anteriores	filaments
auricular n., great [general sensory]	n. auricularis magnus	anterior and posterior branches
auricular n., posterior [motor, general sensory]	n. auricularis posterior	occipital branch
auriculotemporal n. [general sensory]	n. auriculotemporalis	anterior auricular n., n. of external acoustic meatus, parotid branches, branch to tympanic membrane, branch communicating with facial n.; terminal branches superficial temporal to scalp
axillary n. [motor, general sensory]	n. axillaris	lateral superior brachial cutaneous n., muscular branches
buccal n. [general sensory]	n. buccalis	
cardiac n., cervical, inferior [sympathetic (accelerator), visceral afferent (chiefly pain)]	n. cardiacus cervicalis inferior	to cardiac plexus
cardiac n., cervical, middle [sympathetic (accelerator), visceral afferent (chiefly pain)]	n. cardiacus cervicalis medius	to deep cardiac plexus
cardiac n., cervical, superior [sympathetic (accelerator)]	n. cardiacus cervicalis superior	to cardiac plexus

TABLE OF NERVES — continued

Common Name [Modality]	NA Designation	Branches
cardiac n., inferior. *See* cardiac n., cervical, inferior		
cardiac n., middle. *See* cardiac n., cervical, middle		
cardiac n., superior. *See* cardiac n., cervical, superior		
cardiac n's, thoracic [sympathetic (accelerator), visceral afferent (chiefly pain)]	nn. cardiaci thoracici	together with tympanic n. forms tympanic plexus
caroticotympanic n's [sympathetic]	nn. caroticotympanici	help form tympanic plexus
carotid n's, external [sympathetic]	nn. carotici externi	filaments
carotid n., internal [sympathetic]	n. caroticus internus	filaments
cavernous n's of clitoris [parasympathetic, sympathetic, visceral afferent]	nn. cavernosi clitoridis	filaments
cavernous n's of penis [sympathetic, parasympathetic, visceral afferent]	nn. cavernosi penis	filaments
cerebral n's. *See* cranial n's		

Table continued on following page

T A B L E   O F   N E R V E S -- continued

Common Name [Modality]	NA Designation	Branches
cervical n's; The 8 pairs of n's whose nuclei of origin arise from cervical segments of the spinal cord	nn. cervicales	ventral branches of upper 4 unite to form cervical plexus; those of lower 4 with branch of first thoracic n. form brachial plexus
cervical n., transverse [general sensory]	n. transversus colli	superior and inferior branches
ciliary n's, long [sympathetic, general sensory]	nn. ciliares longi	filaments
ciliary n's, short [parasympathetic, sympathetic, general sensory]	nn. ciliares breves	filaments
clunial n's, inferior [general sensory]	nn. clunium inferiores	filaments
clunial n's, middle [general sensory]	nn. clunium medii	filaments
clunial n's, superior [general sensory]	nn. clunium superiores	filaments
coccygeal n.	n. coccygeus	
cochlear n. See vestibulocochlear n.		
cranial n's: The 12 pairs of nerves attached to the base of the brain	nn. craniales	
cubital n. See ulnar n.		

TABLE OF NERVES -- continued

Common Name [Modality]	NA Designation	Branches
cutaneous n. of arm, lateral, inferior [general sensory]	n. cutaneus brachii lateralis inferior	filaments
cutaneous n. of arm, lateral, superior [general sensory]	n. cutaneus brachii lateralis superior	filaments
cutaneous n. of arm, medial [general sensory]	n. cutaneus brachii medialis	filaments
cutaneous n. of arm, posterior [general sensory]	n. cutaneus brachii posterior	filaments
cutaneous n. of calf, lateral [general sensory]	n. cutaneus surae lateralis	sural n's
cutaneous n. of calf, medial [general sensory]	n. cutaneus surae medialis	sural n's
cutaneous n., dorsal, inter-mediate [general sensory]	n. cutaneus dorsalis intermedius	dorsal digital n's of foot
cutaneous n., dorsal, lateral [general sensory]	n. cutaneus dorsalis lateralis	filaments
cutaneous n., dorsal, medial [general sensory]	n. cutaneus dorsalis medialis	filaments
cutaneous n. of forearm, lateral [general sensory]	n. cutaneus antebrachii lateralis	filaments
cutaneous n. of forearm, medial [general sensory]	n. cutaneus antebrachii medialis	anterior and ulnar branches
cutaneous n. of forearm, posterior [general sensory]	n. cutaneus antebrachii posterior	filaments

Table continued on following page

TABLE OF NERVES -- continued

Common Name [Modality]	NA Designation	Branches
cutaneous n. of thigh, lateral [general sensory]	n. cutaneus femoris lateralis	anterior, posterior branches
cutaneous n. of thigh, posterior [general sensory]	n. cutaneus femoris posterior	inferior clunial n's, perineal branches
digital n's, dorsal, radial. *See* digital n's of radial n., dorsal		
digital n's, dorsal, ulnar. *See* digital n's of ulnar n., dorsal		
digital n's of foot, dorsal [general sensory]	nn. digitales dorsales pedis	
digital n's of lateral plantar n., plantar, common [general sensory]	nn. digitales plantares communes nervi plantaris lateralis	medial n. gives rise to 2 proper plantar digital n's
digital n's of lateral plantar n., plantar, proper [motor, general sensory]	nn. digitales plantares proprii nervi plantaris lateralis	proper plantar n's
digital n's of lateral surface of great toe and medial surface of second toe, dorsal [general sensory]	nn. digitales dorsales hallucis lateralis et digiti secundi medialis	filaments
digital n's of medial plantar n., plantar, common [motor, general sensory]	nn. digitales plantares communes nervi plantaris medialis	muscular and proper plantar digital n's
digital n's of medial plantar n., plantar, proper [general sensory]	nn. digitales plantares proprii nervi plantaris medialis	proper plantar n's
digital n's of median n., palmar, common [motor, general sensory]	nn. digitales palmares communes nervi mediani	

T A B L E O F N E R V E S -- continued

Common Name [Modality]	NA Designation	Branches
digital n's of median n., palmar, proper [motor, general sensory]	nn. digitales palmares proprii nervi mediani	filaments
digital n's of radial n., dorsal [general sensory]	nn. digitales dorsales nervi radialis	filaments
digital n's of ulnar n., dorsal [general sensory]	nn. digitales dorsales nervi ulnaris	proper plantar n's
digital n's of ulnar n., palmar, common [general sensory]	nn. digitales palmares communes nervi ulnaris	proper palmar digital n's
digital n's of ulnar n., palmar, proper [general sensory]	nn. digitales palmares proprii nervi ulnaris	filaments
dorsal n. of clitoris [general sensory, motor]	n. dorsalis clitoridis	filaments
dorsal n. of penis [general sensory, motor]	n. dorsalis penis	filaments
dorsal scapular n. [motor]	n. dorsalis scapulae	
ethmoidal n., anterior [general sensory]	n. ethmoidalis anterior	internal, external, lateral, and medial nasal branches
ethmoidal n., posterior [general sensory]	n. ethmoidalis posterior	filaments
n. of external acoustic meatus [general sensory]	n. meatus acustici externi	

Table continued on following page

TABLE OF NERVES -- continued

Common Name [Modality]	NA Designation	Branches
facial n. (7th cranial) [motor, parasympathetic, general sensory, special sensory]. *See* also intermediate n.	n. facialis	stapedius n.; posterior auricular n.; parotid plexus; digastric, temporal, zygomatic, buccal, lingual, marginal mandibular, and cervical branches, and communicating branch with tympanic plexus
femoral n. [general sensory, motor]	n. femoralis	saphenous n., muscular and anterior cutaneous branches
fibular n. *See* entries under peroneal n.	n. fibularis (NA alternative for n. peroneus)	
frontal n. [general sensory]	n. frontalis	supraorbital and supratrochlear n's
genitofemoral n. [general sensory, motor]	n. genitofemoralis	genital and femoral branches
glossopharyngeal n. (9th cranial) [motor, parasympathetic, general sensory, special sensory, visceral sensory]	n. glossopharyngeus	tympanic n., pharyngeal, stylopharyngeal, tonsillar, and lingual branches, branch to carotid sinus, communicating branch with auricular branch of vagus n.
gluteal n., inferior [motor]	n. gluteus inferior	
gluteal n., superior [motor, general sensory]	n. gluteus superior	superior filaments
hemorrhoidal n's, inferior. *See* rectal n's, inferior		
hypogastric n.	n. hypogastricus (dexter et sinister)	filaments
hypoglossal n. (12th cranial) [motor]	n. hypoglossus	lingual branches

T A B L E   O F   N E R V E S   — continued

Common Name [Modality]	NA Designation	Branches
iliohypogastric n. [motor, general sensory]	n. iliohypogastricus	lateral and anterior cutaneous branches
ilioinguinal n. [general sensory]	n. ilioinguinalis	anterior scrotal or labial branches
infraoccipital n. See suboccipital n.		
infraorbital n. [general sensory]	n. infraorbitalis	middle and anterior superior alveolar, inferior palpebral, internal and external nasal, and superior labial branches
infratrochlear n. [general sensory]	n. infratrochlearis	palpebral branches
intercostobrachial n's [general sensory]	nn. intercostobrachiales	filaments
intermediate n. [parasympathetic, special sensory]	n. intermedius	greater petrosal n., chorda tympani
interosseous n. of forearm, anterior [motor, general sensory]	n. interosseous [antebrachii] anterior	
interosseous n. of forearm, posterior [motor, general sensory]	n. interosseous [antebrachii] posterior	muscular, articular branches
interosseous n. of leg [general sensory]	interosseous cruris	filaments
ischiadic n. See sciatic n.		
jugular n.	n. jugularis	filaments

Table continued on following page

T A B L E   O F   N E R V E S -- continued

Common Name [Modality]	NA Designation	Branches
labial n's, anterior [general sensory]	nn. labiales anteriores	filaments
labial n's, posterior [general sensory]	nn. labiales posteriores	filaments
lacrimal n. [general sensory]	n. lacrimalis	superior and palpebral branches
laryngeal n., inferior [motor]	n. laryngeus inferior	filaments
laryngeal n., recurrent [parasympathetic, visceral afferent, motor]	n. laryngeus recurrens	inferior laryngeal n., tracheal, esophageal, and inferior cardiac branches
laryngeal n., superior [motor, general sensory, visceral afferent, parasympathetic]	n. laryngeus superior	external, internal, and communicating branches
lingual n. [general sensory]	n. lingualis	sublingual n., lingual branch, branch to isthmus of fauces, branch communicating with hypoglossal n. and chorda tympani
lumbar n's: The 5 pairs of n's that arise from lumbar segments of the spinal cord	nn. lumbales	ventral, dorsal branches
mandibular n. (third division of trigeminal n.) [general sensory, motor]	n. mandibularis	meningeal branch, masseteric, deep temporal, lateral and medial pterygoid, buccal, auriculotemporal, lingual and inferior alveolar n's

TABLE OF NERVES -- continued

Common Name [Modality]	NA Designation	Branches
masseteric n. [motor, general sensory]	n. massetericus	filaments
maxillary n. (second division of trigeminal n.) [general sensory]	n. maxillaris	meningeal branch, zygomatic n., posterior superior alveolar branches, infraorbital n., pterygopalatine n's, and indirectly branches of pterygopalatine ganglion
median n. [general sensory]	n. medianus	anterior interosseous n. of forearm, common palmar digital n's, and muscular and palmar branches, and a communicating branch with ulnar n.
mental n. [general sensory]	n. mentalis	mental and inferior labial branches
musculocutaneous n. [general sensory, motor]	n. musculocutaneus	lateral cutaneous n. of forearm, muscular branches
mylohyoid n. [motor]	n. mylohyoideus	filaments
nasociliary n. [general sensory]	n. nasociliaris	long ciliary, posterior ethmoidal, anterior ethmoidal, and infratrochlear n's and a communicating branch to ciliary ganglion
nasopalatine n. [parasympathetic, general sensory]	n. nasopalatinus	filaments
obturator n. [general sensory, motor]	n. obturatorius	anterior, posterior, and muscular branches
occipital n., greater [general sensory, motor]	n. occipitalis major	muscular branches
occipital n., lesser [general sensory]	n. occipitalis minor	auricular branches

Table continued on following page

T A B L E   O F   N E R V E S -- continued

Common Name [Modality]	NA Designation	Branches
occipital n., third [general sensory]	n. occipitalis tertius	
oculomotor n. (3rd cranial) [motor, parasympathetic]	n. oculomotorius	superior and inferior branches
olfactory n's (1st cranial) [special sensory]	nn. olfactorii	
ophthalmic n. (first division of trigeminal n.) [general sensory]	n. ophthalmicus	tentorial branches, frontal, lacrimal, naso-ciliary n's
optic n. (2nd cranial) [special sensory]	n. opticus	
palatine n., anterior. *See* palatine n., greater		
palatine n., greater [parasympathetic, sympathetic, general sensory]	n. palatinus major	posterior inferior [lateral] nasal branches
palatine n's, lesser [parasympathetic, sympathetic, general sensory]	nn. palatini minores	
perineal n's [general sensory, motor]	nn. perineales	muscular branches and posterior scrotal or labial nerves
peroneal n., common [general sensory, motor]	n. peroneus communis	supplies short head of biceps femoris muscle while still incorporated in sciatic nerve, gives off lateral sural cutaneous n., and divides into superficial and deep peroneal n's

T A B L E   O F   N E R V E S   -- continued

Common Name [Modality]	NA Designation	Branches
peroneal n., deep [general sensory, motor]	n. peroneus profundus	gives off muscular branches to tibialis anterior, extensor hallucis longus, extensor digitorum longus, and peroneus tertius muscles; lateral terminal division supplies extensor digitorum brevis muscle and tarsal joints
peroneal n., superficial [general sensory, motor]	n. peroneus superficialis	divides into muscular branches and medial and intermediate dorsal cutaneous n's
petrosal n., deep [sympathetic]	n. petrosus profundus	pterygoid canal n.
petrosal n., greater [parasympathetic, general sensory]	n. petrosus major	filaments
petrosal n., lesser [parasympathetic]	n. petrosus minor	ganglionic branches
phrenic n. [general sensory, motor]	n. phrenicus	pericardial and phrenicoabdominal branches
phrenic n's, accessory	nn. phrenici accessorii	join phrenic n's
plantar n., lateral [general sensory, motor]	n. plantaris lateralis	muscular, superficial, and deep branches
plantar n., medial [general sensory, motor]	n. plantaris medialis	common plantar digital n's and muscular branches
pneumogastric n. See vagus n.		
pterygoid n., lateral [motor]	n. pterygoideus lateralis	
pterygoid n., medial [motor]	n. pterygoideus medialis	tensor veli palatini, tensor tympani

Table continued on following page

TABLE OF NERVES -- continued

Common Name [Modality]	NA Designation	Branches
n. of pterygoid canal [parasympathetic, sympathetic]	n. canalis pterygoidei	
pterygopalatine n's [general sensory]	nn. pterygopalatini	orbital, greater palatine, posterior superior nasal, pharyngeal
pudendal n. [general sensory, motor, parasympathetic]	n. pudendus	enters pudendal canal, gives off inferior rectal n., then divides into perineal n. and dorsal n. of penis (clitoris)
radial n. [general sensory, motor]	n. radialis	posterior cutaneous and inferior lateral cutaneous n's of arm, posterior cutaneous n. of forearm, muscular, deep, and superficial branches
rectal n's, inferior [general sensory, motor]	nn. rectales inferiores	filaments
recurrent n. See laryngeal n., recurrent		
saccular n.	n. saccularis	
sacral n's	nn. sacrales	
saphenous n. [general sensory]	n. saphenus	infrapatellar and medial crural cutaneous
sciatic n. [general sensory, motor]	n. ischiadicus	divides into common peroneal and tibial n's, usually in lower third of thigh
scrotal n's, anterior [general sensory]	nn. scrotales anteriores	filaments
scrotal n's, posterior [general sensory]	nn. scrotales posteriores	filaments

TABLE OF NERVES 399

T A B L E   O F   N E R V E S -- continued

Common Name [Modality]	NA Designation	Branches
spinal n's: The 31 pairs of n's that arise from the spinal cord and pass between vertebrae	nn. spinales	
splanchnic n., greater [preganglionic sympathetic, visceral afferent]	n. splanchnicus major	filaments
splanchnic n., lesser [preganglionic sympathetic, visceral afferent]	n. splanchnicus minor	renal branch
splanchnic n., lowest [sympathetic, visceral afferent]	n. splanchnicus imus	filaments
splanchnic n's, lumbar [preganglionic sympathetic, visceral afferent]	nn. splanchnici lumbales	filaments
splanchnic n's, pelvic [preganglionic parasympathetic, visceral afferent]	nn. splanchnici pelvini	filaments
splanchnic n's, sacral [preganglionic sympathetic, visceral afferent]	nn. splanchnici sacrales	filaments
stapedius n. [motor]	n. stapedius	filaments
subclavian n. [motor, general sensory]	n. subclavius	articular branches
subcostal n. [general sensory, motor]	n. subcostalis	filaments

Table continued on following page

TABLE OF NERVES -- continued

Common Name [Modality]	NA Designation	Branches
sublingual n. [parasympathetic, general sensory]	n. sublingualis	filaments
suboccipital n. [motor]	n. suboccipitalis	filaments
subscapular n. [motor]	n. subscapularis	superior, inferior branches
supraclavicular n's, anterior. See supraclavicular n's, medial		
supraclavicular n's, intermediate [general sensory]	nn. supraclaviculares intermedii	filaments
supraclavicular n's, lateral [general sensory]	nn. supraclaviculares laterales	filaments
supraclavicular n's, medial [general sensory]	nn. supraclaviculares mediales	filaments
supraclavicular n's, middle. See supraclavicular n's, intermediate		
supraclavicular n's, posterior. See supraclavicular n's, lateral		
supraorbital n. [general sensory]	n. supraorbitalis	lateral and medial branches
suprascapular n. [motor, general sensory]	n. suprascapularis	supraspinous, infraspinous, articular branches

T A B L E   O F   N E R V E S -- continued

Common Name [Modality]	NA Designation	Branches
supratrochlear n. [general sensory]	n. supratrochlearis	filaments
sural n. [general sensory]	n. suralis	lateral dorsal cutaneous n. and lateral calcaneal branches
temporal n's, deep [motor]	nn. temporales profundi	
n. of tensor tympani [motor]	n. tensoris tympani	filaments
n. of tensor veli palatini [motor]	n. tensoris veli palatini	filaments
thoracic n's: The 12 pairs of nerves that arise from thoracic segments of the spinal cord	nn. thoracici	dorsal, ventral branches
thoracic n., long [motor]	n. thoracicus longus	filaments
thoracodorsal n. [motor]	n. thoracodorsalis	filaments
tibial n. [general sensory, motor]	n. tibialis	interosseous n. of leg, medial cutaneous n. of calf, sural and medial and lateral plantar n's, and muscular and medial calcaneal branches
trigeminal n. (5th cranial) [general sensory, motor]	n. trigeminus	
trochlear n. (4th cranial) [motor]	n. trochlearis	filaments

Table continued on following page

T A B L E   O F   N E R V E S -- continued

Common Name [Modality]	NA Designation	Branches
tympanic n. [general sensory, para- sympathetic]	n. tympanicus	helps form tympanic plexus
ulnar n. [general sensory, motor]	n. ulnaris	muscular, dorsal, palmar, superficial, and deep branches
utricular n.	n. utricularis	filaments
utriculoampullary n.	n. utriculoampullaris	
vaginal n's [sympathetic, parasym- pathetic]	nn. vaginales	filaments
vagus n., (10th cranial) [parasympathetic, visceral afferent, motor, general sensory]	n. vagus	superior and recurrent laryngeal n's, meningeal, auricular, pharyngeal cardiac, bronchial, gastric, hepatic, celiac, and renal branches, pharyngeal, pulmonary, and esophageal plexuses, and anterior and posterior trunks
vertebral n. [sympathetic]	n. vertebralis	meningeal branches
vestibulocochlear n. (8th cranial)	n. vestibulocochlearis	medial and lateral branches
vidian n. See n. of pterygoid canal		
vidian n., deep. See petrosal n., deep		
zygomatic n. [general sensory]	n. zygomaticus	zygomaticofacial and zygomaticotemporal branches

TABLE OF VEINS

Common Name	NA Designation	Receives Blood from or is Formed by	Drains into, Joins, or Continues as
accompanying v. of hypoglossal nerve	v. comitans nervi hypoglossi	formed by union of profunda linguae v. and sublingual v.	facial, lingual, or internal jugular
adrenal v's. See suprarenal v., left and right			
anastomotic v., inferior	v. anastomotica inferior	interconnects superficial middle cerebral v. and transverse sinus	
anastomotic v., superior	v. anastomotica superior	interconnects superficial middle cerebral v. and superior sagittal sinus	
angular v.	v. angularis	formed by union of supratrochlear v. and supraorbital v.	continues inferiorly as facial v.
antebrachial v., median	v. mediana antebrachii	a palmar venous plexus	cephalic v. and/or basilic v., or median cubital v.
appendicular v.	v. appendicularis		joins anterior and posterior cecal v's to form ileocolic v.
v. of aqueduct of vestibule	v. aqueductus vestibuli	internal ear	superior petrosal sinus
arcuate v's of kidney	vv. arcuatae renis	formed by union of interlobular v's and venules of kidney	interlobar v's

NOTES: v. = vein; v's = veins; v.[L] = vena; vv.[L] = venae.

Table continued on following page

TABLE OF VEINS — continued

Common Name	NA Designation	Receives Blood from or is Formed by	Drains into, Joins, or Continues as
auditory v's, internal. *See* labyrinthine v's			
auricular v's, anterior	vv. auriculares anteriores		superficial temporal v.
auricular v., posterior	v. auricularis posterior	a plexus on side of head	joins retromandibular v. to form external jugular v.
axillary v.	v. axillaris	formed at lower border of teres major muscle by junction of basilic v. and brachial v.	at lateral border of first rib is continuous with subclavian v.
azygos v.	v. azygos	ascending lumbar v.	superior vena cava
azygous v., left. *See* hemiazygos v.			
azygos v., lesser superior. *See* hemiazygos v., accessory			
basal v.	v. basalis	anterior perforated substance	internal cerebral v.
basilic v.	v. basilica	ulnar side of dorsal rete of hand	joins brachial v's to form axillary v.
basilic v., median	v. mediana basilica		basilic v.
basivertebral v's	vv. basivertebrales	venous sinuses in cancellous tissue of bodies of vertebrae, which communicate with venous plexus on anterior surface of vertebrae and with external and internal vertebral plexuses	
brachial v's	vv. brachiales		join basilic v. to form axillary v.

T A B L E   O F   V E I N S -- continued

Common Name	NA Designation	Receives Blood from or is Formed by	Drains into, Joins, or Continues as
brachiocephalic v's	vv. brachiocephalicae (dextra et sinistra)	head, neck, and upper limbs; formed at root of neck by union of ipsilateral internal jugular and subclavian v's	unite to form superior vena cava
bronchial v's	vv. bronchiales	larger subdivisions of bronchi	azygos v. on left; hemiazygos or superior intercostal v. on right
v. of bulb of penis	v. bulbi penis	bulb of penis	internal pudendal v.
v. of bulb of vestibule	v. bulbi vestibuli	bulb of vestibule of vagina	internal pudendal v.
cardiac v's, anterior	vv. cordis anteriores	anterior wall of right ventricle	right atrium of heart, or lesser cardiac v.
cardiac v., great	v. cordis magna	anterior surface of ventricles	coronary sinus
cardiac v., middle	v. cordis media	diaphragmatic surface of ventricles	coronary sinus
cardiac v., small	v. cordis parva	right atrium and ventricle	coronary sinus
cardiac v's, smallest	vv. cordis minimae	numerous small veins arising in myocardium, draining independently into cavities of heart and most readily seen in the atria	
carotid v., external. See retromandibular v.			
cavernous v's of penis	vv. cavernosae penis	corpora cavernosa	deep v's and dorsal v. of penis
central v's of liver	vv. centrales hepatis	liver substance	hepatic v.

Table continued on following page

TABLE OF VEINS -- continued

Common Name	NA Designation	Receives Blood from or is Formed by	Drains into, Joins, or Continues as
central v. of retina	v. centralis retinae		superior ophthalmic v.
central v. of suprarenal gland	v. centralis glandulae suprarenalis	the large single vein into which the various veins within the substance of the gland empty, and which continues at the hilus as the suprarenal v.	
cephalic v.	v. cephalica	radial side of dorsal rete of hand	axillary v.
cephalic v., accessory	v. cephalica accessoria	dorsal rete of hand	joins cephalic v. just above elbow
cephalic v., median	v. mediana cephalica		cephalic v.
cerebellar v's, inferior	vv. cerebelli inferiores	inferior surface of cerebellum	transverse, sigmoid, and inferior petrosal sinuses, or occipital sinus
cerebellar v's, superior	vv. cerebelli superiores	upper surface of cerebellum	straight sinus and great cerebral v., or transverse and superior petrosal sinuses
cerebral v., anterior	v. cerebri anterior		basal v.
cerebral v., great	v. cerebri magna	formed by union of the 2 internal cerebral veins	continues as or drains into straight sinus
cerebral v's, inferior	vv. cerebri inferiores	veins that ramify on base and inferolateral surface of brain, those on inferior surface of frontal lobe draining into inferior sagittal sinus and cavernous sinus; those on temporal lobe into superior petrosal sinus and transverse sinus; and those on occipital lobe into straight sinus	
cerebral v's, internal (2)	vv. cerebri internae	formed by union of thalamostriate v. and choroid v.; collect blood from basal ganglia	unite at splenium or corpus callosum to form great cerebral v.

TABLE OF VEINS -- continued

Common Name	NA Designation	Receives Blood from or is Formed by	Drains into, Joins, or Continues as
cerebral v., middle, deep	v. cerebri media profunda		basal v.
cerebral v., middle, superficial	v. cerebri media superficialis	lateral surface of cerebrum	cavernous sinus
cerebral v's, superior	vv. cerebri superiores	about 12 veins draining superolateral and medial surfaces of cerebrum toward longitudinal fissure	superior sagittal and medial surfaces of cerebrum toward longitudinal fissure
cervical v., deep	v. cervicalis profunda	a plexus in suboccipital triangle	vertebral v. or brachiocephalic v.
cervical v's, transverse	vv. transversae colli		subclavian v.
choroid v.	v. choroidea	choroid plexus, hippocampus, fornix, corpus callosum	joins thalamostriate v. to form internal cerebral v.
ciliary v's	vv. ciliares	arise in eyeball by branches from ciliary muscle; anterior ciliary v's also receive branches from sinus venosus, sclerae, episcleral v's and conjunctiva of eyeball	superior ophthalmic v., posterior ciliary v's empty also into inferior ophthalmic v.
circumflex femoral v's, lateral	vv. circumflexae femoris laterales		femoral v. or profunda femoris v.
circumflex femoral v's, medial	vv. circumflexae femoris mediales		femoral v. or profunda femoris v.
circumflex iliac v., deep	v. circumflexa ilium profunda	a common trunk formed by veins accompanying deep circumflex iliac artery	

Table continued on following page

TABLE OF VEINS -- continued

Common Name	NA Designation	Receives Blood from or is Formed by	Drains into, Joins, or Continues as
circumflex iliac v., superficial	v. circumflexa ilium superficialis		great saphenous v.
v. of cochlear canal	v. canaliculi	cochlea	superior bulb of internal jugular v.
colic v., left	v. colica sinistra		inferior mesenteric v.
colic v., middle	v. colica media		superior mesenteric v.
colic v., right	v. colica dextra		superior mesenteric v.
conjunctival v's	vv. conjunctivales	conjunctiva	superior ophthalmic v.
coronary v's. *See* entries under cardiac v's.			
cubital v., median	v. mediana cubiti		basilic v.
cutaneous v.	v. cutanea	one of the small veins that begin in papillae of skin, form subpapillary plexuses, and open into the subcutaneous veins	
cystic v.	v. cystica	gallbladder	right branch of portal v.
deep v's of clitoris	vv. profundae clitoridis	clitoris	vesical venous plexus
deep v's of penis	vv. profundae penis	penis	dorsal v. of penis
digital v's of foot, dorsal	vv. digitales dorsales pedis		unite at clefts to form dorsal metatarsal v's
digital v's, palmar	vv. digitales palmares		superficial palmar venous arch
digital v's, plantar	vv. digitales plantares		unite at clefts to form plantar metatarsal v's

TABLE OF VEINS -- continued

Common Name	NA Designation	Receives Blood from or is Formed by	Drains into, Joins, or Continues as
diploic v., frontal	v. diploica frontalis	frontal bone	supraorbital v. externally, or superior sagittal sinus internally
diploic v., occipital	v. diploica occipitalis	occipital bone	occipital v. or transverse sinus
diploic v., temporal, anterior	v. diploica temporalis anterior	lateral portion of frontal bone, anterior part of parietal bone	sphenoparietal sinus internally, or a deep temporal v. externally
diploic v., temporal, posterior	v. diploica temporalis posterior	parietal bone	transverse sinus
dorsal v. of clitoris, deep	v. dorsalis clitoridis profunda	clitoris, subcutaneously	vesical plexus
dorsal v's of clitoris, superficial	vv. dorsales clitoridis superficiales	clitoris, subcutaneously	external pudendal v.
dorsal v. of penis, deep	v. dorsalis penis profunda	the single median vein lying subfascially in penis between the dorsal arteries; it begins in small veins around corona of glans, is joined by deep veins of penis as it passes between arcuate pubic and transverse perineal ligaments, where it divides into a left and a right vein to join prostatic plexus	
dorsal v's of penis, superficial	vv. dorsales penis superficiales	penis, subcutaneously	external pudendal v.
dorsal v's of tongue. See lingual v's, dorsal	vv. dorsales linguae		
emissary v., condylar	v. emissaria condylaris	a small vein running through condylar canal of skull, connecting sigmoid sinus with vertebral v. or internal jugular v.	
emissary v., mastoid	v. emissaria mastoidea	a small vein passing through mastoid foramen of skull, connecting sigmoid sinus with occipital v. or posterior auricular v.	

Table continued on following page

T A B L E   O F   V E I N S -- continued

Common Name	NA Designation	Receives Blood from or is Formed by	Drains into, Joins, or Continues as
emissary v., occipital	v. emissaria occipitalis	an occasional small vein running through a minute foramen in occipital protuberance of skull, connecting confluence of sinuses with occipital v.	
emissary v., parietal	v. emissaria parietalis	a small vein passing through parietal foramen of skull, connecting superior sagittal sinus with superficial temporal v's	
epigastric v., inferior	v. epigastrica inferior		external iliac v.
epigastric v., superficial	v. epigastrica superficialis		great saphenous v. or femoral v.
epigastric v's, superior	vv. epigastricae superiores		internal thoracic v.
episcleral v's	vv. episclerales		ciliary v's
esophageal v's	vv. esophageae	esophagus	hemiazygos v. and azygos v., or left brachiocephalic v.
ethmoidal v's	vv. ethmoidales		superior ophthalmic v.
facial v.	v. facialis	the vein beginning at medial angle of eye as angular v., descending behind facial artery, and usually ending in internal jugular v.; sometimes joins retromandibular v. to form a common trunk	
facial v., deep	v. faciei profunda	pterygoid plexus	facial v.
facial v., posterior. *See* retromandibular v.			
facial v., transverse	v. transversa faciei		retromandibular v.
femoral v.	v. femoralis	continuation of popliteal v.	at inguinal ligament becomes external iliac v.

T A B L E   O F   V E I N S -- continued

Common Name	NA Designation	Receives Blood from or is Formed by	Drains into, Joins, or Continues as
femoral v., deep	v. profunda femoris		femoral v.
fibular v's. *See* peroneal v's.	vv. fibulares (NA alternative for vv. peroneae)		
gastric v., left	v. gastrica sinistra		portal v.
gastric v., right	v. gastrica dextra		portal v.
gastric v's, short	vv. gastricae breves	left portion of greater curvature of stomach	splenic v.
gastroepiploic v., left	v. gastroepiploica sinistra		splenic v.
gastroepiploic v., right	v. gastroepiploica dextra		superior mesenteric v.
genicular v's	vv. genus		popliteal v.
gluteal v's, inferior	vv. gluteae inferiores	subcutaneous tissue of back of thigh, muscles of buttock	internal iliac v.
gluteal v's, superior	vv. gluteae superiores	muscles of buttock	internal iliac v.
hemiazygos v.	v. hemiazygos	ascending lumbar v.	azygos v.
hemiazygos v., accessory	v. hemiazygos accessoria	the descending intercepting trunk for upper, often fourth through eighth, left posterior intercostal v's; it lies on left side and at eighth thoracic vertebra joins hemiazygos v. or crosses to right side to join azygos v. directly	
hemorrhoidal v's. *See* entries under rectal v's.			

Table continued on following page

TABLE OF VEINS -- continued

Common Name	NA Designation	Receives Blood from or is Formed by	Drains into, Joins, or Continues as
hepatic v's	vv. hepaticae	central v's of liver	inferior vena cava on posterior aspect of liver
hypogastric v. *See* iliac v., internal.			
ileal v's. *See* jejunal and ileal v's.			
ileocolic v.	v. ileocolica		superior mesenteric v.
iliac v., common	v. iliaca communis	arises at sacroiliac joint by union of external and internal iliac v's	unites with fellow of opposite side to form inferior vena cava
iliac v., external	v. iliaca externa	continuation of femoral v.	joins internal iliac v. to form common iliac v.
iliac v., internal	v. iliaca interna	formed by union of parietal branches	joins external iliac v. to form common iliac v.
iliolumbar v.	v. iliolumbalis		internal iliac v. and/or common iliac v.
innominate v's. *See* brachiocephalic v's.			
intercapital v's	vv. intercapitales	veins at clefts of fingers that pass between heads of metacarpal bones and establish communication between dorsal and palmar venous systems of hand	
intercostal v's, anterior (12 pairs)	vv. intercostales anteriores		internal thoracic v's
intercostal v., highest	v. intercostalis suprema		brachiocephalic, vertebral, or superior intercostal v.

TABLE OF VEINS -- continued

Common Name	NA Designation	Receives Blood from or is Formed by	Drains into, Joins, or Continues as
intercostal v's, posterior, IV and XI	vv. intercostales posteriores (IV et XI)		azygos v. on right; hemiazygos or accessory hemiazygos v. on left
intercostal v., superior, left	v. intercostalis superior sinistra	formed by union of second, third, and sometimes fourth posterior intercostal v's	
intercostal v., superior, right	v. intercostalis superior dextra	formed by union of second, third, and sometimes fourth posterior intercostal v's	azygos v.
interlobar v's of kidney	vv. interlobares renis	venous arcades of kidney	join to form renal v.
interlobular v's of kidney	vv. interlobulares renis	capillary network of renal cortex	venous arcades of kidney
interlobular v's of liver	vv. interlobulares hepatis	liver	portal v.
interosseous v's of foot, dorsal. See metatarsal v's, dorsal.			
intervertebral v.	v. intervertebralis	vertebral venous plexuses	in neck, vertebral v.; in thorax, intercostal v's; in abdomen, lumbar v's; in pelvis, lateral sacral v's
jejunal v's. See jejunal and ileal v's.			
jejunal and ileal v's	vv. jejunales et ilei	jejunum and ileum	superior mesenteric v.
jugular v., anterior	v. jugularis anterior		external jugular v. or subclavian v., or jugular venous arch

Table continued on following page

TABLE OF VEINS -- continued

Common Name	NA Designation	Receives Blood from or is Formed by	Drains into, Joins, or Continues as
jugular v., external	v. jugularis externa	formed by union of retromandibular v. and posterior auricular v.	subclavian v., internal jugular v., or brachiocephalic v.
jugular v., internal	v. jugularis interna	begins as superior bulb, draining much of head and neck	joins subclavian v. to form brachiocephalic v.
labial v's, anterior	vv. labiales anteriores	anterior aspect of labia in female	external pudendal v.
labial v's, inferior	vv. labiales inferiores	region of lower lip	facial v.
labial v's, posterior	vv. labiales posteriores	labia in female	vesical venous plexus
labial v., superior	v. labiales superior	region of upper lip	facial v.
labyrinthine v's	vv. labyrinthi	cochlea	inferior petrosal sinus or transverse sinus
lacrimal v.	v. lacrimalis	lacrimal gland	superior ophthalmic v.
laryngeal v., inferior	v. laryngea inferior	larynx	inferior thyroid v.
laryngeal v., superior	v. laryngea superior	larynx	superior thyroid v.
lingual v.	v. lingualis		internal jugular v.
lingual v., deep	v. profunda linguae	deep aspect of tongue	joins sublingual v. to form accompanying v. of hypoglossal nerve
lingual v's, dorsal	vv. dorsales linguae	veins that unite with a small vein accompanying lingual artery and join main lingual trunk	

TABLE OF VEINS -- continued

Common Name	NA Designation	Receives Blood from or is Formed by	Drains into, Joins, or Continues as
lumbar v's, I and II	vv. lumbales (I et II)		ascending lumbar v.
lumbar v's, III and IV	vv. lumbales (III et IV)		usually, inferior vena cava
lumbar v., ascending	v. lumbalis ascendens	an ascending intercepting vein for lumbar v's on either side; it begins in lateral sacral region and ascends to first lumbar vertebra, where by union with subcostal v. it becomes on right side the azygos v. and on left the hemiazygos v.	
maxillary v's	vv. maxillares	usually form a single short trunk with pterygoid plexus	joins superficial temporal v. in parotid gland to form retro-mandibular v.
mediastinal v's	vv. mediastinales	anterior mediastinum	brachiocephalic v. or azygos v.
meningeal v's	vv. meningeae	dura mater (also communicate with lateral lacunae)	regional sinuses and veins
meningeal v's, middle	vv. meningeae mediae		pterygoid venous plexus
mesenteric v., inferior	v. mesenterica inferior		splenic v.
mesenteric v., superior	v. mesenterica superior		joins splenic v. to form portal v.
metacarpal v's, dorsal	vv. metacarpeae dorsales	veins arising from union of dorsal veins of adjacent fingers and passing proximally to join in forming dorsal venous network of hand	
metacarpal v's, palmar	vv. metacarpeae palmares		deep palmar venous arch
metatarsal v's, dorsal	vv. metatarseae dorsales	arise from dorsal digital v's of toes at clefts of toes	dorsal venous arch
metatarsal v's, plantar	vv. metatarseae plantares	arise from plantar digital v's at clefts of toes	plantar venous arch

Table continued on following page

T A B L E   O F   V E I N S -- continued

Common Name	NA Designation	Receives Blood from or is Formed by	Drains into, Joins, or Continues as
musculophrenic v's	vv. musculophrenicae	parts of diaphragm and wall of thorax and abdomen	internal thoracic v's
nasal v's, external	vv. nasales externae		angular v., facial v.
nasofrontal v.	v. nasofrontalis	supraorbital v.	superior ophthalmic v.
oblique v. of left atrium	v. obliqua atrii sinistri		coronary sinus
obturator v's	vv. obturatoriae	hip joint and regional muscles	internal iliac v. and/or inferior epigastric v.
occipital v.	v. occipitalis		opens under trapezius muscle into suboccipital venous plexus, or accompanies occipital artery to end in internal jugular v.
ophthalmic v., inferior	v. ophthalmica inferior	a vein formed by confluence of muscular and ciliary branches, and running backward to join superior ophthalmic v. or to open directly into cavernous sinus; it sends a communicating branch through inferior orbital fissure to join pterygoid venous plexus	
ophthalmic v., superior	v. ophthalmica superior	a vein beginning at medial angle of eye, where it communicates with frontal, supraorbital, and angular v's, and may be joined by inferior ophthalmic v. at superior orbital fissure before opening into cavernous sinus	
ovarian v., left	v. ovarica sinistra	pampiniform plexus of broad ligament on left	left renal v.
ovarian v., right	v. ovarica dextra	pampiniform plexus of broad ligament on right	inferior vena cava
palatine v., external	v. palatina externa	tonsils and soft palate	facial v.

T A B L E   O F   V E I N S -- continued

Common Name	NA Designation	Receives Blood from or is Formed by	Drains into, Joins, or Continues as
palpebral v's	vv. palpebrales		superior ophthalmic v.
palpebral v's, inferior	vv. palpebrales inferiores	lower eyelid	facial v.
palpebral v's, superior	vv. palpebrales superiores	upper eyelid	angular v.
pancreatic v's	vv. pancreaticae	pancreas	splenic v., superior mesenteric v.
pancreaticoduodenal v's	vv. pancreaticoduodenales	4 veins that drain blood from pancreas and duodenum, closely following pancreaticoduodenal arteries, a superior and an inferior vein originating from an anterior and a posterior venous arcade; anterior superior v. joins right gastro-epiploic v., and posterior superior v. joins portal v.; anterior and posterior inferior v's join uppermost jejunal v. or superior mesenteric v.	
paraumbilical v's	vv. paraumbilicales	veins that communicate with portal v. above and descend to anterior abdominal wall to anastomose with superior and inferior epigastric and superior vesical v's in region of umbilicus	
parotid v's	vv. parotideae	parotid gland	superficial temporal v.
perforating v's	vv. perforantes		profunda femoris v.
pericardiac v's	vv. pericardiacae	pericardium	brachiocephalic, inferior thyroid, and azygos v's, superior vena cava
pericardiacophrenic v's	vv. pericardiaco-phrenicae	pericardium and diaphragm	left brachiocephalic v.
peroneal v's	vv. peroneae		posterior tibial v.

Table continued on following page

T A B L E   O F   V E I N S -- continued

Common Name	NA Designation	Receives Blood from or is Formed by	Drains into, Joins, or Continues as
pharyngeal v's	vv. pharyngeae	pharyngeal plexus	internal jugular v.
phrenic v's, inferior	vv. phrenicae inferiores		on right, enters inferior vena cava; on left, enters left suprarenal or renal v., or inferior vena cava
phrenic v's, superior. *See* pericardiacophrenic v's.			
popliteal v.	v. poplitea	formed by union of anterior and posterior tibial v's	at adductor hiatus becomes femoral v.
portal v.	v. portae	a short, thick trunk formed by union of superior mesenteric and splenic v's behind neck of pancreas; it ascends to right end of porta hepatis, where it divides into successively smaller branches until it forms a capillary-like system of sinusoids that permeates entire substance of liver	
posterior v. of left ventricle	v. posterior ventriculi sinistri cordis	posterior surface of left ventricle	coronary sinus
prepyloric v.	v. prepylorica		right gastric v.
profunda femoris v. *See* femoral v., deep.			
profunda linguae v. *See* lingual v., deep.			
v. of pterygoid canal	v. canalis pterygoidei		pterygoid plexus
pudendal v's, external	vv. pudendae externae		great saphenous v.
pudendal v., internal	v. pudenda interna		internal iliac v.

T A B L E   O F   V E I N S -- continued

Common Name	NA Designation	Receives Blood from or is Formed by	Drains into, Joins, or Continues as
pulmonary v., inferior, left	v. pulmonalis inferior sinistra	lower lobe of left lung	left atrium of heart
pulmonary v., inferior, right	v. pulmonalis inferior dextra	lower lobe of right lung	left atrium of heart
pulmonary v., superior, left	v. pulmonalis superior sinistra	upper lobe of left lung	left atrium of heart
pulmonary v., superior, right	v. pulmonalis superior dextra	upper and middle lobes of right lung	left atrium of heart
pyloric v. See gastric v., right.			
radial v's	vv. radiales		brachial v's
ranine v. See sublingual v.			
rectal v's, inferior	vv. rectales inferiores	rectal plexus	internal pudendal v.
rectal v's, middle	vv. rectales mediae	rectal plexus	internal iliac and superior rectal v's
rectal v., superior	v. rectalis superior	upper part of rectal plexus	inferior mesenteric v.
renal v's	vv. renales	kidneys	inferior vena cava
retromandibular v.	v. retromandibularis	the vein formed in upper part of parotid gland behind neck of mandible by union of maxillary and superficial temporal v's; it passes downward through the gland, communicates with facial v. and, emerging from the gland, joins with posterior auricular v. to form external jugular v.	

Table continued on following page

T A B L E   O F   V E I N S -- continued

Common Name	NA Designation	Receives Blood from or is Formed by	Drains into, Joins, or Continues as
sacral v's, lateral	vv. sacrales laterales		help form lateral sacral plexus; empty into internal iliac v. or superior gluteal v's
sacral v., median	v. sacralis mediana		common iliac v.
saphenous v., accessory	v. saphena accessoria	when present, medial and posterior superficial parts of thigh	great saphenous v.
saphenous v., great	v. saphena magna		femoral v.
saphenous v., small	v. saphena parva		popliteal v.
scrotal v's, anterior	vv. scrotales anteriores	anterior aspect of scrotum	external pudendal v.
scrotal v's, posterior	vv. scrotales posteriores		vesical venous plexus
v. of septum pellucidum	v. septi pellucidi		thalamostriate v.
sigmoid v's	vv. sigmoideae	sigmoid colon	inferior mesenteric v.
spinal v's	vv. spinales		
spiral v. of modiolus	v. spiralis modioli		labyrinthine v's
splenic v.	v. lienalis	formed by union of several branches at hilus of spleen	joins superior mesenteric v. to form portal v.
stellate v's of kidney	venulae stellatae renis	superficial parts of renal cortex	interlobular v's of kidney
sternocleidomastoid v.	v. sternocleidomastidea		internal jugular v.
striate v.	v. striata	anterior perforated substance of brain	basal v.

T A B L E   O F   V E I N S -- continued

Common Name	NA Designation	Receives Blood from or is Formed by	Drains into, Joins, or Continues as
stylomastoid v.	v. stylomastoidea		retromandibular v.
subclavian v.	v. subclavia	continues axillary v. as main venous channel of upper limb	joins internal jugular v. to form brachiocephalic v.
subcostal v.	v. subcostalis		joins ascending lumbar v. to form azygos v. on right, hemiazygos v. on left
subcutaneous v's of abdomen	vv. subcutaneae abdominis		
sublingual v.	v. sublingualis		lingual v.
submental v.	v. submentalis		facial v.
supraorbital v.	v. supraorbitalis		joins supratrochlear v. at root of nose to form angular v.
suprarenal v., left	v. suprarenalis sinistra	left suprarenal gland	left renal v.
suprarenal v., right	v. suprarenalis dextra	right suprarenal gland	inferior vena cava
suprascapular v.	v. suprascapularis		usually into external jugular v.; occasionally into subclavian v.
supratrochlear v's (2)	vv. supratrochleares	venous plexuses high up on forehead	joins supraorbital v. at root of nose to form angular v.
temporal v's, deep	vv. temporales profundae	deep portions of temporal muscle	pterygoid plexus
temporal v., middle	v. temporalis media	arises in substance of temporal muscle	joins superficial temporal v.

Table continued on following page

T A B L E   O F   V E I N S -- continued

Common Name	NA Designation	Receives Blood from or is Formed by	Drains into, Joins, or Continues as
temporal v's, superficial	vv. temporales superficiales	veins that drain lateral part of scalp in frontal and parietal regions, the branches forming a single superficial temporal v. in front of ear, just above zygoma; this descending vein receives middle temporal and transverse facial v's and, entering parotid gland, unites with maxillary v. to form retromandibular v.	
testicular v., left	v. testicularis sinistra	left pampiniform plexus	left renal v.
testicular v., right	v. testicularis dextra	right pampiniform plexus	inferior vena cava
thalamostriate v.	v. thalamostriata	corpus striatum and thalamus	joins choroid v. to form internal cerebral v's
thoracic v's, internal	vv. thoracicae internae	2 veins formed by junction of the veins accompanying internal thoracic artery of either side; each continues along the artery to open into brachiocephalic v.	
thoracic v., lateral	v. thoracica lateralis		axillary v.
thoracoacromial v.	v. thoracoacromialis		subclavian v.
thoracoepigastric v's	vv. thoracoepigastricae		superiorly into lateral thoracic v.; inferiorly into femoral v.
thymic v's	vv. thymicae	thymus	left brachiocephalic v.
thyroid v., inferior	v. thyroidea inferior	either of 2 veins, left and right, that drain thyroid plexus into left and right brachiocephalic v's; occasionally they may unite into a common trunk to empty, usually, into left brachiocephalic v.	
thyroid v's, middle	vv. thyroideae mediae	thyroid gland	internal jugular v.
thyroid v., superior	v. thyroidea superior	thyroid gland	internal jugular v., occasionally in common with facial v.

T A B L E   O F   V E I N S -- continued

Common Name	NA Designation	Receives Blood from or is Formed by	Drains into, Joins, or Continues as
tibial v's, anterior	vv. tibiales anteriores		join posterior tibial v's to form popliteal v.
tibial v's, posterior	vv. tibiales posteriores		join anterior tibial v's to form popliteal v.
tracheal v's	vv. tracheales	trachea	brachiocephalic v.
tympanic v's	vv. tympanicae	small veins from middle ear that pass through petrotympanic fissure and open into the plexus around temporomandibular joint	
ulnar v's	vv. ulnares		join radial v's at elbow to form brachial v's
umbilical v.	v. umbilicalis (formerly)	in the early embryo, either of the paired veins that carry blood from chorion to sinus venosus and heart; they later fuse and become left umbilical v. of fetus	
umbilical v. of fetus, left	v. umbilicalis sinistra	the vein formed by fusion of atrophied right umbilical v. with the left umbilical v., which carries all the blood from placenta to ductus venosus	
uterine v's	vv. uterinae	uterine plexus	internal iliac v's
vena cava, inferior	vena cava inferior	the venous trunk for the lower limbs and for pelvic and abdominal viscera; it begins at level of fifth lumbar vertebra by union of common iliac v's and ascends on right of aorta	
vena cava, superior	vena cava superior	the venous trunk draining blood from head, neck, upper limbs, and thorax; it begins by union of 2 brachiocephalic v's and passes directly downward	

PART III

APPENDICES

Useful Data

APPENDIX 1
Symbols and Metric Prefixes

Symbol	Meaning	Symbol	Meaning
Ⓛ	left	σ	1/100 of a second, standard deviation
®	right, trademark	χ^2	chi square (test)
Ⓜ	murmur	τ	life (time)
⊙	start of operation	$\tau\frac{1}{2}$	half-life (time)
⊗	end of operation	?	question of, questionable, possible
□	male	>	greater than
○	female	≯	not greater than
♂	male	≥	greater than or equal to
♀	female	<	less than
*	birth	≮	not less than
†	death	≤	less than or equal to
α	alpha particle, is proportional to	~	approximate
Δ	prism diopter	$\simeq$	approximately equal to
Δt	time interval	±	not definite, plus/minus
ΔA	change in absorbance	(+)	significant
ΔpH	change in pH	(−)	insignificant
Ω	ohm	(±)	possibly significant
π	3.1416−ratio of circumference of a circle to its diameter	↓	decreased, depression
		↑	elevation, increased

Symbols consisting of letters of the alphabet appear in Part I, Vocabulary.

⇡	up	2×	twice
↑V	increase due to *in vivo* effect	×2	twice
↓V	decrease due to *in vivo* effect	′	foot, minute, primary accent, univalent
↑C	increase due to chemical interference during the assay	″	inch, second, secondary accent, bivalent
↓C	decrease due to chemical interference during the assay	⊓̈	two
→	causes, no change, transfer to	/	of, per
←	is due to	:	ratio (is to)
⇌	reversible reaction	::	equality between ratios, "as"
⊖	normal	∴	therefore
√c̄	check with	+	plus, positive, present
φ	none	−	minus, negative, absent
∨	systolic blood pressure	÷	divided by
∧	diastolic blood pressure	=	equals
#	gauge, number, weight, pound(s)	≠	does not equal, not equal to
		≅	approximately equals
℞	recipe, take	%	per cent
°	degree	℥	ounce
24°	24 hours	f℥	fluid ounce
1°	primary	℈	scruple
2°	secondary	♏	minim
2d	second	ℨ	drachm, dram
2ndry	secondary	f℈	fluidrachm, fluidram
1×	once	√	root, square root, radical
		∛̸	square root

$\sqrt[3]{}$	cube root	606	arsphenamine
∞	infinity	914	neoarsphenamine
$\bigcirc$	combined with		

Prefixes for Metric System Multiples and Submultiples

Symbol	Name	Value
T	tera	10^{12}
G	giga	10^{9}
M	mega	10^{6}
my	myria	10^{4}
k	kilo	10^{3}
h	hecto	10^{2}
dk	deka	10
d	deci	10^{-1}
c	centi	10^{-2}
m	milli	10^{-3}
μ	micro	10^{-6}
n	nano	10^{-9}
p	pico	10^{-12}
f	femto	10^{-15}
a	atto	10^{-18}

APPENDIX 2
Medically Significant Prefixes and Suffixes

A hyphen appears following a prefix (as in ante-)
and precedes a suffix (as in -agra).

a-	not, without: *a*typical, *an*odontia (*n* is added to the prefix before words beginning with a vowel)	auri-	ear: *auri*nasal
		auto-	self: *auto*intoxication
		bi-	twice: *bi*lateral
		bili-	bile: *bili*ary
		bio-	life: *bio*genous
ab-	away from: *ab*ducent	blasto-	formation of cells: *blasto*derm
abdomin(o)-	abdomen: *abdomin*algia, *abdomino*cystic	-blast	an immature cell: histio*blast*
actino-	ray, radium: *actino*genesis	blephar(o)-	eyelid or eyelash: *blephar*edema, *blepharo*adenoma
ad-	toward: *ad*duct		
aden(o)-	gland: *aden*itis, *adeno*pharyngitis	brachy-	short: *brachy*cephalic
		brady-	slow: *brady*cardia
aer(o)-	air: *aer*emia, *aero*cele	bronch-,	windpipe: *bronch*itis,
-agogue	leading, inducing: galact*agogue*	bronchi-, bronchio-	*bronchi*ectasis, *broncho*malacia
alb-	white: *alb*umin	calor-	heat: *calor*imeter
-algia	pain: neur*algia*	carbo-	coal, charcoal: *carbo*hydrate
ambi-	both: *ambi*lateral		
an-	see *a*	cardi(o)-	heart: *cardi*asthenia, *cardio*cele
ante-	before: *ante*flexion		
anti-	against: *anti*pyogenic	cata-	down, lower: *cata*crotism
antro-	cavern: *antro*dynia		
arachn(o)-	spider: *arachn*idism, *arachno*dactyly	caud(o)-	tail: *caud*ate, *caudo*cephalad
arteri(o)-	artery: *arteri*ectasis, *arterio*sclerosis	-cele	tumor, hernia: cysto*cele*
		centi-	hundred, hundredth part: *centi*meter
arthr(o)-	joint: *arthr*ectomy, *arthro*cele	cephal(o)-	cranium, head: *cephal*hydrocele, *cephalo*thoracic
-asis, -esis, -iasis, -osis	state or condition: metast*asis*, metath*esis*, cholelith*iasis*, trichin*osis*		
		cerebro-	brain: *cerebro*spinal

430

cervic(o)-	neck: *cervic*itis, *cervico*vesical	digit-	finger, toe: *digit*ate
chol-, chole-, cholo-	bile: *chol*angitis, *chole*cystitis, *cholo*lith	diplo-	double: *diplo*pia
		dis-	absence, reversal, separation: *dis*location
chondro-	cartilage: *chondro*malacia	dolicho-	long: *dolicho*cephaly
cili-	eyelid: *cili*ary;	dorsi-, dorso-	back: *dorsi*spinal, *dorso*lumbar
circum-	around: *circum*ferential	-duct	draw, lead: ovi*duct*
cleid(o)-	hook, clavicle: *cleid*arthritis, *cleido*mastoid	dys-	difficult, painful, bad, disordered: *dys*trophy
colp(o)-	bosom or fold; vagina: *colp*ectomy, *colpo*dynia	ec-	out of: *ec*centric
		ect(o)-	out of, away from: *ect*iris, *ecto*pic
contra-	against: *contra*indication	-ectomy	surgical removal of: cholecyst*ectomy*
cortico-	bark, rind: *cortico*steroid	em-, en-	in: *em*bolism, *en*capsulated
costo-	rib: *costo*chondral	end(o)-	inward, within: *end*aural, *endo*carditis
cox(o)-	hip, hip joint: *cox*algia, *coxo*dynia	enter(o)-	intestines: *enter*itis, *entero*cele
crani(o)-	cranium: *crani*ectomy, *cranio*cele	ep-, epi-	on, upon, above, over: *ep*axial, *epi*dermis
cry(o)-	cold: *cry*esthesia, *cryo*pathy	eso-	inside, within: *eso*phoria
crypt(o)-	hidden, obscure: *crypt*esthesia, *crypto*empyema	eu-	well, good, easily: *eu*crasia
cut-	skin: *cut*aneous	ex-	out, away from: *ex*cretion
cyst-, cysti-, cystido-, cysto-	bladder: *cyst*itis, *cysti*cercoid, *cystido*laparotomy, *cysto*myxoma	exo-	outside, extra: *exo*toxin
		extra-	beyond, in addition: *extra*cellular
		-facient	making: cale*facient*
cyt(o)-	cell: *cyt*ase, *cyto*clasis	fasci-	band: *fasci*culus
dacry(o)-	tears: *dacry*adenitis, *dacryo*lith	febr-	fever: *febr*ile
		fil-	thread: *fil*iform
derma-, dermat-, dermato-, dermo-	skin: *derma*brasion, *dermat*algia, *dermato*phytosis, *dermo*blast	-flect	bend, divert: de*flect*
		-form	shape: ossi*form*
		galact(o)-	milk: *galact*emia, *galacto*phoritis
dextr(o)-	right side: *dextr*al, *dextro*cardia	gam(o)-	marriage or sexual union: *gam*etophyte, *gamo*genesis
di-	two: *di*morphic		
dia-	throughout, completely: *dia*kinesis	gangli(o)-	ganglion, knot: *gangli*al, *ganglio*neuroma

gastr(o)-	stomach: *gastr*itis, *gastro*duodenal	homo-, homeo-, homoio-	same, common, similar: *homo*geneous, *homeo*pathic, *homoio*thermy
gelat-	freeze, congeal: *gelat*inous	hydr(o)-	water or hydrogen: *hydr*amnios, *hydro*cephalus
-genic	producing, productive of: osteo*genic*	hyper-	above, beyond, extreme: *hyper*trophy
genio-	chin: *genio*plasty	hypno-	sleep: *hypno*tic
genito-	relationship to organs of reproduction: *genito*crural	hypo-	beneath, under deficient: *hypo*chondrium
geno-	reproduction or sex: *geno*type	hypso-	height: *hypso*kinesis
-glia	glue: neuro*glia*	hyster(o)-	womb: *hyster*ectomy, *hystero*salpingostomy
gloss(o)-	tongue: *gloss*itis, *glosso*dynia	-iasis	morbid or diseased condition: elephant*iasis*
glyc-	sweet: *glyc*emia	iatro-	relation to physician or to medicine: *iatro*physics
-gram	write, record: encephalo*gram*		
-graph	scratch, write, record: cardio*graph*	-id	having the shape of, resembling: dermatophyt*id*
gymno-	naked: *gymno*cyte		
gyn-, gyne-, gyneco-, gyno-	woman, female sex: *gyn*atresia, *gyne*phobia, *gyneco*mastia, *gyno*pathy	-ide	a binary chemical compound: chlor*ide*
		idio-	self: *idio*pathic
		ileo-	ileum: *ileo*cecal
gyro-	round, ring, circle: *gyro*spasm	ilio-	ilium or flank: *ilio*pubic
		im- or in-	in, within, into: *im*mersion, *in*jection
hema-, hemo-, hemato-	blood: *hema*pheresis, *hemo*globin, *hemato*cele		
		infra-	beneath, below: *infra*clavicular
hemi-	one half: *hemi*plegia	inter-	occurring between: *inter*capillary
hepat(o)-	liver: *hepat*itis, *hepato*megaly	intra-	occurring within: *intra*nasal
heter(o)-	other, different: *heter*adenia, *hetero*genous	ischio-	hip, haunch: *ischio*pubic
		ischo-	suppressed: *ischo*gyria
hex(a)-	six: *hex*ose, *hexa*chromic	-ism	state, condition, or fact of being: magnet*ism*
hidr(o)-	sweat: *hidr*adenitis, *hidro*cystoma	-ites	dropsy: tympan*ites*
histio-, histo-	web, tissue: *histio*cytoma, *histo*genesis	-itis	inflammation: arth*ritis*
		jejuno-	jejunum: *jejuno*ileal

juxta-	near, close by, adjoining: *juxta*position	meno-	menses: *meno*rrhagia
labio-	lip: *labio*gingival	mento-	chin: *mento*labial
laparo-	flank, loin: *laparo*gastroscopy	mero-	part, one of similar parts: *mero*diastolic
laryng(o)-	larynx, windpipe: *laryng*itis, *laryngo*cele	meso-	middle, medium, moderate: *meso*cardium
leuc(o)- or leuk(o)-	white: *leuk*emia, *leuko*blast	meta-	change or transformation, beyond, over: *meta*basis
levo-	left: *levo*cardia	metra-,	uterus: *metra*tonia,
lien(o)-	spleen: *lien*ectomy, *lieno*pancreatic	metro-	*metro*malacia
lig-	tie, bind: *lig*ation	micr(o)-	small size: *micr*encephalon,
linguo-	tongue: *linguo*cervical		*micro*biology
lipo-	relationship to fat or lipids: *lipo*adenoma	mio-	smaller, less: *mio*pragia
		mogi-	difficult: *mogi*phonia
litho-	stone or calculus: *litho*nephritis	mono-	one or single, limited to one part: *mono*clonal
-lith	concretion or calculus: phlebo*lith*	-morph	form or shape: meso*morph*
loco-	place: *loco*motor	muco-	mucus: *muco*lipidosis
logo-	speech, words: *logo*rrhea	multi-	many: *multi*cellular
lymph(o)-	water: *lymph*adenosis, *lympho*matosis	myc-, mycet-, myco-	fungus: *myc*elium, *mycet*oma, *myco*phage
lyso-	dissolution, lysis: *lyso*staphin	-myces	fungus: myelo*myces*
lysso-	rabies: *lysso*dexis	myel(o)-	marrow: *myel*itis, *myelo*cyte
macro-	large, long, of abnormal size: *macro*blast	my(o)-	muscle: *my*itis, *myo*blast
mal-	ill, bad: *mal*adjustment	myria-	a great number: *myria*pod
mammo-	breast, mammary gland: *mammo*gram	myx(o)-	mucus or slime: *myx*adenoma, *myxo*cystitis
mast(o)-	breast or mastoid process: *mast*adenoma, *masto*plasia	naso-	nose: *naso*lacrimal
		necro-	death: *necro*lysis
mega-	big, great: *mega*cephalic	neo-	new or strange: *neo*genesis
megal(o)-	great size: *megal*erythema, *megalo*blast	nephelo-	cloudiness or mistiness: *nephelo*pia
-megaly	enlargement: spleno*megaly*	nephr(o)-	kidney: *nephr*itis, *nephro*megaly
meio-	small, decreasing: *meio*sis	neur(o)-	a nerve or the nervous system: *neur*algia, *neuro*cytoma
meningo-	membrane: *meningo*cele		

nitro-	presence of the group —NO$_2$: *nitro*benzene	patho-	disease: *patho*genesis
noto-	the back: *noto*chord	-pathy	morbid condition or disease: cardio*pathy*
ob-	against, in front of, toward: *ob*elion	-penia	poverty, need, reduction in number: leuko*penia*
octa-, octi-, octo-	eight: *octa*decanoate, *octi*para, *octo*genarian	peri-	around, near: *peri*cystitis
oculo-	the eye: *oculo*facial	-petal	directed, moving toward a center: cortici*petal*
odonto-	tooth or teeth: *odonto*genesis	-pexy	fixing, putting together: entero*pexy*
-ology	a science or branch of knowledge: radi*ology*	phaco-	lentil-shaped object: *phaco*glaucoma
-oma	tumor or neoplasm: carcin*oma*	-phagia, -phagy	perversion of appetite: aero*phagia*, aero*phagy*
onco-	tumor, swelling, or mass: *onco*lysis	pharmaco-	relation to drug or medicine: *pharmaco*logic
oophor(o)-	ovary: *oophor*algia, *oophoro*salpingitis	phleb(o)-	vein or veins: *phleb*itis, *phlebo*pexy
ophthalm(o)-	the eye: *ophthal*malgia, *ophthalmo*plegia	phon(o)-	voice, sound: *phon*ation, *phono*cardiogram
orchi-, orchido-, orchio-	the testes: *orchi*dic, *orchido*ptosis, *orchio*cele	phot(o)-	relationship to light: *phot*esthesis, *photo*allergic
oro-	mouth: *oro*lingual	phren(o)-	diaphragm or mind: *phren*algia, *phreno*hepatic
orrho-	serum: *orrho*meningitis		
ortho-	straight, normal, correct: *ortho*gnathia	physio-	nature: *physio*nomy
-osis	a disease or morbid process: scler*osis*	physo-	air or gas: *physo*cephaly
osteo-	bone or bones: *osteo*arthritis	phyto-	plant or plants: *phyto*chrome
-ostomy	mouth or opening: gastroentero*stomy*	picro-	bitter: *picro*geusia
ot(o)-	ear: *ot*itis, *oto*laryngology	-piesis	pressure: oto*piesis*
-otomy	surgical incision: cholecysto*tomy*	plasmo-	plasma or substance of a cell: *plasmo*cyte
ovi-, ovo-	egg or ova: *ovi*gerous, *ovo*testis	-plasty	shaping or surgical formation: peritoneo*plasty*
oxy-	sharp, quick, or sour: *oxy*chloride	platy-	broad or flat: *platy*coria
pachy-	thick: *pachy*onychia	-plegia	paralysis, stroke: para*plegia*
pan-	all: *pan*arthritis	pleur(o)-	pleura, rib: *pleur*isy, *pleuro*dynia
para-	beside, beyond, accessory to: *para*thyroid		

-plexy	stroke or seizure: apo*plexy*	rachi(o)-	spine: *rachi*algia, *rachio*myelitis
pluri-	several, more: *pluri*visceral	radio-	ray or radiation: *radio*plastic
-pnea	breathing: ortho*pnea*	re-	back, again: *re*activation
pneuma-, pneumato-	air, gas, or respiration: *pneuma*tic, *pneumato*dyspnea	retro-	backward, located behind: *retro*sternal
pod-, podo-	foot: *pod*iatry, *podo*dynia	-rhage	breaking, bursting forth: hemor*rhage*
polio-	relationship to gray matter: *polio*dystrophy	-rhaphy	joining in a seam, suture of a part: blpharor*rhaphy*
poly-	many, much: *poly*articular	-rhea	flow: gonor*rhea*
post-	after: *post*partum	rheo-	relationship to electric current, flow: *rheo*stat
pre-	before: *pre*natal		
pro-	forward, in front of, or precursor: *pro*collagen	rhin(o)-	nose: *rhin*encephalon, *rhino*plasty
proct(o)-	rectum: *proct*itis, *procto*scope	rhizo-	root: *rhizo*meningomyelitis
proso-	forward, anterior: *proso*palgia	rhodo-	red: *rhodo*phylaxis
		sacro-	sacrum: *sacro*iliac
prosopo-	relationship to the face: *prosopo*plegic	salpingo-	relationship to a tube, uterine or auditory: *salpingo*cele
prostat(o)-	prostate: *prostat*ic, *prostato*cystitis	sangui-	blood: *sangui*neous
psammo-	sand or sandlike: *psammo*sarcoma	sarco-	flesh: *sarco*matoid
		scapho-	boat-shaped: *scapho*cephalic
pseud(o)-	false or spurious: *pseud*albuminuria, *pseudo*bulbar	scato-	fecal matter: *scato*scopy
		schizo-	divided, division: *schizo*phrenia
psych(o)-	psyche, mind: *psychi*atric, *psycho*motor	scirrho-	hard cancer or scirrhous carcinoma: *scirrho*phthalmia
-ptosis	downward displacement: cardio*ptosis*	sclero-	hard: *sclero*derma
		scolio-	twisted, crooked: *scolio*sis
pyel(o)-	pelvis, usually the renal pelves: *pyel*itis, *pyelo*nephritis	-scope	instrument for examining: sigmoido*scope*
pyloro-	pylorus: *pyloro*plasty		
py(o)-	pus: *py*uria, *pyo*nephrosis	-scopy	act of examining: procto*scopy*
quadri-	four, fourfold: *quadri*plegia	semi-	one half, partly: *semi*membranous

sial(o)-	saliva, salivary glands: *sial*adenosis, *sialo*lithiasis	sulfo-	indicating presence of a divalent sulfur: *sulfo*namide
sidero-	iron: *sidero*blast	super-	above or in excess: *super*genual, *super*numerary
sinistro-	left, left side: *sinistro*cerebral		
skia-	shadows by roentgen rays: *skia*scopy	syndesmo-	connective tissue or ligaments: *syndesmo*rrhaphy
spasmo-	spasm: *spasmo*lysant	tachy-	swift, rapid: *tachy*cardia
spermato-,	seed, specifically male: *spermato*cele, *spermo*lith	tarso-	edge of eyelid; instep of the foot: *tarso*cheiloplasty, *tarso*clasis
spermo-			
spheno-	wedge-shaped: *spheno*temporal	tauto-	same: *tauto*meral
spir(o)-	coil, spiral; breath or breathing: *spir*adenoma, *spiro*graphy	tele-	end, distance, far away: *tele*fluoroscopy
		telo-	end: *telo*dendron
splen(o)-	spleen: *splen*emia, *spleno*renal	teno-,	tendon: *teno*nitis, *tenonto*plasty
		tenonto-	
spondyl(o)-	vertebra, or spinal column: *spondyl*algia, *spondylo*desis	tera-	three, threefold: *tera*curie
		tetra-	four: *tetra*chirus
staphyl(o)-	resemblance to a bunch of grapes: *staphyl*edema, *staphylo*coccus	therm(o)-	heat: *therm*algia, *thermo*dynamics
		thio-	sulfur: *thio*cyanate
stearo-,	fat: *stearo*pten, *steato*lytic	thoraco-	chest: *thoraco*stenosis
steato-		-thrix	hair: endo*thrix*
stereo-	solid, three dimensional: *stereo*cineflurography	thyro-	thyroid gland: *thyro*cele
		toco-	childbirth or labor: *toco*graphy
steth(o)-	chest: *steth*algia, *stetho*scope	tomo-	cutting, slicing: *tomo*graphy
stomato-	mouth or ostium uteri: *stomato*gastric	-tomy	cutting, incising: colo*tomy*
-stomy	surgical creation of an artifical opening: gastroentero*stomy*	tono-	tone, tension: *tono*graphy
		toxo-	toxin, poison: *toxo*plasmosis
streph(o)-	twisted: *streph*enopodia, *strepho*symbolia	tracheo-	trachea: *tracheo*bronchitis
strepto-	twisted: *strepto*coccus	trans-	through, across, beyond: *trans*duction
stylo-	stake, pole: *stylo*mastoid	tri-	three, thrice: *tri*angular
sub-	under, near, almost: *sub*dural	tropho-	food or nourishment: *tropho*chromidia

-tropin	affinity for structure or thing denoted by stem: gonado*tropin*	varico-	twisted and swollen: *varico*cele
typhlo-	cecum: *typhlo*colitis	ventro-	pertaining to the belly or located anteriorly: *ventro*inguinal, *ventro*dorsal
ulo-	gingivae: *ulo*rrhagia		
ultra-	excess, beyond: *ultra*sonogram		
uni-	one: *uni*locular	vivi-	life: *vivi*fication
urethro-	urethra: *urethro*cele	xeno-	strange, foreign: *xeno*phthalmia
-uria	urine: olig*uria*		
ur-, uro-, urono-	urine, urinary tract, urination: *ur*inate, *uro*bilinuria, *urono*phile	xero-	dryness: *xero*derma

APPENDIX 3
Tables of Weights and Measures*

Measures of Mass

AVOIRDUPOIS WEIGHT

GRAINS	DRAMS	OUNCES	POUNDS	METRIC EQUIVALENTS, GRAMS
1	0.0366	0.0023	0.00014	0.0647989
27.34	1	0.0625	0.0039	1.772
437.5	16	1	0.0625	28.350
7000	256	16	1	453.5924277

APOTHECARIES' WEIGHT

GRAINS	SCRUPLES Ә	DRAMS ℨ	OUNCES ℥	POUNDS(LB.)	METRIC EQUIVALENTS, GRAMS
1	0.05	0.0167	0.0021	0.00017	0.0647989
20	1	0.333	0.042	0.0035	1.296
60	3	1	0.125	0.0104	3.888
480	24	8	1	0.0833	31.103
5760	288	96	12	1	373.24177

*Courtesy of Miller, B. F., and Keane, C. B.: Encyclopedia and Dictionary of Medicine, Nursing, and Allied Health, 2nd ed. Philadelphia. W. B. Saunders Company, 1978.

TROY WEIGHT

GRAINS	PENNYWEIGHTS	OUNCES	POUNDS	METRIC EQUIVALENTS, GRAMS
1	0.042	0.002	0.00017	0.0647989
24	1	0.05	0.0042	1.555
480	20	1	0.083	31.103
5760	240	12	1	373.24177

METRIC WEIGHT

MICROGRAM	MILLIGRAM	CENTIGRAM	DECIGRAM	GRAM	DECAGRAM	HECTOGRAM	KILOGRAM	EQUIVALENTS	
								AVOIRDUPOIS	APOTHECARIES'
1	...	...	...	...	...	...	...	0.000015 grains	
10^3	1	...	...	...	...	...	...	0.015432 grains	
10^4	10	1	...	...	...	...	...	0.154323 grains	
10^5	10^2	10	1	...	...	...	...	1.543235 grains	
10^6	10^3	10^2	10	1	...	...	...	15.432356 grains	
10^7	10^4	10^3	10^2	10	1	...	...	5.6438 dr.	7.7162 scr.
10^8	10^5	10^4	10^3	10^2	10	1	...	3.527 oz.	3.215 oz.
10^9	10^6	10^5	10^4	10^3	10^2	10	1	2.2046 lb.	2.6792 lb.
10^{12}	10^9	10^8	10^7	10^6	10^5	10^4	10^3	2204.6223 lb.	2679.2285 lb.

Measures of Length

Metric Measure

MICRON	MILLI-METER	CENTI-METER	DECI-METER	METER	DEKA-METER	HECTO-METER	KILO-METER	MYRIA-METER	MEGA-METER	EQUIVALENTS	
1	0.001	10^{-4}	…	…	…	…	…	…	…	0.000039	inch
10^3	1	10^{-1}	…	…	…	…	…	…	…	0.03937	inch
10^4	10	1	…	…	…	…	…	…	…	0.3937	inch
10^5	10^2	10	1	…	…	…	…	…	…	3.937	inch
10^6	10^3	10^2	10	1	…	…	…	…	…	39.37	inch
10^7	10^4	10^3	10^2	10	1	…	…	…	…	10.9361	yards
10^8	10^5	10^4	10^3	10^2	10	1	…	…	…	109.3612	yards
10^9	10^6	10^5	10^4	10^3	10^2	10	1	…	…	1093.6121	yards
10^{10}	10^7	10^6	10^5	10^4	10^3	10^2	10	1	…	6.2137	miles
10^{11}	10^8	10^7	10^6	10^5	10^4	10^3	10^2	10	1	62.1370	miles

Measures of Capacity

APOTHECARIES' (WINE) MEASURE

MINIMS	FLUID DRAMS	FLUID OUNCES	GILLS	PINTS	QUARTS	GALLONS	CUBIC INCHES	EQUIVALENTS		
								MILLI-LITERS	CUBIC CENTIMETERS	
1	0.0166	0.002	0.0005	0.00013			0.00376	0.06161	0.06161
60	1	0.125	0.0312	0.0078	0.0039		0.22558	3.6967	3.6967
480	8	1	0.25	0.0625	0.0312	0.0078	1.80468	29.5737	29.5737
1920	32	4	1	0.25	0.125	0.0312	7.21875	118.2948	118.2948
7680	128	16	4	1	0.5	0.125	28.875	473.179	473.179
15360	256	32	8	2	1	0.25	57.75	946.358	946.358
61440	1024	128	32	8	4	1	231	3785.434	3785.434

Measures of Capacity (continued)

	METRIC MEASURE								EQUIVALENTS (APOTHECARIES' FLUID)
MICROLITER	MILLILITER	CENTILITER	DECILITER	LITER	DEKALITER	HECTOLITER	KILOLITER	MYRIALITER	
1	...	...	...	...	...	...	...	...	0.01623108 min.
10^3	1	...	...	...	...	...	...	...	16.23 min.
10^4	10	1	...	...	...	...	...	...	2.7 fl. dr.
10^5	10^2	10	1	...	...	...	...	...	3.38 fl. oz.
10^6	10^3	10^2	10	1	...	...	...	...	2.11 pts.
10^7	10^4	10^3	10^2	10	1	...	...	...	2.64 gal.
10^8	10^5	10^4	10^3	10^2	10	1	...	...	26.418 gal.
10^9	10^6	10^5	10^4	10^3	10^2	10	1	...	264.18 gal.
10^{10}	10^7	10^6	10^5	10^4	10^3	10^2	10	1	2641.8 gal.

1 liter = 2.113363738 pints (Apothecaries').

Conversion Tables

AVOIRDUPOIS—METRIC WEIGHT		APOTHECARIES'—METRIC LIQUID MEASURE	
Ounces	Grams	Minims	Milliliters
1/16	1.772	1	0.06
1/8	3.544	2	0.12
1/4	7.088	3	0.19
1/2	14.175	4	0.25
1	28.350	5	0.31
2	56.699	10	0.62
3	85.049	15	0.92
4	113.398	20	1.23
5	141.748	25	1.54
6	170.097	30	1.85
7	198.447	35	2.16
8	226.796	40	2.46
9	255.146	45	2.77
10	283.495	50	3.08
11	311.845	55	3.39
12	340.194	60 (1 fl.dr.)	3.70
13	368.544		
14	396.893	Fluid drams	
15	425.243	1	3.70
16 (1 lb.)	453.59	2	7.39
		3	11.09
Pounds		4	14.79
1 (16 oz.)	453.59	5	18.48
2	907.18	6	22.18
3	1360.78 (1.36 kg.)	7	25.88
4	1814.37 (1.81 ″)	8 (1 fl.oz.)	29.57
5	2267.96 (2.27 ″)		
6	2721.55 (2.72 ″)	Fluid ounces	
7	3175.15 (3.18 ″)	1	29.57
8	3628.74 (3.63 ″)	2	59.15
9	4082.33 (4.08 ″)	3	88.72
10	4535.92 (4.54 ″)	4	118.29
		5	147.87
		6	177.44
		7	207.01
		8	236.58
		9	266.16
		10	295.73
		11	325.30
		12	354.88
		13	384.45
		14	414.02
METRIC—AVOIRDUPOIS WEIGHT		15	443.59
		16 (1 pt.)	473.18
GRAMS	OUNCES	32 (1 qt.)	946.36
0.001 (1 mg.)	0.000035274	128 (1 gal.)	3785.43
1	0.035274		
1000 (1 kg.)	35.274 (2.2046 lb.)		

METRIC—APOTHECARIES' LIQUID MEASURE

MILLILITERS	MINIMS	MILLILITERS	FLUID DRAMS	MILLILITERS	FLUID OUNCES
1	16.231	5	1.35	30	1.01
2	32.5	10	2.71	40	1.35
3	48.7	15	4.06	50	1.69
4	64.9	20	5.4	500	16.91
5	81.1	25	6.76	1000 (1 L.)	33.815
		30	7.1		

Conversion Tables (*continued*)

APOTHECARIES'—METRIC WEIGHT		METRIC—APOTHECARIES' WEIGHT	
Grains	Grams	Milligrams	Grains
1/150	0.0004	1	0.015432
1/120	0.0005	2	0.030864
1/100	0.0006	3	0.046296
1/80	0.0008	4	0.061728
1/64	0.001	5	0.077160
1/50	0.0013	6	0.092592
1/48	0.0014	7	0.108024
1/30	0.0022	8	0.123456
1/25	0.0026	9	0.138888
1/16	0.004	10	0.154320
1/12	0.005	15	0.231480
1/10	0.006	20	0.308640
1/9	0.007	25	0.385800
1/8	0.008	30	0.462960
1/7	0.009	35	0.540120
1/6	0.01	40	0.617280
1/5	0.013	45	0.694440
1/4	0.016	50	0.771600
1/3	0.02	100	1.543240
1/2	0.032		
1	0.065	Grams	
1 1/2	0.097 (0.1)	0.1	1.5432
2	0.12	0.2	3.0864
3	0.20	0.3	4.6296
4	0.24	0.4	6.1728
5	0.30	0.5	7.7160
6	0.40	0.6	9.2592
7	0.45	0.7	10.8024
8	0.50	0.8	12.3456
9	0.60	0.9	13.8888
10	0.65	1.0	15.4320
15	1.00	1.5	23.1480
20 (1϶)	1.30	2.0	30.8640
30	2.00	2.5	38.5800
Scruples		3.0	46.2960
1	1.296 (1.3)	3.5	54.0120
2	2.592 (2.6)	4.0	61.728
3 (1ʒ)	3.888 (3.9)	4.5	69.444
Drams		5.0	77.162
1	3.888	10.0	154.324
2	7.776		
3	11.664		Equivalents
4	15.552	10	2.572 drams
5	19.440	15	3.858 "
6	23.328	20	5.144 "
7	27.216	25	6.430 "
8 (1ʒ)	31.103	30	7.716 "
Ounces		40	1.286 oz.
1	31.103	45	1.447 "
2	62.207	50	1.607 "
3	93.310	100	3.215 "
4	124.414	200	6.430 "
5	155.517	300	9.644
6	186.621	400	12.859 "
7	217.724	500	1.34 lb.
8	248.828	600	1.61 "
9	279.931	700	1.88 "
10	311.035	800	2.14 "
11	342.138	900	2.41 "
12 (1 lb.)	373.242	1000	2.68

Metric Doses With Approximate Apothecary Equivalents*

These *approximate* dose equivalents represent the quantities usually prescribed, under identical conditions, by physicians trained, respectively,in the metric or in the apothecary system of weights and measures. In labeling dosage forms in both the metric and the apothecary system, if one is the approximate equivalent of the other, the approximate figure shall be enclosed in parentheses.

When prepared dosage forms such as tablets, capsules, pills, etc., are prescribed in the metric system, the pharmacist may dispense the corresponding *approximate* equivalent in the apothecary system, and vice versa, as indicated in the following table.

Caution—For the conversion of specific quantities in a prescription which requires compounding, or in converting a pharmaceutical formula from one system of weights or measures to the other, *exact* equivalents must be used.

METRIC	LIQUID MEASURE APPROX. APOTHECARY EQUIVALENTS	METRIC	LIQUID MEASURE APPROX. APOTHECARY EQUIVALENTS
1000 ml.	1 quart	3 ml.	45 minims
750 ml.	1 1/2 pints	2 ml.	30 minims
500 ml.	1 pint	1 ml.	15 minims
250 ml.	8 fluid ounces	0.75 ml.	12 minims
200 ml.	7 fluid ounces	0.6 ml.	10 minims
100 ml.	3 1/2 fluid ounces	0.5 ml.	8 minims
50 ml.	1 3/4 fluid ounces	0.3 ml.	5 minims
30 ml.	1 fluid ounce	0.25 ml.	4 minims
15 ml.	4 fluid drams	0.2 ml.	3 minims
10 ml.	2 1/2 fluid drams	0.1 ml.	1 1/2 minims
8 ml.	2 fluid drams	0.06 ml.	1 minim
5 ml.	1 1/4 fluid drams	0.05 ml.	3/4 minim
4 ml.	1 fluid dram	0.03 ml.	1/2 minim

METRIC	WEIGHT APPROX. APOTHECARY EQUIVALENTS	METRIC	WEIGHT APPROX. APOTHECARY EQUIVALENTS
30 Gm.	1 ounce	30 mg.	1/2 grain
15 Gm.	4 drams	25 mg.	3/8 grain
10 Gm.	2 1/2 drams	20 mg.	1/3 grain
7.5 Gm.	2 drams	15 mg.	1/4 grain
6 Gm.	90 grains	12 mg.	1/5 grain
5 Gm.	75 grains	10 mg.	1/6 grain
4 Gm.	60 grains (1 dram)	8 mg.	1/8 grain
3 Gm.	45 grains	6 mg.	1/10 grain
2 Gm.	30 grains (1/2 dram)	5 mg.	1/12 grain
1.5 Gm.	22 grains	4 mg.	1/15 grain
1 Gm.	15 grains	3 mg.	1/20 grain
0.75 Gm.	12 grains	2 mg.	1/30 grain
0.6 Gm.	10 grains	1.5 mg.	1/40 grain
0.5 Gm.	7 1/2 grains	1.2 mg.	1/50 grain
0.4 Gm.	6 grains	1 mg.	1/60 grain
0.3 Gm.	5 grains	0.8 mg.	1/80 grain
0.25 Gm.	4 grains	0.6 mg.	1/100 grain
0.2 Gm.	3 grains	0.5 mg.	1/120 grain
0.15 Gm.	2 1/2 grains	0.4 mg.	1/150 grain
0.12 Gm.	2 grains	0.3 mg.	1/200 grain
0.1 Gm.	1 1/2 grains	0.25 mg.	1/250 grain
75 mg.	1 1/4 grains	0.2 mg.	1/300 grain
60 mg.	1 grain	0.15 mg.	1/400 grain
50 mg.	3/4 grain	0.12 mg.	1/500 grain
40 mg.	2/3 grain	0.1 mg.	1/600 grain

Note—A milliliter (ml.) is the approximate equivalent of a cubic centimeter (cc.).

*Adopted by the latest Pharmacopeia, National Formulary, and New and Nonofficial Remedies, and approved by the Federal Food and Drug Administration.

APPENDIX 4
Table of Elements

NAME	SYMBOL	AT. NO.	AT. WT.*
Actinium	Ac	89	(227)
Aluminum	Al	13	26.982
Americium	Am	95	(243)
Antimony	Sb	51	121.75
Argon	Ar	18	39.948
Arsenic	As	33	74.922
Astatine	At	85	(210)
Barium	Ba	56	137.34
Berkelium	Bk	97	(247)
Beryllium	Be	4	9.012
Bismuth	Bi	83	208.980
Boron	B	5	10.811
Bromine	Br	35	79.909
Cadmium	Cd	48	112.40
Calcium	Ca	20	40.08
Californium	Cf	98	(249)
Carbon	C	6	12.011
Cerium	Ce	58	140.12
Cesium	Cs	55	132.905
Chlorine	Cl	17	35.453
Chromium	Cr	24	51.996
Cobalt	Co	27	58.933
Copper	Cu	29	63.54
Curium	Cm	96	(247)
Dysprosium	Dy	66	162.50
Einsteinium	Es	99	(254)
Erbium	Er	68	167.26
Europium	Eu	63	151.96
Fermium	Fm	100	(253)
Fluorine	F	9	18.998
Francium	Fr	87	(223)
Gadolinium	Gd	64	157.25
Gallium	Ga	31	69.72
Germanium	Ge	32	72.59
Gold	Au	79	196.967
Hafnium	Hf	72	178.49
Hahnium	Ha	105	(260)
Helium	He	2	4.003
Holmium	Ho	67	164.930
Hydrogen	H	1	1.008
Indium	In	49	114.82
Iodine	I	53	126.904
Iridium	Ir	77	192.2
Iron	Fe	26	55.847
Krypton	Kr	36	83.80
Lanthanum	La	57	138.91
Lawrencium	Lw	103	(257)
Lead	Pb	82	207.19
Lithium	Li	3	6.939
Lutetium	Lu	71	174.97
Magnesium	Mg	12	24.312
Manganese	Mn	25	54.938
Mendelevium	Md	101	(256)

*Atomic weights are corrected to conform with the 1961 values of the Commission on Atomic Weights, expressed to the fourth decimal point, rounded off to the nearest thousandth. The numbers in parentheses are the mass numbers of the most stable or most common isotope.

Table of Elements (*continued*)

NAME	SYMBOL	AT. NO.	AT. WT.*
Mercury	Hg	80	200.59
Molybdenum	Mo	42	95.94
Neodymium	Nd	60	144.24
Neon	Ne	10	20.183
Neptunium	Np	93	(237)
Nickel	Ni	28	58.71
Niobium	Nb	41	92.906
Nitrogen	N	7	14.007
Nobelium	No	102	(253)
Osmium	Os	76	190.2
Oxygen	O	8	15.999
Palladium	Pd	46	106.4
Phosphorus	P	15	30.974
Platinum	Pt	78	195.09
Plutonium	Pu	94	(242)
Polonium	Po	84	(210)
Potassium	K	19	39.102
Praseodymium	Pr	59	140.907
Promethium	Pm	61	(147)
Protactinium	Pa	91	(231)
Radium	Ra	88	(226)
Radon	Rn	86	(222)
Rhenium	Re	75	186.2
Rhodium	Rh	45	102.905
Rubidium	Rb	37	85.47
Ruthenium	Ru	44	101.07
Rutherfordium	Rf	104	(261)
Samarium	Sm	62	150.35
Scandium	Sc	21	44.956
Selenium	Se	34	78.96
Silicon	Si	14	28.086
Silver	Ag	47	107.870
Sodium	Na	11	22.990
Strontium	Sr	38	87.62
Sulfur	S	16	32.064
Tantalum	Ta	73	180.948
Technetium	Tc	43	(99)
Tellurium	Te	52	127.60
Terbium	Tb	65	158.924
Thallium	Tl	81	204.37
Thorium	Th	90	232.038
Thulium	Tm	69	168.934
Tin	Sn	50	118.69
Titanium	Ti	22	47.90
Tungsten	W	74	183.85
Uranium	U	92	238.03
Vanadium	V	23	50.942
Xenon	Xe	54	131.30
Ytterbium	Yb	70	173.04
Yttrium	Y	39	88.905
Zinc	Zn	30	65.37
Zirconium	Zr	40	91.22

*Atomic weights are corrected to conform with the 1961 values of the Commission on Atomic Weights, expressed to the fourth decimal point, rounded off to the nearest thousandth. The numbers in parentheses are the mass numbers of the most stable or most common isotope.

APPENDIX 5
Eponymic Diseases and Syndromes

Aarskog-Scott s.
Aarskog's s.
Aase's s.
Abercrombies's s.
Achard s.
Achard-Thiers s.
Acosta's d.
Adair-Dighton s.
Adams' d.
Adams-Stokes d.
Addison's d.
Addison-Biermer d.
Addison-Scholz d.
addisonian s.
Adie's s.
Ahumada–del Castillo s.
Aicardi's s.
Akureyri d.
Albarrán's d.
Albers-Schönberg d.
Albert's d.
Albright-McCune-Sternberg s.
Albright's s.
Aldrich's s.
Ale-Calo s.
Alexander's d.
Alezzandrini's s.
Alibert's d.
Allen-Masters s.
Almeida's d.
Alper's d.
Alport's s.
Alström's s.
Alzheimer's d.
amniotic infection s. of Blane

Anders' d.
Andersen's d., s.
Andes d.
André's s.
Andrews' d.
Angelucci's s.
Anton's s.
Apert-Crouzon d.
Apert's d., s.
Aran-Duchenne d.
Argonz–del Castillo s.
Armstrong's d.
Arndt-Gottron s.
Arnold-Chiari s.
Arnold's nerve reflex cough s.
Ascher's s.
Asherman's s.
Ashley's s.
Aufrecht's d.
Aujeszky's d.
Avellis' s.
Axenfeld's s.
Ayerza's d., s.
Baastrup's d.
Babinski-Fröhlich s.
s. of Babinski-Nageotte
Babinski's s.
Babinski-Vaquez s.
Baelz's d.
Bäfverstedt's s.
Balfour's d.
Balint's s.
Baller-Gerold s.
Ballet's d.
Ballingall's d.

Baló's d.
Bamberger-Marie d.
Bamberger's d.
Bamle d.
Bang's d.
Bannister's d.
Banti's d., s.
Barclay-Baron d.
Barcoo d.
Bardet-Biedl s.
Barlow's d., s.
Barraquer's d.
Barré-Guillain s.
Barrett's s.
Barter's s.
Barthélemy's d.
Bartter's s.
Basedow's d.
Basel d.
Bassen-Kornzweig s.
Bateman's d.
Batten-Mayou d.
Batten's d.
Bayle's d.
Bazin's d.
Beard's d.
Beau's d., s.
Beauvais' d.
Bechterew's (Bekhterev's) d.
Becker's d.
Beck's d.
Beckwith's s.
Beckwith-Wiedemann s.
Begbie's d.
Béguez César d.
Behçet's s.
Behr's d.
Beigel's d.
Bekhterev's d.
Bell's d.
s. of Benedikt
Benson's d.
Bergeron's d.
Berger's d.
Berlin's d.
Bernard-Horner s.

Bernard-Sergent s.
Bernard-Soulier s.
Bernard's s.
Bernhardt-Roth s.
Bernhardt's d.
Bernheim's s.
Bertolotti's s.
Besnier-Boeck d.
Besnier-Boeck-Schaumann d., s.
Best's d.
Bianchi's s.
Biedl's d.
Bielschowsky-Jansky d.
Bielschowsky's d.
Biemond's s.
Biermer's d.
Biett's d.
Bilderbeck's d.
Bilginturan's s.
Billroth's d.
Binswanger's d.
Bird's d.
Björnstad's s.
Blatin's s.
Bloch-Sulzberger s.
Blocq's d.
Bloodgood's d.
Bloom's s.
Blount-Barber d.
Blount's d.
Blum's s.
body of Luys s.
Boeck's d.
Boerhaave's s.
Bogaert's d.
Bonnet-Dechaume-Blanc s.
Bonnevie-Ullrich s.
Bonnier's s.
Böök's s.
Börjeson-Forssman-Lehmann s.
Börjeson's s.
Bornholm's d.
Bostock's d.
Bouchard's d.
Bouchet-Gsell d.
Bouillaud's d., s.

Bourneville-Pringle d.
Bourneville's d.
Bouveret's d., s.
Bowen's d.
Brachmann–de Lange s.
Bradley's d.
Brailsford-Morquio d.
Breda's d.
Breisky's d.
Brennemann's s.
Bretonneau's d.
Bright's d.
Brill's d.
Brill-Symmers d.
Brill-Zinsser d.
Brinton's d.
Brion-Kayser d.
Briquet's s.
Brissaud-Marie s.
Brissaud's d.
Brissaud-Sicard s.
Bristowe's s.
Brock's s.
Brocq's d.
Brodie's d.
Brooke's d.
Brown-Séquard d., s.
Brown's vertical retraction s.
Brown-Symmers d.
Bruck's d.
Brugsch's s.
Bruns' s.
Brunsting's s.
Brushfield-Wyatt d., s.
Bruton's d.
Budd-Chiari s.
Budd's d.
Buerger's d.
Buhl's d.
Bürger-Grütz s.
Burnett's s.
Bury's d.
Buschke-Ollendorff s.
Buschke's d.
Busquet's d.
Buss d.

Busse-Buschke d.
Byler's d.
Bywaters' s.
Cacchi-Ricci d.
Caffey-Kenny s.
Caffey's d., s.
Caffey-Silverman s.
Calvé-Perthes d.
Camurati-Engelmann d.
Canada-Cronkhite s.
Canavan's d.
Cantú s.
Capdepont's d.
Capgras' s.
Caplan's s.
Caroli's d.
Carpenter's s.
Carrión's d.
Castellani's d.
Catel-Hempel s.
Cavare's d.
Cazenave's d.
s. of Cestan-Chenais
Cestan-Raymond s.
Cestan's s.
Chabert's d.
Chagas-Cruz d.
Chagas' d.
Championniére's d.
Charcot-Marie-Tooth d.
Charcot's d., s.
Charcot-Weiss-Barker s.
Charlin's s.
Charlouis' d.
Charrin's d.
Chauffard's s.
Chauffard-Still s.
Cheadle's d.
Chédiak-Higashi s.
Chédiak-Steinbrinck-Higashi s.
Cheney's s.
Cherchevski's d.
Chester's d.   *Chilaiditi's S.*
Chiari-Arnold s.
Chiari-Budd s.
Chiari-Frommel s.

Chiari II s.
Chiari's s.
Chilaiditi's s.
Chotzen's s.
Christensen-Krabbe d.
Christian's d., s.
Christian-Weber d.
Christmas d.
Christ-Siemens s.
Christ-Siemens-Touraine s.
Churg-Strauss s.
Ciarrocchi's d.
Citelli's s.
Civatte's d.
Clarke-Hadfield s.
Claude Bernard–Horner s.
Claude's s.
Clérambault-Kandinsky s.
Clough and Richter's s.
Clouston's s.
Coats' d.
Cockayne's s.
Coffin-Lowry s.
Coffin-Siris s.
Cogan's s.
Cohen's s.
Collet-Sicard s.
Collet's s.
Concato's d.
Conn's s.
Conor and Bruch's d.
Conradi's d., s.
Cooley's d.
Cooper's d.
Corbus' d.
Cori's d.
Cornelia de Lange's s.
Corrigan's d.
Corvisart's d.
Costen's s.
Cotard's s.
Cottunius' d.
Cotugno's d.
Courvoisier-Terrier s.
Cowden's d.
Crandall's s.

Creutzfeldt-Jakob d., s.
Crigler-Najjar s.
Crocq's d.
Crohn's d.
Cronkhite-Canada. s.
Cronkhite's s.
Crouzon's d.
Cruveilhier-Baumgarten s.
Cruveilhier's d.
Cruz-Chagas d.
Csillag's d.
Curschmann's d.
Curtius' s.
Cushing's d., s.
Cyriax's s.
Czerny's d.
Daae-Finsen d.
Daae's d.
DaCosta's d., s.
Dalrymple's d.
Danbolt-Closs s.
Dandy-Walker s.
Danielssen-Boeck d.
Danielssen's d.
Danlos' s.
Darier's d.
Darling's d.
David's d.
Debré-Sémélaigne s.
de Clerambault s.
Degos' d., s.
Déjérine-Klumpke s.
s. of Déjérine-Roussy
Déjérine's d., s.
Déjérine-Sottas d., s.
de Lange's s.
del Castillo s.
Dennie-Marfan s.
de Quervain's d.
Dercum's d.
De Sanctis-Cacchione
de Toni–Fanconi s.
Deutschländer's d.
Devergie's d.
Devic's d.
DiFerrante's s.

DiGeorge's s.
Dighton-Adair s.
Di Guglielmo d., s.
Dimitri's d.
Döhle d.
Donohue's s.
Down's s.
Dresbach's s.
Dressler's s.
Duane's s.
Dubini's d.
Dubin-Johnson s.
Dubin-Sprinz d., s.
Dubois' d.
Dubreuil-Chambardel s.
Duchenne-Aran d.
Duchenne-Erb s.
Duchenne-Griesinger d.
Duchenne's d., s.
Duhring's d.
Dukes' d.
Duplay's s.
Dupré's s.
Dupuytren's d.
Durand-Nicolas-Favre d.
Durand's d.
Durante's d.
Duroziez's d.
Dutton's d.
Dyggve-Melchior-Clausen s.
Dyke-Davidoff s.
Eagle s.
Eales's d.
Eaton-Lambert s.
Ebstein's d.
Economo's d.
Eddowes' s.
Edsall's d.
Edwards-Patau s.
Edwards' s.
Ehlers-Danlos s.
Eichstedt's d.
Eisenlohr's s.
Eisenmenger's s.
Ekbom s.
Ellis–van Creveld s.

Engelmann-Camurati d.
Engelmann's d.
Engel-Recklinghausen d.
English d.
Engman's d.
Epstein's d., s.
Erb-Charcot d.
Erb-Goldflam d.
Erb-Landouzy d.
Erb's d., s.
Erdheim d.
Eulenburg's d.
Ewing's d.
Faber's s.
Fabry's d.
Fahr's d.
Fahr-Volhard d.
Fallot's s.
Fanconi's s.
Farber's d., s.
Farber-Uzman s.
Fauchard's d.
Favre-Durand-Nicholas d.
Favre-Racouchot s.
Fede's d.
Feer's d.
Felty's s.
Fenwick's d.
Fiedler's d.
Fiessinger-Leroy-Reiter s.
Feissinger's s.
Figueira's s.
Filatov-Dukes d.
Filatov's d.
Fisher's s.
Fitz-Hugh-Curtis s.
Fitz's s.
Flajani's d.
Flatau-Schilder d.
Fleischner's d.
Flynn-Aird s.
Foong's s.
Foix's s.
Fölling's d.
Forbes-Albright s.
Forbes' d.

Fordyce's d.
Forestier-Certonciny s.
Forestier-Rotés-Querol s.
Forney's s.
Forssman's carotid s.
Förster's d.
Foster Kennedy s.
Fothergill's d.
Fournier's d.
Foville's s.
Fox-Fordyce d.
Fraley s.
Franceschetti-Jadassohn s.
Franceschetti s.
Francis' d.
François' s.
Frankl-Hochwart's d.
Franklin's d.
Fraser's s.
Freeman-Sheldon s.
Frei's d.
Freiberg-Kohler's d.
Freiberg's d.
Frenkel's anterior ocular traumatic s.
Frey's s.
Frias' s.
Friderichsen-Waterhouse s.
Friedländer's d.
Friedmann's d.
Friedmann's vasomotor s.
Friedreich's d.
Friend d.
Fröhlich's s.
Froin's s.
Frommel-Chiari s.
Frommel's d.
Fuchs' s.
Fürstner's d.
Gailliard's s.
Gairdner's d.
Gaisböck's d.
Gamna's d.
Gamstorp's d.
Gandy-Nanta d.
Ganser's s.
Gardner-Diamond s.

Gardner's s.
Garré's d.
Gasser's s.
Gaucher's d.
Gee-Herter d.
Gee-Herter-Heubner d.
Gee's d.
Gee-Thaysen d.
Gélineau's s.
Gensoul's d.
Gerhardt's d., s.
Gerlier's d.
Gerstmann's s.
Gianotti-Crosti s.
Gibert's d.
Gibney's d.
Giedion s.
Gierke's d.
Gilbert's d., s.
Gilchrist's d.
Gilles de la Tourette's s.
Glanzmann-Riniker s.
Glanzmann's d.
Glasser's d.
Glénard's d.
Glisson's d.
Goldberg-Maxwell s.
Goldenhar's s.
Goldflam-Erb d.
Goldflam's d.
Goldscheider's d.
Goldstein-Reichmann s.
Goldstein's d.
Goltz-Gorlin s.
Goltz's s.
Goodman's s.
Goodpasture's s.
Good's s.
Gopalan's s.
Gordon's s.
Gorham's d.
Gorlin-Chaudhry-Moss s.
Gorlin-Goltz s.
Gorlin-Psaume s.
Gorlin's s.
Gougerot and Blum d.

Gougerot-Carteaud s.
Gougerot-Nulock-Houwer s.
Gougerot-Sjögren d.
Gowers' s.
Gradenigo's s.
Graefe's d.
Graham Little s.
Graves' d.
Greenfield's d.
Greenhow's d.
Greig's s.
Griesinger's d.
Grönblad-Strandberg s.
Gross's d.
Grover's d.
Gruber's s.
Gubler's s.
di Guglielmo's d.
Guillain-Barré s.
Guinon's d.
Gull's d.
Gull-Sutton d.
Gunn's s.
Günther's d.
Habermann's d.
Haber's s.
Hadfield-Clarke s.
Haff d.
Haglund's d.
Hagner's d.
Hailey-Hailey d.
Hajdu-Cheney s.
Hakim's s.
Hakola's s.
Hallermann-Streiff s.
Hallermann-Streiff-Francois s.
Hallervorden s.
Hallervorden-Spatz d., s.
Hallgren's s.
Hallopeau's d.
Hallopeau-Siemens s.
Hall's d., s.
Hamman-Rich s.
Hamman's d.
Hammond's d.
Hand-Schüller-Christian d.

Hand's d.
Hanhart's s.
Hanot-Chauffard s.
Hanot's d.
Hansen's d.
d. of the Hapsburgs
Harada's s.
Hare's s.
Harris' s.
Hartnup d., s.
Hashimoto's d.
Hassin's s.
Hayem-Widal s.
Heberden's d.
Hebra's d.
Heerfordt's d., s.
Hegglin's s.
Heidenhaim's s.
Heine-Medin d.
Heiner's s.
Heller-Döhle d.
Helweg-Larssen s.
Hench-Rosenberg s.
Henderson-Jones d.
Henoch-Schönlein s.
Herrmann's s.
Hers' d.
Herter-Heubner d.
Herter's d.
Heubner's d.
Hildenbrand's d.
Hines-Bannick s.
Hippel-Lindau d.
Hippel's d.
Hirschfeld's d.
Hirschsprung's d.
His's d.
His-Werner d.
Hjärre's d.
Hodara's d.
Hodgkin's d.
Hodgson's d.
Hoffa's d.
Hoffmann-Werdnig s.
Hollister-Hollister s.
Holmes-Adie s.

Holt-Oram s.
Homén's s.
Hoppe-Goldflam d.
Horner-Bernard s.
Horner's s.
Horton's d., s.
Houssay s.
Huchard's d.
Hünermann's d.
Hunter-Fraser s.
Hunter-Hurler s.
Hunter's s.
Huntington's d.
Hunt's d., s.
Hurler-Pfaundler s.
Hurler's d., s.
Hutchinson-Boeck d.
Hutchinson-Gilford d.
Hutchinson's d.
Hutchison s.
Hutinel's d.
Hyde's d.
Irvine's s.
Isambert's d.
Ivemark's s.
Ives-Houston s.
Ivic's s.
Jaccoud's s.
Jackson's s.
Jacod's s.
Jadassohn-Lewandowsky s.
Jaffe-Lichtenstein d., s.
Jahnke's s.
Jakob-Creutzfeldt d.
Jakob's d.
Jaksch's d.
Janet's d.
Jansen's d.
Jansky-Bielschowsky d.
Jensen's d.
Jervell and Lange-Nielsen s.
Jeune's d., s.
Job's s.
Johne's d.
Johnson-Stevens d.
Jourdain's d.

Juberg-Hayward s.
Jüngling's d.
juvenile Paget's d.
Kahlbaum's d.
Kahler's d.
Kaiserstuhl d.
Kalischer's d.
Kallmann's s.
Kanner's s.
Kartagener's s.
Kasabach-Merritt s.
Kashin-Beck d.
Kast's s.
Kawasaki d.
Kayser's d.
Kearns' s.
Kedani d.
Kennedy's s.
Keutel's s.
Kienböck's d.
Kiloh-Nevin s.
Kimmelstiel-Wilson s.
Kimura's d.
Kinnier Wilson d.
Kinsbourne s.
Kirkland's d.
Klauder's s.
Klebs' d.
Klein-Waardenburg s.
Kleine-Levin s.
Klemperer's d.
Klinefelter's s.
Klippel-Feil s.
Klippel's d.
Klippel-Trenaunay s.
Klippel-Trenaunay-Weber s.
Klumpke-Déjérine s.
Klüver-Bucy s.
Kneist s.
Kocher-Debré-Sémélaigne s.
Kocher's s.
Koenig's s.
Koenig-Wichman d.
Koerber-Salus-Elschnig s.
Köhler-Pellegrini-Stieda d.
Köhler's bone d.

Köhlmeier-Degos d.
Kokka d.
König's s.
Korsakoff's d., s.
Koshevnikoff's d.
Krabbe's d., s.
Krause's s.
Krishaber's d.
Kufs' d.
Kugelberg-Welander d.
Kuhnt-Junius d.
Kümmell's d.
Kümmell-Verneuil d.
Kunkel's s.
Kuskokwim s.
Kussmaul-Maier d.
Kussmaul's d.
Kyrle's d.
Laband's s.
Labbé's neurocirculatory s.
Ladd's s.
Laennec's d.
Lafora's d.
Lambert-Eaton s.
Lancereaux-Mathieu d.
Landouzy's d.
Landry's d., s.
Lane's d.
Langdon-Down's d.
Langer-Giedion s.
Larrey-Weil d.
Larsen-Johansson d.
Larsen's d., s.
Laségue's d.
Lauber's d.
Laubry-Soulle s.
Launois' s.
Launois-Cléret s.
Laurence-Biedl s.
Laurence-Moon s.
Laurence-Moon-Bardet-Biedl s.
Laurence-Moon-Biedl s.
Läwen-Roth s.
Lawford's s.
Lawrence-Seip s.
Leber's d.

Legal's d.
Legg-Calvé d.
Legg-Calvé-Perthes d.
Legg-Calvé-Waldenström d.
Legg's d.
Leigh's d.
Leiner's d.
Leloir's d.
Lenegre's d.
Lennox s.
Lenz's s.
Leredde's s.
Leriche's d., s.
Leri-Weill d., s.
Lermoyez's s.
Leroy's d.
Lesch-Nyhan s.
Letterer-Siwe d.
Lévi's s.
Lev's d.
Lévy-Roussy s.
Lewandowsky-Lutz d.
Leyden-Moebius s.
Leyden's d.
Lhermitte and McAlpine s.
Libman-Sacks d., s.
Lichtheim's d., s.
Liebenberg s.
Lightwood's s.
Lignac-Fanconi d., s.
Lignac's d., s.
Lindau's d.
Lindau–von Hippel d.
Lipschütz's d.
Little's d.
Lobo's d.
Lobstein's d., s.
Löffler's s.
Looser-Milkman s.
Lorain-Lévi s.
Lorain's d.
Louis-Bar s.
Lowe's d., s.
Lowe-Terrey-MacLachlan s.
Lown-Ganong-Levine s.
Lucas-Championniére d.

Lucey-Driscoll s.
Luft's d.
Lutembacher's s.
Lutz-Splendore-Almeida d.
Lyell's d., s.
MacKenzie's d., s.
MacLean-Maxwell d.
Macleod's s.
Madelung's d.
Maffucci's s.
Magitot's d.
Maher's d.
Majocchi's d.
Malassez's d.
Malherbe's d.
Malibu d.
Malin's s.
Mallory-Weiss s.
Manson's d.
Manzke's s.
Marañón's s.
Marburg virus d.
Marchesani's s.
Marchiafava-Bignami d.
Marchiafava-Micheli d.
March's d.
Marcus Gunn's s.
Marek's d.
Marfan's s.
Margolis s.
Marinesco-Garland s.
Marie-Bamberger d., s.
Marie-Robinson s.
Marie's d., s.
Marie-Strümpell d.
Marie-Tooth d.
Marinesco-Sjögren's s.
Marion's d.
Maroteaux-Lamy s.
Marshall's s.
Marshall-Smith s.
Marsh's d.
Martin's d.
Martorell's s.
Mathieu's d.
Mauriac s.

Maxcy's d.
Mayer-Rokitansky-Küster s.
McArdle-Schmid-Pearson d.
McArdle's d.
McCune-Albright s.
McKusick-Kaufman s.
Meckel-Gruber s.
Meckel's s.
Meck's s.
Medin's d.
Meige's d.
Meigs' s.
Meleda d.
Melkersson-Rosenthal s.
Melkersson's s.
Melnick-Needles s.
Ménétrier's d., s.
Mengert's shock s.
Meniere's d., s.
Menkes' s.
Merzbacher-Pelizaeus d.
Meyenburg-Altherr-Uehlinger s.
Meyenburg's d.
Meyer-Betz d.
Meyer-Schwickerath and Weyers s.
Meyer's d.
Mibelli's d.
Miescher's d.
Mikulicz's d., s.
Milkman's s.
Millard-Gubler s.
Miller's d.
Mills' d.
Milroy's d.
Milton's d.
Minamata d.
Minkowski-Chauffard s.
Minor's d.
Minot–von Willebrand s.
Mitchell's d.
Möbius' d., s.
Moeller-Barlow d.
Mohr's s.
Molten's d.
Monakow's s.
Mondor's d.

Monge's d.
Moore's s.
Morel-Kraepelin d.
Morel's s.
Morgagni-Adams-Stokes s.
Morgagni's d., s.
Morgagni-Stewart-Morel s.
Morquio-Brailsford d.
Morquio's s.
Morquio-Ullrich s.
Morris' s.
Morton's d., s.
Morvan's d., s.
Moschcowitz's d.
Mosse's s.
Mounier-Kuhn s.
Mozer's d.
Mseleni's d.
Mucha-Habermann d., s.
Mucha's d.
Muckle-Wells s.
Munchausen's s.
Munchmeyer's d.
Murchison-Sanderson s.
Myá's d.
Nadia d.
Naegeli's s.
Naffziger's s.
Nager's s.
Neftel's d.
Nelson's s.
Netherton's s.
Neumann's d.
Nezelof's s.
Nicolas-Favre d.
Nidoko d.
Nieden's s.
Niemann-Pick d.
Niemann's d.
Nierhoff-Huebner s.
Noack's s.
Nonne-Milroy-Meige s.
Nonne's s.
Noonan's s.
Nordau's d.
Norrie's d.

Norum's d.
Nothnagel's s.
Novy's rat d.
Ogilvie's s.
Oguchi's d.
Ohara's d.
Ollier's d.
Olmer's d.
Opitz's d.
Oppenheim's d., s.
Ormond's d.
Osgood-Schlatter d.
Osler's d.
Osler-Vaquez d.
Osler-Weber-Rendu d.
Ostrum-Furst s.
Otto's d.
Owren's d.
Paas's d.
Paget's d.
Paget's d., extramammary
Pallister-Hall s.
Pancoast's s.
Panner's d.
Papillon-Léage and Psaume s.
Papillon-Lefévre s.
Parinaud's oculoglandular s.
Parinaud's s.
Parkes Weber s.
parkinsonian s.
Parkinson's d.
Parrot's d.
Parry-Romberg s.
Parry's d.
Parsons' d.
Patau's s.
Patella's d.
Paterson-Brown-Kelly s.
Paterson-Kelly s.
Paterson's s.
Patterson's s.
Pauzat's d.
Pavy's d.
Payr's d.
Pel-Ebstein d.
Pelizaeus-Merzbacher d.

Pellegrini's d.
Pellegrini-Stieda d.
Pellizzi's s.
Pena-Shokeir I s.
Pendred's s.
Pepper s.
Perrin-Ferraton d.
Perthes' d.
Pette-Döring d.
Peutz-Jeghers s.
Peutz s.
Peyronie's d.
Pfaundler-Hurler s.
Pfeiffer's d., s.
Phocas' d.
Picchini's s.
Pick's d.
pickwickian s.
Pictou d.
Pierre Robin s.
Pinkus' d.
Plummer's d.
Plummer-Vinson s.
Poland's s.
Polhemus-Schafer-Ivemark s.
Pompe's d.
Poncet's d.
Porter's d.
Posada's d.
Posada-Wernicke d.
Potter's s.
Pott's d.
Poulet's d.
Prader-Willi s.
Preiser's d.
Pringle's d.
Profichet's s.
pseudo-Turner's s.
Purtscher's d.
Putnam-Dana s.
Pyle's d.
Quervain's d.
Quie's s.
Quincke's d.
Quinquaud's d.
Raeder's paratrigeminal s.

Ramsay Hunt s.
Ranikhet d.
Rayer's d.
Raymond-Cestan s.
Raynaud's d.
Recklinghausen-Applebaum d.
Recklinghausen's d.
Recklinghausen's d. of bone
Reclus' d.
Reed-Hodgkin d.
Refetoff s.
Refsum's d.
Reichmann's d., s.
Reifenstein's s.
Reiter's d., s.
Rendu-Osler d.
Rendu-Osler-Weber d.
Renpenning's s.
Reye's s.
Ribas-Torres d.
Ribbing's d.
Richards-Rundle s.
Richter's s.
Riedel's d.
Rieger's s.
Riga-Fede d.
Riga's d.
Riggs' d.
Riley-Day s.
Riley-Smith s.
Ritter's d.
Roaf's s.
Robert's s.
Robinow's s.
Robinson's d.
Robin's s.
Robles' d.
Roger's d., s.
Rokitansky-Küster-Hauser s.
Rokitansky's d.
Romano-Ward s.
Romberg's d., s.
Rose d.
Rosenbach's s.
Rosenthal-Kloepfer s.
Rosenthal's s.

Rosewater's s.
Rossbach's d.
Rot-Bernhardt d., s.
Roth-Bernhardt d., s.
Rothmann-Makai s.
Rothmund s.
Rothmund-Thomson s.
Roth's d., s.
Rotor's s.
Rot's d., s.
Rotter's s.
Rougnon-Heberden d.
Roussy-Déjérine s.
Roussy-Lévy's d., s.
Rovsing s.
Rubarth's d.
Rubinstein's s.
Rubinstein-Taybi s.
Rud's s.
Rüdiger s.
Rummo's d.
Russell's s.
Rust's d., s.
Ruvalcaba s.
Ruysch's d.
Sabin-Feldman s.
Sachs' d.
Saethre-Chotzen s.
St. Agatha's d.
St. Aignon's d.
St. Anthony's d.
St. Appolonia's d.
St. Avertin's d.
St. Avidus' d.
St. Blasius' d.
St. Dymphna's d.
St. Erasmus' d.
St. Fiacre's d.
St. Gervasius' d.
St. Gotthard's tunnel d.
St. Hubert's d.
St. Job's d.
St. Mathurin's d.
St. Modestus' d.
St. Roch's d.
St. Sement's d.

St. Valentine's d.
St. Zachary's d.
Saldino-Mainzer. s.
Sanchez Salorio s.
Sander's d.
Sanders' d.
Sandhoff's d.
Sandifer s.
Sanfilippo's s.
Saunders' d.
Savill's d.
Say's s.
Say-Gerald s.
Schafer's s.
Schamberg's d.
Schanz's d., s.
Schaumann's d., s.
Scheie's s.
Schenck's d.
Scheuermann's d.
Schilder's d.
Schimmelbusch's d.
Schinzel-Giedion s.
Schinzel s.
Schirmer's s.
Schlatter-Osgood d.
Schlatter's d.
Schmid-Fraccaro s.
Schmidt's s.
Schmorl's d.
Scholz's d.
Schönlein-Henoch d., s.
Schönlein's d.
Schottmüller's d.
Schridde's d.
Schroeder's d., s.
Schüller-Christian d., s.
Schüller's d., s.
Schultz s.
Schultz's d.
Schwartz-Jampel s.
Schwartz s.
Schwediauer's d.
Schweninger-Buzzi d.
Seckel's s.
Seitelberger's d.

Selter's d.
Selye s.
Senear-Usher s.
Sertoli-cell–only s.
Sever's d.
Sézary reticulosis s.
Sézary s.
Shaver's d.
Sheehan's s.
Shichito d.
Shokeir's s.
Shwachman s.
Shwachman-Diamond s.
Shy-Drager s.
Sicard's s.
Silverskiöld's s.
Silver's s.
Silvestrini-Corda s.
Simmonds' d.
Simons' d.
Simpson's s.
Singleton-Merten s.
Sipple's s.
Sjögren-Larsson s.
Sjögren's d., s.
Skevas-Zerfus d.
Sluder's s.
Sly's d.
Smith-Lemli-Opitz s.
Smith's d.
Smith-Strang d.
Smythe's s.
Sneddon-Wilkinson d.
Sohval-Soffer s.
Sorsby's s.
Sotos' s.
Sotos' s. of cerebral gigantism
Spencer's d.
Spens's s.
Speransky-Richen-Siegmund s.
Spielmeyer-Stock d.
Spielmeyer-Vogt d.
Sprinz-Dubin s.
Sprinz-Nelson s.
Spurway s.
Stanton's d.

Stargardt's d.
Steele-Richardson-Olszewski s.
Steinbrocker's s.
Steiner's s.
Steinert's d.
Stein-Leventhal s.
Sterbe d.
Sternberg's d.
Stevens-Johnson s.
Stewart-Morel-Moore s.
Stewart-Morel s.
Stewart-Treves s.
Sticker's d.
Stickler s.
Stieda's d.
Still-Chauffard s.
Stilling s.
Stilling-Turk-Duane s.
Still's d.
Stokes-Adams d.
Stokes' d.
Stokvis' d.
Stokvis-Talma s.
Strümpell-Leichtenstern d.
Strümpell-Lorrain d.
Strümpell-Marie d.
Strümpell's d.
Strümpell-Westphal d.
Stryker-Halbeisen s.
Stühmer's d.
Sturge-Kalischer-Weber s.
Sturge's s.
Sturge-Weber s.
Sudeck-Leriche s.
Sudeck's d.
Sulzberger-Garbe s.
Sutton and Gull's d.
Sutton's d.
Swediaur's d.
Sweet's d., s.
Swift-Feer d.
Swift's d.
Swyer-James s.
Sydenham's d.
Sylvest's d.
Symmers' d.

Tabatznik's s.
Takahara's d.
Takayasu's d., s.
Talfan d.
Talma's d.
Tangier d.
Tapia's s.
Tar's s.
Taussig-Bing s.
Tay-Sachs d.
Tay's d.
Taybi's s.
Taybi-Linder s.
Terry's s.
Teschen d.
Thaysen's d.
Theiler's d.
Thibierge-Weissenbach s.
Thiele s.
Thiemann's d.
Thomsen's d.
Thomson's d.
Thorn's s.
Thornwaldt's d., s.
Thygeson's d.
Tietze's s.
Tillaux's s.
Timme's s.
Tolosa-Hunt s.
Tommaselli's d.
Tooth d.
Tornwaldt's d.
Torre's s.
Torsten-Sjögren's s.
Touraine-Solente-Golé s.
Tourette's d.
Townes' s.
Treacher Collins s.
Trevor's d.
Troisier's s.
Trousseau's s.
Turcot s.
Turner's s.
Tyzzer's d.
Uehlinger's s.
Ullrich-Feichtiger s.

Ullrich-Turner s.
Ulysses s.
Underwood's d.
Unna's d.
Unverricht's d.
Urbach-Oppenheim d.
Urbach-Wiethe d.
Usher's s.
van Bogaert's d.
van Buchem's d., s.
van Buren's d.
van der Hoeve's s.
Van der Woude's s.
Vaquez-Osler d.
Vaquez's d.
Verner-Morrison s.
Vernet's s.
Verneuil's d.
Verse's d.
Vidal's d.
Villaret's s.
Vincent's d.
Vinson-Plummer s.
Vinson's s.
Virchow's d.
Virchow-Seckel s.
Vogt-Koyanagi s.
Vogt-Spielmeyer d.
Vogt's s.
Volkmann's d., s.
Voltolini's d.
von Bechterew's (Bekhterev's) d.
von Economo's d.
von Gierke's d.
von Hippel–Lindau d.
von Hippel's d.
von Jaksch's d.
von Meyenburg's d.
von Recklinghausen's d.
von Willebrand's d., s.
Voorhoeve's d.
Vrolik's d.
Waardenburg's s.
Wagner's d.
Waldenström's d.
Wallenberg's s.

Wardrop's d.
Wartenberg's d.
Washburn-Mason s.
Wassilieff's d.
Waterhouse-Friderichsen s.
Weaver's s.
s. of Weber
Weber-Christian d.
Weber-Cockayne s.
Weber-Dimitri d.
Weber-Dubler s.
Weber's d.
Wegener's s.
Wegner's d.
Weill-Marchesani s.
Weil's d., s.
Weir Mitchell's d.
Weissenbacher-Zweymüller s.
Wenckebach's d.
Werdnig-Hoffmann d., s.
Werlhof's d.
Wermer's s.
Werner-His d.
Werner-Schultz d.
Werner's s.
Wernicke-Korsakoff s.
Wernicke's d., s.
Wesselsbron d.
Westphal's d.
Westphal-Strümpell d.
West's s.
Weyers' oligodactyly s.
Weyers-Thier s.
Whipple's d.
White's d.
Whitfield's s.
Whitmore's d.

Whytt's d.
Widal s.
Wildervanck s.
Wilkie's d.
Willebrand's s.
Williams-Campbell s.
William s.
Willis' d.
Wilson-Mikity s.
Wilson's d., s.
Winchester's s.
Winckel's d.
Windscheid's d.
Winiwarter-Buerger d.
Winkler's d.
Winter's s.
Winton d.
Wiskott-Aldrich s.
Witkop's d.
Witkop–Von Sallmann d.
Wohlfart-Kugelberg-Welander d.
Wolff-Parkinson-White s.
Wolf-Hirschhorn s.
Wolfram s.
Wolf's s.
Wolman's d.
Woringer-Kolopp d.
Wright's s.
Wyburn-Mason s.
Young's s.
Zahorsky's d.
Zellweger s.
Ziehen-Oppenheim d.
Zieve s.
Zimmermann-Labaud s.
Zollinger-Ellison s.

APPENDIX 6
Greek Alphabet

The Greek alphabet has 24 letters:			
Printed			
Capital	*Small*	**Names of Letters**	
Α	α	Ἄλφα	alpha
Β	β	Βῆτα	beta
Γ	γ	Γάμμα	gamma
Δ	δ	Δέλτα	delta
Ε	ε	Ἔψιλον	epsilon
Ζ	ζ	Ζῆτα	zeta
Η	η	Ἦτα	eta
Θ	θ	Θῆτα	theta
Ι	ι	Ἰῶτα	iota
Κ	κ	Κάππα	kappa
Λ	λ	Λάμβδα	lambda
Μ	μ	Μῦ	mu
Ν	ν	Νῦ	nu
Ξ	ξ	Ξῦ	xi
Ο	ο	Ὄμικρον	omicron
Π	π	Πῖ	pi
Ρ	ρ	Ῥῶ	rho
Σ	σ, ς	Σίγμα	sigma
Τ	τ	Ταῦ	tau
Υ	υ	Ὕψιλον	upsilon
Φ	φ	Φῖ	phi
Χ	χ	Χῖ	khi
Ψ	ψ	Ψῖ	psi
Ω	ω	Ὠμέγα	omega